SOCIAL DEMOGRAPHY

STUDIES IN POPULATION

Under the Editorship of: H. H. WINSBOROUGH

Department of Sociology
University of Wisconsin
Madison, Wisconsin

SOCIAL DEMOGRAPHY

Edited by

Karl E. Taeuber
Larry L. Bumpass
James A. Sweet

Center for Demography and Ecology
University of Wisconsin—Madison
Madison, Wisconsin

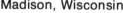

ACADEMIC PRESS   New York   San Francisco   London
A Subsidiary of Harcourt Brace Jovanovich, Publishers

ACADEMIC PRESS, INC.
111 Fifth Avenue, New York, New York 10003

United Kingdom Edition published by
ACADEMIC PRESS, INC. (LONDON) LTD.
24/28 Oval Road, London NW1 7DX

Library of Congress Cataloging in Publication Data

Conference on Social Demography, Madison, Wis., 1975.
    Social demography.

    (Studies in population)
    "Based on the proceedings of a Conference on Social
Demography, held in Madison, Wisconsin, July 1975;
co–sponsored by the Center for Demography and Ecology,
University of Wisconsin, and the Center for Population
Research, National Institute of Child Health and Human
Development."
    Includes bibliographies.
    1.   Fertility, Human––Congresses.   2.   Population
density––Congresses.   3.   Social mobility––Congresses.
4.   Population research––Congresses.   I.   Taeuber,
Karl E.   II.   Bumpass, Larry L.   III.   Sweet, James A.
IV.   Wisconsin.   University––Madison.   Center for
Demography and Ecology.   V.   United States.   National
Institute of Child Health and Human Development.   Center
for Population Research.   VI.   Title.   VII.   Series.
HB849.C62   1975   301.32   78–606153
ISBN   0–12–682650–1

Contents

2
The Pervasiveness of Postwar Fertility Trends in the United States

RONALD R. RINDFUSS and JAMES A. SWEET

3
Age and the Sociology of Fertility: How Old Is Too Old?

RONALD R. RINDFUSS and LARRY L. BUMPASS

4
Couples' Decision-Making Processes Regarding Fertility

LINDA J. BECKMAN

II
SPATIAL DISTRIBUTION

8
The New Pattern of Nonmetropolitan Population Change

157

CALVIN L. BEALE and GLENN V. FUGUITT

III
SOCIAL MOBILITY

9
Mobility and Stratification: An Overview

181

DAVID D. McFARLAND

10
Changes in the Socioeconomic Stratification of the Races

197

DAVID L. FEATHERMAN and ROBERT M. HAUSER

11
Statistical Histories of the Life Cycle of Birth Cohorts: The Transition from Schoolboy to Adult Male   231

HALLIMAN H. WINSBOROUGH

12
Some Methodological Issues in the Analysis of Longitudinal Surveys   261

BURTON SINGER and SEYMOUR SPILERMAN

IV
EMERGING ISSUES

13
The Next Fifteen Years in Demographic Analysis   299

SAMUEL H. PRESTON

LIST OF CONTRIBUTORS

Numbers in parentheses indicate the pages on which the authors' contributions begin.

Calvin L. Beale (157), Economic Research Service, Department of Agriculture, Washington, D.C. 20560

Linda J. Beckman (61), Department of Psychiatry, University of California at Los Angeles, Los Angeles, California 90024

Larry L. Bumpass (45), Center for Demography and Ecology, University of Wisconsin—Madison, Madison, Wisconsin 53706

David L. Featherman (197), Department of Rural Sociology, University of Wisconsin—Madison, Madison, Wisconsin 53706

Glenn V. Fuguitt (157), Department of Rural Sociology, University of Wisconsin—Madison, Madison, Wisconsin 53706

Omer R. Galle (95), Population Research Center, University of Texas at Austin, Austin, Texas 78705

Walter R. Gove (95), Department of Sociology, Vanderbilt University, Nashville, Tennessee 37235

Robert M. Hauser (197), Department of Sociology, University of Wisconsin—Madison, Madison, Wisconsin 53706

Amos H. Hawley (91), Department of Sociology, University of North Carolina, Chapel Hill, North Carolina 27514

David D. McFarland (181), Department of Sociology University of California at Los Angeles, Los Angeles, California 90024

Samuel H. Preston* (299), Center for Studies in Demography and Ecology, University of Washington, Seattle, Washington 98195

Ronald R. Rindfuss (15, 45), Department of Sociology, University of North Carolina, Chapel Hill, North Carolina 27514

Norman B. Ryder (3), Office of Population Research, Princeton University, Princeton, New Jersey 08540

Burton Singer (261), Department of Mathematical Statistics, Columbia University, New York, New York 10027

Seymour Spilerman† (261), Department of Sociology, University of Wisconsin—Madison, Madison, Wisconsin 53706

James A. Sweet (15), Center for Demography and Ecology, University of Wisconsin—Madison, Madison, Wisconsin 53706

Franklin D. Wilson (133), Center for Demography and Ecology, University of Wisconsin—Madison, Madison, Wisconsin 53706

Halliman H. Winsborough (231, 315), Center for Demography and Ecology, University of Wisconsin—Madison, Madison, Wisconsin 53706

* Present address: Population Division, United Nations, New York, New York 10017.
† Present address: Russell Sage Foundation, 230 Park Avenue, New York, New York 10017.

Preface

Governmental sponsorship of social research on a large scale is a recent phenomenon. In the 1950s the National Science Foundation gradually expanded its mandate beyond the physical and biological sciences to include portions of the social sciences. Population research was early identified as a scientific topic of great interest. To guide formulation of policy and program, the foundation commissioned an inventory and appraisal of the state of the discipline. Philip M. Hauser and Otis Dudley Duncan edited the report of that inventory, *The Study of Population* (Chicago: University of Chicago Press, 1959). As graduate students, Taeuber studied with both Hauser and Duncan, and Bumpass and Sweet studied with Duncan. When the Center for Population Research expressed an interest in devoting one of its annual conferences to behavioral science aspects of demography, our first thoughts were of ways to update *The Study of Population*. We quickly realized that such an endeavor was beyond the time and resources available to us. The 1975 conference, held at the University of Wisconsin—Madison, June 15–16, was the first devoted to social and behavioral research. As conference organizers, we sought to indicate to a scientific audience something of the nature of current research in social demography.

In a short conference (1½ days) there could be no serious attempt to provide comprehensive coverage of all types of social science research on population. We chose instead to focus on selected topics. In addition to the plenary session, which assessed some emerging issues in demographic analysis and research, three substantive sessions were held, each with three research papers and an overview paper. All papers from the substantive sessions and two papers from the plenary session are included (the author of a third plenary paper chose not to offer it for publication in this volume). In an effort to assist in the transition from conference presentation to publishable chapter each author was given time for revision, and we took an active role in making editorial suggestions. Several papers were completely rewritten, in some cases with substantial change in content. In one instance (Featherman and Hauser), a composite of material presented at the conference and subsequent work is included. In another instance (Singer and Spilerman), the chapter included in this volume is completely different from the paper summarized orally at the conference.

The first 4 chapters (three research papers preceded by an overview) pertain to fertility, the second 4 pertain to spatial distribution, and the third set of chapters pertains to social mobility. Mortality, migration, and many other topics on which social scientists are conducting demographic research are entirely omitted, and, although demography is at least as much a set of analytic tools as a substantive discipline, only 1 chapter among these 12 is primarily methodological. Thus, the book focuses on selected topics at the cost of a broader sampling of subject matter and analytic style.

Federal agencies do have a tendency, even in their programs of support for basic research, to focus on current national policy issues. There is a persistent danger that the definitions of issues and of needed research will become very narrow and topical. The combination of reproductive biology with demography in a single Center for Population Research, under the umbrella of the National Institutes of Health, poses a particularly persistent tendency to identify population policy with the regulation of fertility through contraceptive intervention. Our choice of topics and chapters represents a deliberate effort to demonstrate that many other issues of profound national policy interest require study with high-quality social science research and illumination with a demographic perspective. The chapters on fertility, for example, demonstrate the virtue of sophisticated trend analysis, explore the sociological meaning of age, and delineate the complex social–psychological processes by which couples make decisions regarding their reproductive behavior.

The chapters on spatial aspects of population include a report on the remarkable "nonmetropolitan turnaround"; this chapter is another example of the improved understanding that flows from careful trend analysis. Also included is a systematic review of the evidence on possible pathological consequences of excessively high or low population density, and an intricate analysis of certain aspects of the spatial organization of metropolitan activities. The redistribution of population is the goal of some national policies and one result of many other policies. None of these chapters is intended directly as policy analysis, but each augments understanding of basic structural change in American society.

One of the noteworthy contributions of the 1959 Hauser and Duncan appraisal, *The Study of Population,* was a definition of *demography* that gave a legitimate place to the study of social mobility: "Demography is the study of the size, territorial distribution, and composition of population, changes therein, and the components of such changes, which may be identified as natality, mortality, territorial movement, and social mobility (change of status) [p. 31]." The study of social mobility is by no means an exclusive domain of demographers, but social demographers have important contributions to make. One social mobility chapter included here addresses one of the fundamental political issues of our time, the changing racial stratification. One chapter seeks to characterize many types of social change in terms of their impact on successive generations of people. The third chapter, taking cognizance of the reliance that many studies of social mobility place on repeated (longitudinal) population surveys, raises some methodological issues that should affect not only the way future scholars analyze such data, but also the way such data systems are designed and implemented.

In the years since publication of *The Study of Population* there has been a veritable revolution in the quantity and character of demographic data. The computer has expanded enormously the capabilities for production of data and the techniques for analysis of data. There has been a severalfold increase in the number of population researchers and in the quantity of scholarly demographic research that is published each year. Design of a strategy for organization and funding of demographic research is less dependent now on an inventory and appraisal of the status of demography as science, and more dependent on an assessment of what holds promise for the future. The topics, the analytic methods, and the data bases common today differ from those of the 1950s, and there is every reason to expect continual change in demographic research. In the plenary session, two young demographers, accomplished at both scholarly writing and research administration, were asked to consider not the "whence" of demography but the "whither." These two chapters challenge all those concerned with social demography and particularly, we hope, the sponsors of this volume, to contemplate the future of research in social demography.

I
FERTILITY

1

Some Problems of Fertility Research

NORMAN B. RYDER

Survey research on fertility began nearly four decades ago with the for-midable Indianapolis Study. Although by now we have learned a great deal, our grasp of the subject remains tentative and uncertain. The pur-pose of this chapter is to identify some difficulties of measurement and conceptualization that call for resolution in our future work on fertility. These reflections on the state of the art have been prompted by participa-tion in the planning of the World Fertility Survey and the 1975 National Fertility Study. The account begins with a discussion of the dependent variable, partly as a matter of convenience of presentation, but partly from the conviction that we must learn how to make accurate and mean-ingful measurements of variations in reproductive behavior before begin-ning the search for explanations of those variations.

Behavioral Data

The elementary information that represents the raw materials for defin-ing our dependent variable comprises the following: the respondent's

3

Social Demography

birthdate; the number and dates of her fertile pregnancies; and the date the information is obtained. Note first that we have two rather different kinds of definition of the universe about which we are attempting to make inferences. If the data source is a system of vital registration for a population, then, like all populations, it experiences continual metabolism, that is, flows of individuals into and out of the system. If, on the other hand, the data source is a set of retrospective histories furnished by the survivors of the respective cohorts included in the sampling frame, we have succeeded in suppressing the effects of that metabolism, but only at the cost of introducing selectivity; characteristics associated with survival are unlikely to be randomly related to reproduction. For populations like that of the United States, such a consideration is fortuitously of little empirical significance, but it may be quite important in some of the countries covered by the World Fertility Survey, where selectivity attributable to both mortality and migration may be substantial over the course of the reproductive life cyle.

A second problem concerns the accuracy of the raw data. In terms of contribution to the understanding of international differences in fertility, it is probably the case that the data with the largest potential yield come from those populations that have the highest proportions illiterate and innumerate. In designing the World Fertility Survey questionnaire, we were highly sensitive to the fact that underreporting of the number of fertile pregnancies is commonplace and substantial. We attempted to cover some of the exigencies believed to produce such underreporting by employing a battery of questions that asked separately about categories of birth by gender, by survival, and by residence. The problem is not simply one of ignorance or faulty memory, but also one of differing sociocultural definitions of the situation. As a simple generalization, international trends and differentials in fertility will reflect not only the reality that is the object of the exercise, but also the sophistication of respondents, the extent of correspondence of their definitions with ours, and the quality of effort put into the collection process.

If we make the assumption that the data are sufficiently complete to warrant analysis, the next question concerns the optimal approach to their summarization. Measurement procedures to this end have been developed primarily from experience with official registration and enumeration statistics. The recommended strategy is to calculate fertility rates (ratios of number of occurrences to number of person-years of exposure to risk of those occurrences) to as high a level of specificity as the data base allows. This yields a surface of rates for the entire range of exposure, sliced in various ways. Indices of the quantity or time pattern of fertility then may be developed using real or synthetic cohort constructions. This approach has served us well, even though it typically provides only a slim ecological clue to explanation.

What is unresolved is the conundrum of how to compare cumulated values for differentially incomplete reproductive histories. Changes in the quantity and tempo of reproduction are interpenetrating in such records; indeed there is, while a cohort is in reproductive transit, a kind of artificiality to the distinction between quantity and tempo. The customary way this difficulty is met is by truncating the longer of the two histories being compared down to the length of the shorter record; however, the resultant comparison of difference in quantity is satisfactory only if the time distributions are the same, and the resultant comparison of difference in tempo is satisfactory only if the quantity is the same. Although this has been a bitter pill for demographers to swallow, we are now beginning to realize that no defensible assertion can be made about either the current level or the current time pattern of fertility. The statements we are seduced into making on these matters from time to time imply models and projections as well as evidence, and models and projections are very much matters of taste and judgment.

Because measurements of the level of fertility and, a fortiori, of changes in the level require joint consideration of the time pattern of births, we need to pay due attention to the accuracy of reports of that time pattern as well as to the possibility of underreporting of the number of births. We know rather little about how respondents may misreport the significant dates of their lives. Are past events shifted forward or backward in time, as a rule? Do such shifts depend to some extent on how long ago the events occurred? If the dates are obtained seriatim, does the respondent perform the necessary arithmetical calculations by estimating the intervals between successive events? Are such interval lengths ordinarily understated or overstated? Different habits in temporal reporting produce different fertility configurations and therefore different appearances of trend in the quantity of fertility. Much ingenuity has been devoted to devising analytic procedures for assessing the plausibility of reported data, essentially by comparing them with what one expects to find. While such procedures are a worthwhile precaution against dispensing misinformation, they have the fundamental flaw of reliance on the knowledge that it is the purpose of research to obtain.

It is customary to process survey data as if they were the product of a registration procedure, and therefore amenable to the same summarizing tactics developed for such data. Given the form in which reproductive histories are provided by the respondent, that approach seems unnatural and unwise. It would seem much more fitting to develop for this purpose the appropriate analogues to the measurement style used in the microanalysis of pregnancy intervals. The form of calculation would be the production of estimates of parameters for each interval in the history of a cohort, as a contingent sequence. Requisite to such calculations are data for successive pairs of events where, with each pair, the former event is necessary to but not sufficient for the occurrence of the latter event. If one locates the former event in time, that is, identifies it as a member of a parity cohort, the results are accessible to time series analysis. Multiple decrement procedures are available to summarize the distribution of lengths of closed and open intervals in the form of a survival curve, indexed (up to some arbitrary truncation length) by the employment of familiar life table measures. In recognition of the ubiquitous problem of age censoring in a cross-sectional survey, it is important to make such calculations separately for respondents of different ages at the beginning of the interval.

The proposed approach has the following advantages. It is isomorphic with the conventional microanalytic approaches to the measurement of fecundability and contraceptive efficacy. It is a parsimonious solution to the censoring problem. It places proper emphasis on the probabilistic character of the reproductive process. It displays the progressive selectivity of parity and of interval length. Finally, the proposed approach does not beg the question of whether the eventual outcome (completed parity) is to be considered as an approximation to some initial target or merely the upshot of a series of ad hoc decisions annd actions in successive time intervals. Although the approach is theoretically feasible with registration data—provided they are specific for parity, interval length, and age— there are substantial practical complexities to the estimation of suitable exposure bases. The reproductive histories collected in a survey, on the contrary, display exposure and occurrence straightforwardly and in natural order.

The survival curves that are the outputs of such a procedure are, from another standpoint, epiphenomena: They may be thought of as revealing the working out of an underlying distribution of respondents by propensity to give birth. If one is prepared to postulate an appropriate distributional family and to assume that the propensity for an individual respondent is invariant over the interval, then ways are available to estimate from the survival curves the parameters of the initiating distributions. In a sense, the life table procedure is a way of combining the distribution of lengths of closed intervals, for some women, with the lengths of open intervals, for the rest, in a way that avoids the well-known biases when either type of interval is considered alone.

We turn now to the subject of refinement of the dependent variable through more precise observations of both occurrences and exposure. As a behavioral record, a dated list of fertile pregnancies is but a crude beginning. The information needed for refinement is straightforward to specify but difficult to obtain with precision. One would like to have a dated list of infertile as well as fertile pregnancies, together with lengths of associated "dead time" before and after delivery. Also, one would want to exclude from gross exposure all segments of noncopulation. We customarily tackle the latter problem by distinguishing between those who are currently married at any time, whom we assume to be copulating, and those who are currently unmarried, whom we assume to be chaste. This approach has regrettable measurement consequences. Substantial copulation among the unmarried inhibits our efforts to calculate a defensible measure of fertility or fecundability or contraceptive efficacy for the earliest pregnancy within any marriage. Even if we could obtain a copulatory record for nonmarried segments, the information might not lend itself to the conventional life table procedures since they rely on the convenient implicit assumption of continual exposure, whereas it is not unlikely that much of nonmarital copulation is sporadic. The less familiar counterpart of this well-known difficulty is the phenomenon of noncopulation among the married. In the 1975 National Fertility Study, we have attempted to obtain a month-by-month exposure record for the time since the beginning of 1970, but we are not confident about the quality of the data because of recall error and outright suppression.

The convenience of the assumption that marriage is both necessary and sufficient for copulation tempts us to insert marital status into our universe definition in the interests of research economy. That practice has two unfortunate consequences. First, to exclude the never-married is tantamount to omitting nuptiality from its proper place in the reproductive sequence. Second, research strategies are inevitably complicated whenever some facet of the dependent variable is lodged within the universe definition. The basic principle of demographic inquiry is observation of all exposure to risk of occurrence of the event of interest, as opposed to research in which individuals select themselves for inclusion in the study by virtue of experiencing the events that are our objects of study.

Determination of segments of nonovulation requires information about the lengths of pregnancy and puerperium for each pregnancy—which can be ascertained or estimated with sufficient precision for most purposes— and also an accurate count of the number of infertile pregnancies—which can be neither ascertained nor estimated. It would appear that many of the spontaneous abortions are forgotten and that many of the induced abortions are concealed. In planning the World Fertility Survey questionnaire, we decided to include a record of infertile pregnancies—to guard against the possibility that some live births might have been misclassified as stillbirths; our recommendation is that subsequent analysis be oriented to birth intervals rather than pregnancy intervals.

The final behavioral data required for fertility analysis are the activities and conditions that intervene, at any point in the sequence that begins with copulation and proceeds through ovulation and conception to birth, to reduce the probability that the sequence will end in birth. The conventional approach, which inquires into the practices of contraception, sterilization and abortion, has several difficulties. For example, nonmarriage or delay of marriage are excluded from the category of intervention or fertility regulation. Second, the catalogue of practices emphasizes intentional interference. In effect, one is asking the respondent two questions at the same time: Did the activity take place? *and* Did the actor intend to modify the probability of a birth? One reason for our behavioral records being incomplete with respect to intervening activities and conditions is the mixture of action and motive in the questioning procedure. The issue may be of particular importance in populations in which most couples do not ostensibly engage in fertility regulation.

During the closing phases of the 1970 National Fertility Study, the writer spent many months attempting to estimate fecundability by studying the distribution of waiting times in pregnancy intervals devoid of reported intervention. The experience was chastening because the outcome was quite implausible. It would appear, taking the data at face value, that the chances of becoming pregnant are not much greater for a nonuser than for a user. Two circumstances underlie this result. First, the nonuser in the United States, particularly beyond the first or second interval, is in a small minority, presumably self-selected on the basis of previous experience in the direction of subfecundity. Second, there is a large amount of unreported contraception and abortion. In the United States we can now afford to ignore the experience of nonusers because they are so few, but in the World Fertility Survey, nonuse will be the norm. It is important in such contexts to extend the rubric of intervening activities well beyond purposive fertility regulation as defined by the respondent. We know little about the determinants of so-called unregulated fertility.

Motivational Data

Fertility surveys in the United States by and large are designed in terms of a voluntaristic model of reproductive behavior. The underlying premise is that couples continually are making reproductive decisions and ordinarily are behaving in ways appropriate to the implementation of those decisions. Such a premise is required to justify our practice of asking (and expecting an unequivocal answer) what the couple's intention had been at any point in their reproductive life cycle. If we get answers, and mostly we do, we proceed to distinguish two areas of inquiry: differences in intention and differences in the extent to which the outcome corresponds with the intention.

Many types of behavior that have reproductive consequences tend to get short shrift in such a model. Some behavior is the outcome of a decision process, but with a goal other than the modification of the probability of a birth. Mixed motives may be more the rule than the exception: Interventions may occur because of the reproductive consequences, or because those are congruent with other desired outcomes, or even despite the reproductive consequences. We have become painfully familiar with the douche for cleanliness only and the pill for medical reasons only, and, above all, whether to get married or stay married. It is obvious on both the individual and the collective levels that nuptiality is an important influence on fertility. Some part of the motivation for formation of marriages belongs in the category of fertility regulation. We can say little with confidence about the determinants of the probability of getting married for an individual, or as a cultural attribute, or about the determinants of age at first marriage, or the probability of remarriage, and so on. There are many studies of nuptiality, but ordinarily these are not designed to consider nuptiality as an intermediate variable in fertility analysis. It is difficult to specify the kinds of questions to ask about exposure to risk of marriage. We tend to regard the event as nonpurposive in obeisance to the romantic ethos—not precisely a chance occurrence but one that is somehow improper to approach from a deterministic standpoint. Methodologically there are very difficult problems because conventional demographic measures are oriented to the characteristics of individuals exposed to risk, whereas nuptiality is a joint event that requires an entirely different approach. This remains the Achilles' heel of the stable population model. Finally, on practical grounds, the premarital population is very large, difficult to sample on the conventional household basis, and shielded from scrutiny as part of the system of social control of the not-quite-adult.

Research in this area is of substantial importance for understanding fertility. One suggestion for the design of inquiry is that we should pursue simultaneously the set of transitions from youth to adulthood (termination of schooling, entry into the labor force, household and family formation) because there are independent determinants of each, and yet they are interdependent. A continuing and continually freshened panel of males and females as they pass from age 15 to age 25, say, would be of great benefit to our knowledge.

Within that subset of fertility regulation covered by the conventional survey, the most difficult problems of conceptualization arise just at the point at which the results have the highest intrinsic interest and importance, namely in the classification of intentions. Our current practice is to use a threefold code: termination, delay, and nondelay. There are several fundamental difficulties within this approach. First, responsible reproductive behavior requires that a couple have an answer to the question: Do you want to become pregnant this month? Those who answer "Yes" are codable as nondelay, but a further question is required for the rest, and that question is in effect a forecast: Do you want to become pregnant in any future month? Clearly we should leave ample room in our code for answers to the second question that are neither "Yes" nor "No." Moreover, since any forecast is presumably conditional on subsequent inputs of information and experience, there is no good basis for expecting such a forecast to remain unchanged thenceforth.

A second basic difficulty is related to the first. In collecting our data retrospectively, we are in the position of asking the respondent what her forecast was (in order to classify the intention as termination or delay) after what is being forecast may have already happened. There would seem to be no way out of this box, which does not include a longitudinal design. This is a primary justification for the shape of our 1975 National Fertility Study. We have reinterviewed a substantial part of the 1970 sample, those with the following characteristics: white, currently married, both wife and husband once-married, wife's age at first marriage less than 25 years, and married less than 20 years at first interview. Also we have interviewed (for the first time) respondents with the same characteristics, but married less than 5 years at interview. In a break with the predecessor studies, the temporal format has been oriented to marriage cohorts rather than birth cohorts. Fortuitously, the range of marriage cohorts, from 1951 –1955 through 1971–1975, encompasses the highest and the lowest fertility (to date) of the modern era.

The reinterview process gives us some prospect of establishing intention, action, and outcome in their proper sequence, and of replacing some observations of interdependency with causal chains—at least to the extent of exploiting the insight that something that happens later cannot affect something that happens earlier. We are more than usually excited by the prospects for the 1975 study because of its place in the history of fertility surveys. Following Indianapolis, surveys went in two directions. The Princeton Fertility Study used a longitudinal design with a narrowly defined sample in an effort to develop causal models, whereas the Growth of American Families Studies and the National Fertility Studies aimed at general descriptive parameters for the total population. Now that the National Center for Health Statistics has assumed the latter task, we are taking the opportunity to merge the two directions of effort by using a longitudinal design with a moderately comprehensive universe.

One problem encountered in American fertility surveys is the considerable number of respondents who state an intention that can be fulfilled only by use of some method, but deny any use. Among the relevant factors in an explanation of such irrationality may be the following: We have no measure of the strength of the intention, and there may be considerable unsolicited ambivalence. The respondent may perceive only a small difference in the consequences if a birth comes earlier or later, and even if it occurs at all or not. Such perceptions of small difference would be expected in a context of unpredictability with respect to the relevant future conditions of life, that is, where there is considerable discounting of the future and a short time horizon for planning. Furthermore, the respondent may perceive that use is likely to be no more than moderately effective, and therefore feel that the costs associated with use are unjustified. Because the action derives from a weighing of costs and benefits, it is insufficient to ask whether the individual would perceive some benefit from use. Finally, there is probably a differential capacity to assess situations and act effectively on the basis of that assessment, both in reproductive behavior and in other spheres. It is implausible that such a differential capacity is completely captured by years of schooling completed.

We have attempted in the 1975 National Fertility Study to determine the preferred waiting time for those who intend to have another child and, retrospectively, for those who became pregnant unwittingly. It is at least tenable that the passage of time is more important than any quantitative reproductive target in determining eventual parity. If there were decisions made about the age to have the first child, the age beyond which no further children would occur, and finally about the desirable interval between children, then the eventual parity would be an algebraic consequence. To date our inquiries into intentions have been dominated by the desired number. Maybe we have not been looking at the problem the way couples do.

Normative Data

Because fertility surveys are indeed surveys of individuals, it is natural to think of them as supplying the raw materials for microanalyses, that is, for attempts to explain the variance in reproductive behavior among individuals. By such a criterion our efforts to date have been profoundly unsuccessful. The strongest influences on fertility are ascribed characteristics (those fixed throughout the relevant part of the respondent's life span), such as religion, education, ethnic group, and farm background. Whether these are to be thought of as microanalytic or macroanalytic in a theoretical sense is a moot question. Superficially these too may appear to be pieces of information about the individual, but it is also tenable to consider the respondent as an agent in the process of inquiry, contributing a description of her reproductive behavior to the construction of a macroanalytic probability distribution of fertility, together with a signification of the groups to which she belongs (and thus the aggregates for which it would be meaningful to construct those distributions).

In the writer's judgment, the fundamental reason such characteristics are strong in the explanation of fertility is the fact that fertility is a group attribute. From the standpoint of the welfare of the group as a whole, the fertility of its members, in the aggregate, is of such substantial importance that their actions cannot be permitted to vary with the vagaries of uninstructed individual choice. Population replacement is a problem that requires an institutionalized solution. For an individual the meaning of membership in a group is the process of socialization that made her a member and the process of social control that keeps her a member. The distinctive reproductive patterns of different groups, which one sees when individual histories are aggregated, are reflections of the socialization and social control systems that characterize those groups. From this viewpoint, our principal analytic task is to derive aggregate measures of fertility and relate them to other properties of the groups that produce such fertility.

To avoid the stigma of sociocultural determinism, this statement must to be leavened with a specification of the scope remaining for individual deviations from the averages of the groups to which they belong. In the first place, socialization varies somewhat in content from individual to individual, that is, it is more or less successful, and the individual ordinarily has somewhat competing sources of normative orientation, in an idiosyncratic mixture. Likewise the network of social control has varying degrees of imperfection. The efficacy of these processes is probably itself a group property. Second, individuals differ physiologically, although again much of this variance is "explained" by group membership. Third, there are chance exigencies of the individual life courses that modify their reproductive histories. Yet again the incidence of emergency situations is not random from one group to another, and the processes of socialization and social control, depending on the group involved, are more or less tolerant of departures from the norm in such situations.

Finally, and of strategic importance in research design, degrees of freedom for individual choice are institutionalized: One is taught that there are options one is permitted or even required to exercise in the light of the circumstantial context. In effect one is programmed, through socialization and social control, with a formula to use in determining the proper course of action in a given situation. In that formula, which symbolizes the normative posture of the group, certain kinds of variables are identified as legitimate inputs to the reproductive decision with specified weights. Examples of such variables are income, health, aspirations for a nonmaternal career, and so forth. To the extent that individuals differ in their particular values for such variables because of the ways their particular lives have developed to that point, the application of the common institutionalized formula will yield variant outcomes. This is the level at which it is pertinent to inquire into the relationship between individual behavior, viewed as a deviation from the average for the groups of which she is a member, and achieved characteristics, that is, the legitimated input variables in the group formula.

The research orientation that derives from this model is that the analyst interested in the sources of individual differences in reproductive behavior first examines the group averages to determine the consequences of individual membership in those groups, and then considers individual deviations from those averages in relation to appropriate microanalytic variables within such groups. The macroanalytic counterpart is comparison of the parameters of individual-level regressions on one or another variable from group to group.

Whatever one's judgment about the fruitfulness of a normative orientation to the explanation of fertility, there can be no gainsaying the detrimental effect the existence of reproductive norms has for the kinds of information we try to collect. Responses to behavioral and attitudinal questions tend to be biased in the direction of normative adherence. The extent of misstatement varies directly with the importance of the behavior to the individual and to the society. Differentials in reported behavior represent some unknowable mixture of the real and the ideal. Because ideals differ between cultures and classes, differentials in reported behavior are ordinarily treacherous guides to differentials in real behavior.

In this respect, of course, we are in no substantially different position from any other social scientist who tries to understand human behavior. Such problems are the necessary costs associated with the study of any sociological topic that is important and therefore shrouded in norms.

2

The Pervasiveness of
Postwar Fertility Trends
in the United States[1]

RONALD R. RINDFUSS and JAMES A. SWEET

Regardless of the measure of period fertility used, it is clear that fertility increased substantially during the late 1940s and most of the 1950s and that it declined during the 1960s and 1970s. In 1945 there were 2.7 million births. By 1957 this number had increased to 4.3 million, and by 1974 it had declined to 3.1 million. Similar changes are observed using total fertility rates. In 1945 the period total fertility rate was 2.5. By 1957 it had increased to 3.8, and by 1969 it had again declined to 2.5.

These wide fluctuations in period fertility rates were unprecedented. Prior to 1945 the United States had experienced a long and almost uninterrupted decline in fertility (Coale and Zelnik, 1963; Grabill *et al.*, 1958, Ch. 2). This decline extended back to colonial times. Thus the postwar swings in fertility represent a clear departure from the trends of the previous 2 centuries.

These fluctuations were also unexpected. During the 1930s and early 1940s demographers were predicting a continuing decline in fertility; con-

[1] The analysis reported here was supported, in part, by a NIH grant, No. HD07682, and by a CPR grant No. HD05876 to the Center for Demography and Ecology.

15

cerned citizens talked about such issues as the threat of stagnation, optimum population size, and the use of baby bonuses. During the 1960s, when the babies of the "baby boom" reached childbearing age, an increase in fertility—at least in the crude birth rate—was predicted. These predictions helped fuel the national concern regarding population growth.

The postwar fluctuations in fertility also had important immediate and long-range effects. The immediate effects revolve around the provision of services to new parents and their infants. During the 1950s there were shortages of obstetricians, maternity beds, and pediatricians. These shortages have been remedied. But now obstetricians dispense the pill and focus on menopause; maternity beds are used for abortions or are converted into surgical care beds; and pediatricians are looking for teenage patients. Even Gerber had to diversify.

The longer-range effects of the fluctuations in period fertility stem from the fact that the United States age distribution now has a very large bump in it. Any institution that is age-related will have to cope with this bump; and most of our institutions are age-related. For example, the same educational system that scheduled double sessions because of a lack of space now must close schools because of a lack of students. The Social Security System eventually will have to finance the retirement of those born during the baby boom by taxing those born during the subsequent decline in fertility—perhaps we will see a reversal of the long-standing trend toward earlier retirement. Furthermore, those people added to the size of the population because of the baby boom will continue indefinitely to have an impact on the size of the population through the process of reproduction.

This chapter is a progress report of a project that is examining the social components of the postwar fluctuations in fertility.[2] Previous researchers have examined the demographic components of these fluctuations (for example, see Freedman, 1962 or Ryder, 1969). As might be expected, the two dominant trends were brought about by a number of diverse, and often countervailing, demographic trends. Our main interest here is in the extent to which various racial, ethnic, educational, income, and residential groups participated in these dominant postwar fluctuations in fertility. Detailed examination of this issue became possible with the release of the Public Use Samples from the 1960 and 1970 Censuses.

It was expected that some groups would have participated disproportionately in the postwar fluctuations in fertility, and that some would not have participated at all. Goldberg (1974, p. 8), writing on a somewhat different topic, recently noted:

[2] That project has now been completed and the results are reported in Rindfuss and Sweet, 1977.

> Residence, education, and income typically serve as the starting point in describing the fertility process. We would be puzzled if we encountered data that failed to reveal differences in fertility associated with those variables.

We are indeed puzzled; the same rise and decline in fertility has been found for every group that we have been able to examine. Of course there are minor differences in the timing of the peak, the amount of the increase, or the size of the decline; these differences have been reported elsewhere (Rindfuss, 1974, 1975a, 1975b, 1975c; Rindfuss and Sweet, 1975; Sweet, 1974a, 1974b, 1974c). However, with one exception, the same basic trend is found for every group. Previous analysts have focused attention on differences in rates of increase (or decrease); the similarity and pervasiveness of the postwar fertility trends have not received attention.

Data

The fertility rates used have been obtained from the 1960 and 1970 United States Censuses by using own children data—this depends on the fact that most children reside with their mothers and that the census enumerates households rather than individuals. *Own children* are defined as all children residing with a *mother,* including some adopted children or stepchildren and excluding those that have died or moved away. Age of child and age of mother are used to determine the numerators of annual, age-specific rates; age of woman is used to determine the denominator. The own children technique is described in detail elsewhere (Cho, 1968, 1971; Cho *et al.,* 1970; Grabill and Cho, 1965; Retherford and Cho, 1974). In other papers we have reported some limitations of the data when used in the study of differential fertility (Rindfuss, 1974, 1975a); because of the summary nature of this chapter they will not be repeated. In general we find that even though the levels may be misspecified, own children data accurately estimate trends.

Two variations of own children data are utilized: (1) a rate similar to a general fertility rate, calculated for currently married women and aggregated over a 3-year period (number of own children aged less than 3), and (2) annual age-specific fertility rates calculated for all women rather than currently married women. The former are used to obtain more detailed information on the decline in fertility that occurred in the 1960s. The latter are used to examine overall fertility trends for the entire period since 1945 and to examine trends in the age pattern of fertility.

Fertility Trends

Annual total fertility rates (period age-specific birth rates summed over all ages) for five education groups are plotted in Figure 2.1 for the period 1945 to 1967. The similarity in fertility trends among all five education groups is striking; the following features are found for every group: (1) an immediate postwar rise in fertility, lasting through 1947; (2) a slight decline following the peak levels of 1947; (3) a gradual and sustained increase in fertility that lasted throughout most of the 1950s and, in some cases, into the 1960s; (4) a decline in fertility, beginning in the late 1950s or early 1960s and continuing through 1967—the last year for which we have reliable data.

If the focus is on racial or ethnic groups, the pervasiveness of the principal fertility trends is also evident (see Figure 2.2). Because of the requirement of combining more than one Public Use Sample to obtain reliable rates for some of these groups, Figure 2.2 is limited to data derived from the 1970 Census and thus is restricted to the period 1955–1969. A similar restriction applies to Figure 2.3. (Note that for some groups there is still some unreliability in the annual estimates as evidenced by the random yearly fluctuations.)

Each of the 6 racial or ethnic groups shown in Figure 2.2 experienced a

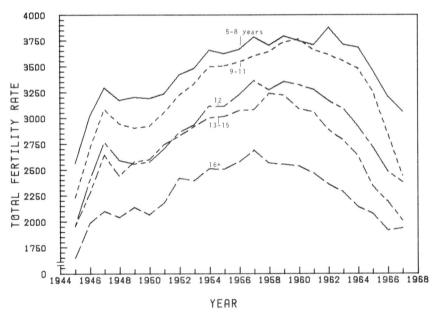

Figure 2.1. Total fertility rates for five education groups: 1945–1967.

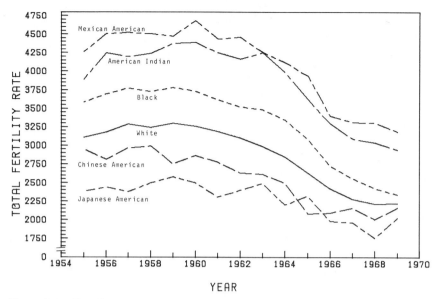

Figure 2.2.   Total fertility rates for six racial or ethnic groups: 1955–1969.

substantial decline (more than 20%) in fertility. This decline began in the late 1950s or early 1960s and continued through 1969. Figure 2.3 shows total fertility rates for Mexican Americans, whites, and blacks for 4 education groups. Again fertility declined for every group. The average decline in fertility from 1957 to 1967 for these 12 groups is 25%, with the smallest decline (13%) recorded for whites with 5–8 years of education and the largest (32%) for blacks with 13+ years of education.

In Table 2.1 we shift to an alternative fertility measure, the number of own children under age 3. When this fertility measure is used, the analysis is confined to currently married women. The annual fertility rates presented in the first three graphs require large numbers of sample cases for their calculations. The own child under 3 measure essentially averages 3 years of fertility exposure, thus reducing the need for larger samples. In addition, since they are calculated from a census for a period as long as 14 years prior to the census, the annual rates cannot be used reasonably for groups of women defined in terms of such characteristics as husband's income, which change in unpredictable ways through time. This is less of a problem when a shorter reference period, that is, 3 years prior to the census, is used. Finally, as we shall show later, this measure is a convenient dependent variable for use in multivariate analyses of fertility differentials. Table 2.1 shows, for a large number of comparatively homogeneous subgroups, a measure of fertility change for the 1960s. The change mea-

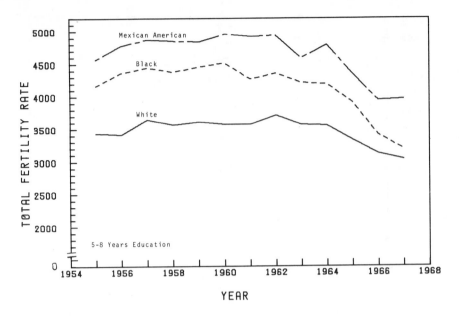

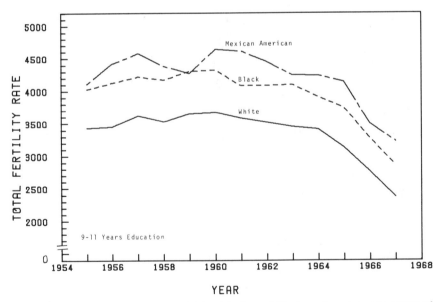

Figure 2.3. Total fertility rates for white, black, and Mexican Americans by years of education: 1955–1967. (Continued on next page.)

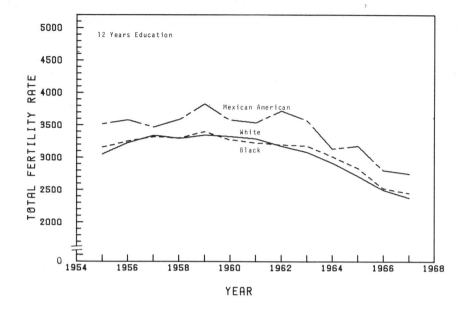

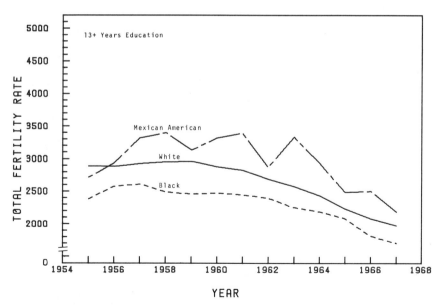

Figure 2.3.   (Continued.)

TABLE 2.1

Standardized[a] Rate of Fertility Decline during the Period 1960–1970 for Currently Married Women by Various Racial, Socioeconomic Status, and Residential Characteristics

| | Standardized rate of decline | | | | Number of women | | | | | | | |
| | | | | | White urban | | Southern rural black | | Non-Southern black | | Spanish surname | |
	White urban	Southern rural black	Non-Southern black	Spanish surname	1960	1970	1960	1970	1960	1970	1960	1970
Education												
Less than 5 years	31.7	42.7	62.2	27.9	144	129	450	131	180	115	728	526
5–8 years	22.3	35.0	42.1	24.5	1409	860	1416	639	1516	720	1312	1202
9–11 years	17.4	39.1	28.9	21.7	2887	2310	900	885	2418	2412	874	1200
12 years	26.5	26.8	29.4	28.8	5622	6255	461	708	2329	3793	807	1411
13–15 years	33.6	29.8	33.7	38.4	1449	1933	65	99	615	978	144	331
16+ years	22.9	−27.3	43.7	23.0	875	1460	63	84	248	469	62	100
Age at marriage												
14–17	27.7	39.6	37.4	30.4	2243	2365	1246	903	1953	2005	1172	1357
18–19	25.8	35.8	32.1	31.7	3320	3916	831	682	1712	2231	1025	1315
20–21	27.6	39.5	31.9	39.0	3154	3357	576	450	1373	1775	738	947
22–24	28.9	37.4	35.3	21.9	2302	2282	421	300	1264	1410	605	734
25–29	40.5	33.9	30.9	21.5	1105	848	216	166	769	807	290	340
30–39	10.7	−4.3	34.7	3.7	262	179	65	45	235	259	97	77
Husband's income (1960 constant dollars)												
Less than $1000	29.4	57.8	22.9	22.3	383	409	432	346	515	546	324	292
$1,000–1,999	24.2	47.4	32.5	34.4	452	487	521	434	570	398	474	326
$2,000–2,999	35.1	41.8	23.7	17.5	555	825	873	698	987	867	644	543
$3,000–3,999	29.4	47.7	32.3	24.1	1031	934	1485	455	1540	1105	631	839
$4,000–4,999	25.1	43.0	37.2	22.0	1134	1291	941	277	1628	1427	643	605
$5,000–7,499	26.6	37.5	36.9	32.4	3962	4807	1308	299	1832	3210	937	1342
$7,500–9,999	27.9	26.6	36.5	36.2	3064	2291	278	24	174	654	197	549
$10,000+	24.3	39.5	33.2	36.7	2366	1903	110	13	60	280	77	274

[a] See text for explanation.

sure is computed by comparing, within a given subgroup, the average number of children under age 3 from the 1960 Census with the average number of children under age 3 from the 1970 Census. In order to control for the possibility of a changing marriage duration distribution, the rates for a given subgroup from the 1970 Census have been standardized on the 1960 marriage duration distribution for that subgroup. Because Public Use Samples have not been released from the 1950 Census, this analysis cannot be performed for the decade of the 1950s.

As can be seen from Table 2.1, the decline in fertility in the 1960s was indeed pervasive. Among the 80 subgroups shown in Table 2.1, increases in fertility were found for only two groups: Southern rural blacks with 16+ years education and Southern rural blacks who first married at ages 30–39. In both cases the base number of women used to calculate the change rates is so small as to render the results suspect. For all the other groups there was a decline—typically over 20%.

The Rural Exception

The only major exception that we have found to the generalization that fertility increased for every social group during the 1950s is found among older (aged 30–44) rural white women.[3] Among these women there was no *net* change in fertility from 1945 to 1957. There certainly were fluctuations as can be seen in the insert of Figure 2.4, but the rate in 1957 was the same as the rate in 1945. (The fertility rates for older women are constructed in the same manner as a conventional total fertility rate except the age limits are 30–44 instead of 15–44.) Comparable urban women, by contrast, experienced a 22% increase during the period. In the 1960s the rate of decline among older rural women (40%) was larger than that among comparable urban women (33%). Thus throughout the entire period, there was a contraction of the rural–urban fertility differential among older women—to the point that during the last few years of the 1960s both groups were reproducing at similar rates.

The main portion of Figure 2.4 shows 2 examples of actual decreases in fertility during the period 1945–1957. For older rural women with only a grade school education and for older rural women who attended, but did not complete, high school, there were absolute declines, albeit small, in the fertility rate between 1945 and 1957 (declines of 3% and 1%, respectively).

[3] In work completed recently, it was found that this exception to the trends of the 1950s among older rural white women was confined to such women residing in the South (Rindfuss, 1978).

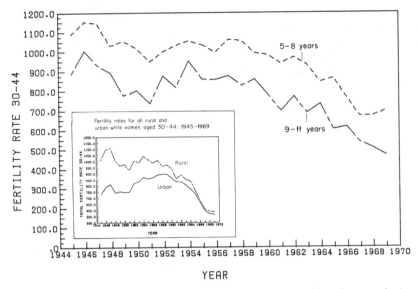

Figure 2.4. Fertility rates for white rural women aged 30–44 with 5–8 years of education and 9–11 years of education: 1945–1969.

Rural women with limited education traditionally have had the highest rates of fertility in the United States. They also would be expected to be among the last to adopt moderately effective methods of birth control. (Unfortunately, fertility surveys were not conducted during the 1940s. However, an indication of this possibility may be gained by looking at the report of the 1955 Growth of American Families Study by Freedman *et al.,* 1959.) It is quite possible that among these women there was increased awareness and utilization of contraception after World War II— in fact, it is possible that the war itself provided an educational opportunity. Increased use of contraception should lead to lower fertility rates, but this may have been offset by the counterbalancing forces leading to the baby boom of the 1950s—thus resulting in moderate fertility declines among older rural women with limited education. Whatever the explanation, these two groups of rural women are the only exceptions that we have found to the generalized pattern of the baby boom; and, it should be noted, both groups participated in the fertility decline of the 1960s.

Marriage Trends

For the United States as a whole, there have been increases, between 1960 and 1974, in the proportion of women never married for each age in the range 18–24 (see Table 2.2). Approximately two-thirds of this increase

TABLE 2.2

Percentage of Women Never Married by Age and Race: 1974 and 1960[a]

Age (in years)	All races		White		Black and other races	
	1974	1960	1974	1960	1974	1960
18	81.9	75.6	81.7	75.5	82.9	76.4
19	68.9	59.7	67.1	59.4	79.7	61.7
20	57.8	46.0	57.1	45.2	61.6	51.4
21	49.0	34.6	47.3	33.7	59.7	41.3
22	37.6	25.6	36.1	24.5	45.7	33.7
23	28.0	19.4	26.4	18.3	38.5	27.0
24	23.4	15.7	22.0	14.6	32.3	23.3

[a] *Source:* U.S. Bureau of the Census, Current Population Reports, Special Studies, Series P-23, No. 51, *Characteristics of American Youth: 1974,* Table 18, p. 16.

occurred between 1960 and 1970 and one-third between 1970 and 1974. Such increases in the percentage single tend to depress period fertility levels by reducing age specific fertility rates at the younger ages. Furthermore, if the age at marriage and fertility relationship holds longitudinally, these increases in age at marriage will reduce completed fertility as well.

A substantial part of the increase in proportions never married by specific ages results from a shift in the education distribution in a direction that favors later marriage. Among urban white women aged 25–29, for example, 33% had less than 12 years of education in 1960, while only 22% fell in that category in 1970. We estimate (Sweet, 1975) that 36% of the 1960–1970 increase in proportions never married by age 18 was due to changing educational composition. For ages 20, 22, and 24, the proportion attributable to changes in the education composition was 60, 68, and 58, respectively.

This increase in the proportion of women never married by various ages pervades all racial and ethnic groups examined (see Table 2.3). For example, among white women 20–24 years of age, there was an increase in the percentage never married from 27.5 to 35.1. Among black women the percentage never married at ages 20–24 rose from 34.9 to 43.6. Increases are found also for the other racial and minority groups.[4]

The United States as a whole also has been experiencing an increase in both the number and rate of divorces. In the late 1950s there were less

[4] Spanish-surname classification is not the best way of studying marriage change for Mexican–Americans, since the size and marital status of the Spanish-surname population is in part a function of marriage patterns and the degree to which Spanish-surname women are marrying men of Spanish surname and the degree to which they are marrying outside this population.

TABLE 2.3

Percentage of Women Never Married by Age and Ethnic Status: 1960 and 1970[a]

	20–24		25–34	
	1960	1970	1960	1970
White	27.5	35.1	8.0	8.9
Black	34.9	43.6	12.6	16.7
Southern rural black	39.4	44.3	13.9	17.8
American Indian	33.3	36.3	11.4	12.3
Chinese American	50.9	68.2	13.8	14.6
Japanese American	51.1	62.4	10.7	14.2
Filipino American	38.9	48.7	14.7	22.3
Puerto Rican American	25.6	28.2	8.7	8.9
Spanish surname	32.5	35.5	10.4	11.5

[a] *Sources:* Census Subject Reports, as follows:

White:	1970 Marital Status, PC(2)-4C, Table 1, pp. 14–17.
	1960 Marital Status, PC(2)-4E, Table 1, pp. 11–13.
Black:	1970 Negro Population, PC(2)-1B, Table 5, p. 40.
	1960 Non-white Population, PC(2)-1C, Table 19, p. 30.
Southern rural black:	1970 Negro Population, PC(2)-1B, Table 5, pp. 54–55.
	1960 Non-white Population, PC(2)-1C, Table 19, p. 37.
American Indian:	1970 American Indian, PC(2)-1F, Table 5, p. 36.
	1960 Non-white Population, PC(2)-1C, Table 20, p. 42.
Chinese American:	1970, PC(2)-1G, Table 5, p. 17; Table 20, p. 76; Table 35, p. 135.
	1960 Non-white Population, PC(2)-1C, Table 22, p. 66.
Japanese American:	1970, PC(2)-1G, Table 5, p. 17; Table 20, p. 76; Table 35, p. 135.
	1960 Non-white Population, PC(2)-1C, Table 21, p. 55.
Filipino American:	1970, PC(2)-1G, Table 5, p. 17; Table 20, p. 76; Table 35, p. 135.
	1960 Non-white Population, PC(2)-1C, Table 23, p. 78.
Puerto Rican American:	1970, Persons of Spanish Origin, Table 6, p. 61.
	1960, Puerto Ricans in the U.S., PC(2)-1D, Table 6, p. 32.
	1970, Puerto Ricans in the U.S., PC(2)-1E, Table 4, p. 38.
Spanish surname:	1970 Spanish Surname, PC(2)-1D, Table 8, p. 24.
	1960 Spanish Surname, PC(2)-1B, Table 7, p. 50.

than 400,000 divorces per year. In 1974 there were 970,000. The crude divorce rate (divorces per 1000 population) rose from around 2.2 in the late 1950s and early 1960s to 4.6 in 1974.

There was also a corresponding increase in the proportion of the population currently separated or divorced.[5] This increase is found among almost all racial and ethnic groups (see Table 2.4). There are, however, a few exceptions; for example, Southern rural blacks aged 20–24 or Filipinos aged 25–34. Data from the Current Population Surveys suggest that

[5] This proportion is a function of rates of first marriage, rates of separation, rates of divorce, and rates of remarriage. In the short run it is difficult to disentangle these various components because data are not available on number of separations, and a constant conditional probability of divorce following separation cannot be assumed.

TABLE 2.4

Percentage of Women Currently Separated or Divorced by Age and Ethnic Status: 1960 and 1974[a]

	20–24		25–34		35–44	
	1960	1970	1960	1970	1960	1970
White	3.3	4.5	4.2	6.4	5.1	7.0
Black	10.1	10.3	22.2	20.3	18.9	22.9
Southern rural black	6.9	6.1	10.8	11.0	10.3	12.1
American Indian	6.2	7.1	8.7	12.2	9.8	14.1
Chinese American	1.2	1.0	1.7	2.7	2.8	3.5
Japanese American	1.1	1.6	2.0	3.7	3.0	4.9
Filipino American	2.7	3.0	3.6	2.9	4.1	5.1
Puerto Rican American	6.7	12.3	10.2	20.6	14.6	29.1
Spanish surname	4.5	5.6	6.5	8.6	9.1	10.1

[a] *Sources:* See Table 2.3.

this trend toward increasing proportions separated and divorced has continued past 1970 (not shown).

Not only have these trends toward later ages at first marriage and toward increasing proportions currently separated and divorced been found among a wide variety of racial and ethnic groups, but also both trends tend to depress period fertility levels. Overall, we estimate that approximately 20% of the 1960 to 1970 decline in current fertility can be attributed to a change in martial status (Sweet, 1975), with the effect being substantially greater at the younger ages than at the older ages.

Trends in the Timing of Fertility

If the focus is on trends in the age pattern of fertility, rather than trends in the level of fertility or proportions marrying, again the same change is found for all groups. In order to examine trends in the age pattern of fertility, the complete fertility schedules will be used rather than aggregating the age-specific fertility rate estimates into total fertility rates.

Conceptually, the issue of fertility timing is a cohort one. However, it was not possible to construct cohort fertility schedules with the limited time series employed here; for this reason, period fertility schedules are used. Thus what is being examined is the proportionate contribution made to a period total fertility rate by women of various ages within the childbearing span. In order to examine differences in the age pattern of fertility without the confounding effect of differences in levels of fertility, the schedules have been standardized such that the total fertility rate of each group is equal to 1.0.

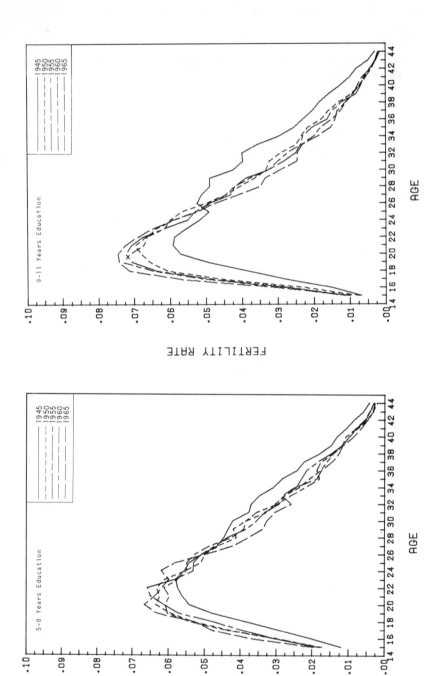

Figure 2.5. Standardized fertility schedules for five education groups: 1945–1965. (Continued on next two pages.)

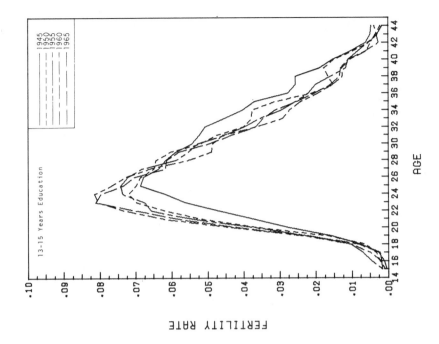

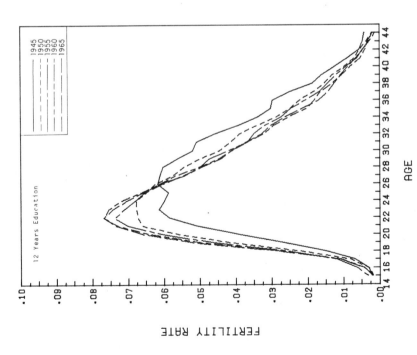

Figure 2.5. (Continued.)

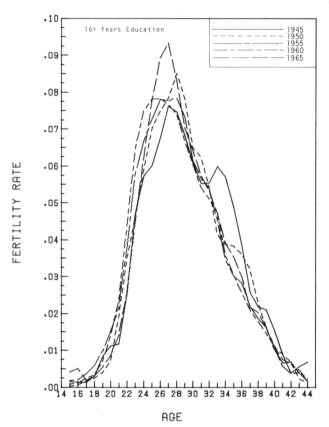

Figure 2.5. (Continued.)

Figure 2.5 shows, for five education groups, standardized fertility schedules for the years 1945, 1950, 1955, 1960, and 1965. Various parameters for these schedules are shown in Table 2.5. Two distinct trends can be observed and these are found within each education group.[6] First, the pattern of fertility has become more compact; that is, an increased proportion of total fertility is now occurring during the prime years of childbearing. Second, there has been a trend toward a younger pattern of fertility. This can be seen by examining the mean age of fertility or the proportion of fertility occurring before various ages. The largest decline in the mean age of the fertility schedule occurred to women with 9–11 years

[6] It should be noted that these changes are somewhat exaggerated because of the unusual nature of period fertility in 1945 (see Rindfuss, 1975c).

TABLE 2.5

Mean Age and Standard Deviation of Fertility Schedule, and Percentage of Total Fertility Occurring before Age 25 and before Age 30 by Education Groups: 1945–1965

Year	Education (in years)				
	5–8	9–11	12	13–15	16+
	Mean age				
1945	26.72	26.76	27.96	28.74	29.76
1950	25.41	25.19	26.91	27.87	29.31
1955	25.62	24.87	26.45	27.43	28.67
1960	25.47	24.78	26.21	27.04	28.60
1965	25.05	24.48	26.21	27.28	28.95
	Standard deviation				
1945	6.72	6.55	5.93	5.76	5.30
1950	6.49	6.27	5.85	5.59	5.05
1955	6.59	6.25	5.86	5.59	5.22
1960	6.55	6.19	5.74	5.48	5.19
1965	6.48	6.24	5.78	5.46	5.02
	Percentage of total fertility occuring before age 25				
1945	43	42	32	26	17
1950	51	53	40	32	18
1955	50	55	44	34	22
1960	50	55	45	38	24
1965	54	58	46	36	18
	Percentage of total fertility occurring before age 30				
1945	67	67	62	58	52
1950	74	76	69	65	56
1955	73	77	71	67	60
1960	74	78	73	70	61
1965	76	79	73	69	59

of education—a decline of more than 2 years. Even among college graduates there was a decline of almost 1 year.

The only exception to the trend toward a younger pattern of fertility occurs among women who attended college. They move in the direction of a younger age pattern of fertility between 1945 and 1960; but between 1960 and 1965, a slight increase in the mean age of fertility is registered. If the series of fertility schedules could be reliably extended past 1965, a similar upturn in the mean age of fertility would be expected for other education groups—the less educated groups experienced declining fertility somewhat later than those who attended college (see Figure 2.1).

For rural whites, urban whites, and blacks a trend toward a younger and a more compact fertility schedule is also found (data not shown). Thus again, the standard explanatory variables do not differentiate with respect to trends. Furthermore, it should be noted that large fluctuations in period fertility rates are more likely if the fertility schedule is comparatively compact. Thus the trend toward a more compact fertility schedule for every group increases the potential for wide fluctuations in period fertility.

Persistence of Cross-Sectional Fertility Differentials

Previous sections have shown that the dominant fertility trends of the 1950s and, especially, of the 1960s can be found within every major social group examined. This section shows that these same social variables do tend to differentiate with respect to cross-sectional fertility levels.

Most of our work examining cross-sectional fertility differentials has been within various racial and ethnic groups. For the purposes of summary, differentials will be presented for three groups: urban whites, non-Southern blacks, and the Spanish-surname population. Differentials in current fertility will be presented for the late 1950s and for the late 1960s. It should be emphasized that these are differentials in current fertility rather than cumulative fertility; as such, for characteristics that change, the effect on current fertility may not be the same as the effect on cumulative fertility—income is the classic example (see Cho *et al.,* 1970). In order to minimize the effects of young children not living with their mothers, the analysis is restricted to differentials in the fertility of currently married women. Even with this restriction, some differentials probably are understated because there is a tendency for fertility levels and the proportion of young children not living with their parents to be directly related. The results presented here show both crude or unadjusted differentials in fertility and adjusted or standardized differentials, that is, differentials that remain after adjusting for the effects of certain potentially confounding variables, by means of a multiple regression analysis.

Table 2.6 shows both unadjusted and adjusted differentials in the number of own children aged less than 3 for the urban white population for three social and economic variables: education, age at marriage, and husband's income. In 1960 there were only small crude differences in fertility among the various education categories. The only exception was women with less than 5 years of schooling—a group that comprises a small proportion of the population. In 1970 there is essentially no crude difference evident among the various education groups. When other factors, including age at marriage, are controlled, the expected inverse relationship

TABLE 2.6

Differentials from the Grand Mean in Recent Fertility by Education, Husband's Income, and Age at First Marriage: Currently Married Urban White Women Aged Less Than 40, 1960 and 1970

	Unadjusted		Adjusted[a]		Number of women	
	1960	1970	1960	1970	1960	1970
Education						
Less than 5 years	.12	.01	.18	.13	144	129
5–8 years	−.05	−.01	−.03	.07	1409	860
9–11 years	−.02	.01	−.01	.06	2887	2310
12 years	.01	.00	−.00	.00	5622	6255
13–15 years	.01	−.03	−.00	−.06	1449	1933
16 + years	.01	.00	−.04	−.05	875	1460
Age at first marriage						
Less than 18	.01	−.02	.08	.04	2243	2365
18–19	.01	.01	.03	.03	3320	3916
20–21	−.01	.00	.00	.00	3154	3357
22–24	−.01	−.01	−.03	−.05	2302	2283
25–29	−.01	.00	−.12	−.10	1105	848
30 +	−.02	.02	−.28	−.15	262	179
Husband's income (1960 constant dollars)						
Less than $1,000	−.09	−.12	−.14	−.13	312	383
$1,000–1,999	−.02	−.04	−.10	−.09	474	452
$2,000–2,999	.06	−.04	−.04	−.12	822	555
$3,000–3,999	.06	.03	−.02	−.04	1399	1031
$4,000–4,999	.02	.04	−.02	−.02	1916	1078
$5,000–7,499	−.00	.02	.01	−.01	4892	4018
$7,500–9,999	−.02	.01	.06	.04	1489	3017
$10,000–14,999	}−.09	−.05	}.05	.04	}1082	1722
$15,000 +		−.07		.09		691
Grand mean	.53	.40				

[a] Variables in model: wife's education, age at marriage, place of residence, husband's occupation, husband's income (1960 constant dollars), region of residence, number of times married, initial parity, and duration since first marriage.

emerges for 1970; but for 1960 this strong differential by education is not found for currently married women. In both 1960 and 1970 there is an age at marriage differential after other confounding factors have been controlled. This inverse relationship between age at marriage and fertility diminished somewhat between 1960 and 1970, but in both time periods the effect is substantial.

In order to examine the relationship between income and fertility in two separate time periods, we simply have converted 1970 incomes into 1960 constant dollars by applying a correction factor, which reflects the decline in the purchasing power of the dollar. For urban white women, there tended to be an inverse zero-order relationship between husband's income and fertility. However, the net or standardized relationship is clearly positive in both years.[7] This reversal between the crude and adjusted pattern occurs because:

1. Higher income men are disproportionately married to women with higher levels of education and higher ages at first marriage. Both of these factors tend to depress fertility.
2. Income increases with age, higher income men are older, have been married longer, and are likely to be beyond the marriage durations at which people typically have children.

If husband's income is categorized in terms of deciles rather than 1960 constant dollars, similar results are obtained.

Among non-Southern blacks, as among urban whites, there was essentially no relationship between education and the fertility of currently married women in 1960; but in 1970 the expected inverse relationship is found (Table 2.7). Similarly, there is a strong inverse relationship between age at marriage and current fertility. The adjusted relationship between income and fertility for non-Southern blacks is weak, but tends to be inverse.

For the final group, the Spanish-surname population, in both years we find an inverse relationship between fertility and both education and age at marriage (Table 2.8). As is the case for urban whites and non-Southern blacks, the relationship between age at marriage and fertility diminished somewhat during the decade. In 1960 we find no systematic relationship between husband's income and fertility. In 1970 there is a tendency for the relationship to be inverse—unlike that found for urban whites and non-Southern blacks.

In order to examine the relationship between such variables as race or residence and current fertility, we have used a total sample and have controlled for various confounding influences by means of a multiple regression analysis. These results are shown in Table 2.9. Fertility differentials among the major racial and ethnic groups in the United States persisted between 1960 and 1970. The Spanish-surname population had very high fertility in comparison with the majority population. If anything, this differential (controlling for the compositional factors also included in

---

[7] This positive income effect is discussed, at length, in Rindfuss and Sweet, 1977, Chapter 4.

TABLE 2.7

Differentials from the Grand Mean in Recent Fertility by Education, Husband's Income, and Age at First Marriage: Currently Married Non-Southern Black Women Aged Less Than 40, 1960 and 1970

	Unadjusted		Adjusted		Number of women	
	1960	1970	1960[a]	1970[b]	1960	1970
Education						
Less than 5 years	−.04	−.11	.00	−.11	181	116
5–8 years	−.05	−.09	.00	−.02	1523	722
9–11 years	.07	.05	.02	.05	2428	2416
12 years	−.02	.01	−.02	−.01	2333	3798
13–15 years	−.03	−.03	−.00	−.03	615	980
16 + years	−.08	−.12	−.01	−.09	249	474
Age at first marriage						
Less than 18	.07	.01	.15	.09	1964	2009
18–19	.06	.08	.08	.08	1719	2235
20–21	−.02	−.01	−.03	−.01	1374	1779
22–24	−.05	−.04	−.09	−.07	1266	1414
25–29	−.13	−.09	−.23	−.17	770	809
30 +	−.23	−.17	−.46	−.35	236	260
Husband's income						
(1960 constant dollars)						
Less than $1000	−.02	.03	−.08	−.02	516	524
$1,000–1,999	.05	.02	−.02	−.04	573	392
$2,000–2,999	.04	.14	−.02	.06	993	526
$3,000–3,999	.05	.05	.03	.02	1546	1272
$4,000–4,999	−.02	.03	.00	.00	1631	1216
$5,000–7,499	−.04	−.03	.01	−.02	1836	3117
$7,500–9,999	−.09	−.06	.02	.00	174	1071
$10,000–14,999	} −.10	−.09	} .01	.01	} 60	306
$15,000 +		.05		.16		82
Grand mean	.60	.41				

[a] Variables in the model: wife's education, age at marriage, husband's occupation, husband's income (1960 constant dollars), number of times married, initial parity, marriage duration, region of birth.

[b] Variables in the model: wife's education, age at marriage, husband's occupation, husband's income (1960 constant dollars), region of birth, initial parity, marriage duration.

the analysis) has increased slightly during the decade. Blacks had a considerably higher level of marital fertility than whites in 1960. By 1970 this differential in the fertility of currently married whites and blacks had been reduced, but not eliminated.

There are persisting fertility differentials with respect to metropolitan

TABLE 2.8

Differentials from the Grand Mean in Recent Fertility by Education, Husband's Income, and Age at First Marriage: Currently Married Spanish Surname Women Aged Less Than 40, 1960 and 1970

	Unadjusted		Adjusted[a]		Number of women	
	1960	1970	1960	1970	1960	1970
Education						
Less than 5 years	.08	.06	.10	.10	728	526
5–8 years	.03	.04	.03	.06	1312	1202
9–11 years	−.02	.03	−.04	.02	874	1200
12 years	−.09	−.06	−.08	−.07	807	1411
13–15 years	−.05	−.10	−.05	−.12	144	331
16 + years	−.19	−.09	−.14	−.11	62	100
Age at first marriage						
Less than 18	.05	.01	.08	.05	1172	1357
18–19	−.02	−.01	.02	.01	1025	1315
20–21	.04	−.04	.04	−.03	738	947
22–24	−.08	.01	−.10	−.03	605	734
25–29	−.02	.08	−.12	−.04	290	340
30 +	−.10	.11	−.40	−.14	97	77
Husband's income (1960 constant dollars)						
Less than $1000	.05	.08	−.03	.00	324	292
$1,000–1,999	.11	.03	.00	−.02	474	326
$2,000–2,999	.10	.17	.02	.10	644	543
$3,000–3,999	.04	.07	.02	.02	631	839
$4,000–4,999	−.00	.07	.02	.06	643	579
$5,000–7,499	−.10	−.07	−.03	−.04	937	1368
$7,500–9,999	−.22	−.12	.00	−.05	197	540
$10,000–14,999	}−.24	−.22	}−.04	−.09	} 77	228
$15,000 +		−.15		.02		55
Grand mean	.78	.55				

[a] Variables in the model: wife's education, age at marriage, husband's occupation, place of residence, husband's income (1960 constant dollars), number of times married, place of birth, initial parity, and marriage duration.

versus nonmetropolitan residence and urban versus farm versus rural nonfarm residence. Within areas identified as metropolitan, the rural non-farm population has the highest fertility level, the urban population has considerably lower fertility levels, and the farm population within metropolitan areas has intermediate levels of reproduction. In the nonmetropol-

TABLE 2.9

Differentials from the Grand Mean in Recent Fertility by "Ethnicity," Residence, and Region: Currently Married Women, 1960 and 1970

	Unadjusted		Adjusted[a]		Number of cases	
	1960	1970	1960	1970	1960	1960
"Ethnicity"						
White, except Spanish sur-name	−.02	−.01	−.02	−.01	17237	17531
White, Spanish surname	.19	.14	.16	.17	392	430
Black	.15	.02	.15	.04	1586	1639
Other races	.09	.01	.03	.02	204	267
Residence						
Metropolitan, urban	−.01	−.01	−.03	−.02	9589	10918
Metropolitan, rural nonfarm	.04	.03	.05	.03	1639	1421
Metropolitan, rural farm	−.04	−.02	.00	.01	173	102
Nonmetropolitan, urban	−.01	−.02	−.01	−.02	2683	3088
Nonmetropolitan, rural non-farm	.00	.04	.01	.03	1711	1426
Nonmetropolitan, rural farm	.01	−.01	.04	.08	648	274
N. A.,[b] urban	.02	.02	.02	.03	1512	1620
N. A., rural nonfarm	.06	.05	.07	.07	856	743
N. A., rural farm	.04	−.01	.08	.09	608	275
Region of residence						
Northeast	−.01	.02	.02	.02	4566	4392
North Central	.02	.02	.02	.02	5629	5558
South	−.01	−.02	−.03	−.02	6071	6388
West	.00	−.02	.00	−.03	3153	3529
Grand mean	.55	.41				

[a] Variables in the model: education, age at marriage, region of residence, initial parity, "ethnicity," residence, husband's income (1960 constant dollars), marriage duration.

[b] Because of confidentiality requirements that no area of less than 250,000 be identi-fied, we can distinguish metropolitan residence for the population of only 25 of the 50 states. The states for which metropolitan residence is not available include predominantly nonmetropolitan states. So what our metropolitan residence variable does is to distinguish first between metropolitan and nonmetropolitan residence in states that have a relatively large metropolitan population. The third category, "Not Ascertained," includes predomi-nantly nonmetropolitan people living in nonmetropolitan states. In 1970 the states for which metropolitan residence was not available are Arizona, Arkansas, Colorado, Delaware, Ha-waii, Idaho, Iowa, Kansas, Kentucky, Louisiana, Maine, Minnesota, Mississippi, Montana, Nebraska, Nevada, New Hampshire, New Mexico, North Dakota, Oklahoma, Oregon, Rhode Island, South Dakota, Utah, and West Virginia.

itan areas, fertility levels are considerably higher for the rural farm population than for the urban or rural nonfarm populations. In 1970 there are
only very small metropolitan and nonmetropolitan fertility differences for
urban and rural nonfarm wives, but a very large metropolitan–nonmetropolitan difference in the fertility of farm wives.

There are also persisting regional differences in fertility net of these
other residential as well as socioeconomic and demographic factors. The
Northeast and North Central regions tend to have higher levels of current
fertility than the South or West.

Summary and Conclusion

To summarize, the vast changes in fertility and fertility-related behavior since World War II were both unprecedented and unpredicted; and
they have had important immediate and long-range effects on American
society. Furthermore, they are pervasive; that is, those social variables
that we have been able to examine with census data, such as race, ethnic
status, education and residence, do not indicate differences with respect
to trends in fertility. Nor do these social variables differentiate trends in
such related phenomena as proportion marrying or the age pattern of fertility. In short, the same trends were found for every group. Yet these
same social and economic variables do tend to differentiate current fertility levels in the cross section.

It might be asked why variables such as race, ethnic status, or education should affect fertility *trends*. The typical time series proposition is
formulated as follows: A change in X implies a change in Y. Here Y is
fertility and X is race, ethnic status, or education. Because race, ethnic
status, and education tend not to change, why should they be expected to
affect changes in fertility? The reason is that race, ethnic status, and education (and other variables, such as income or residence, which are
changeable) are "filter" variables; people tend to live their lives within
groups whose boundaries are defined by these variables. We would expect that any secular change that affects fertility trends would be filtered
through these groups and, therefore, fertility trends would be affected by
the standard social and economic variables. That this is not the case suggests that those factors responsible for changes in period fertility during
the past 25 years were sufficiently powerful to permeate every group; or,
alternatively, that there were a number of factors operating in the same
direction and that some operated on certain social groups and some
operated on others. Undoubtedly, both possibilities are partially true.

It should be noted that the expected "filtering" effect of race and education is different from the more common compositional explanation to which these variables are put. The compositional explanation accounts for changes over time in some dependent variable by showing that the total population is changing with respect to the proportion of the population in each of the various categories of some predictor variable known to be related to the dependent variable. For example, education is inversely related to fertility in the cross section. Thus an upgrading in the educational attainment of the population would be expected to bring about a reduction in fertility. In the present chapter, such a compositional explanation is shown to be partly responsible for the increase in proportion of women never married. But this type of compositional explanation is not applicable to the fertility trends of the past 25 years because the same trend is found *within* each group examined.

Not only were these trends found within every subgroup in the United States, but also many of the same trends can be found in other developed nations as well—albeit with important differences. In general those countries that had comparatively low levels of fertility during the 1930s experienced a sustained postwar surge in fertility in the 1940s and 1950s, followed by declining fertility rates in the 1960s (Campbell, 1974; Teitelbaum, 1973; and Westoff, 1974). The elevation in fertility was most pronounced in the United States, Canada, Australia, and New Zealand; but it was found in numerous European countries as well.

This pervasiveness of fertility trends suggests that the explanations needed must be of a broad and historical nature. "Broad" here refers to factors that cut across boundaries of the social structure, and "historical" implies explanations that refer to specific events or series of events. Such explanations are not uncommon in the literature; examples would include the relative prosperity of the 1950s, the introduction of the pill, or the birth of the women's movement.

The problem with such explanations is that (a) they generally are ex post facto, (b) in the short run there is not sufficient variation to test these explanations, and (c) they tend not to aid in the prediction of future events. (See Spilerman, 1975, for a more detailed discussion of the various problems.) However, the difficulties involved in historical explanations should not dissuade demographers from pursuing them because, as the results of our project to date suggest, historical factors are most likely to be responsible for the recent wide fluctuations in period fertility—fluctuations that have had a substantial impact on virtually every social institution.

ACKNOWLEDGMENTS

The assistance of Barbara Witt is gratefully acknowledged.

References

Campbell, A. A.
1974 "Beyond the demographic transition." *Demography* 11 4: 549–561.
Cho, L. J.
1968 "Income and differentials in current fertility." *Demography* 5: 198–211.
1971 "On estimating annual birth rates from census data on children." *Proceedings of the American Statistical Association, Social Statistics Section.* Pp. 86–96.
Cho, L. J., W. H. Grabill, and D. J. Bogue
1970 *Differential Current Fertility in the United States.* Chicago: University of Chicago Press.
Coale, A. J., and M. Zelnik
1963 *New Estimates of Fertility and Population in the United States.* Princeton, N.J.: Princeton University Press.
Freedman, R.
1962 "American studies of family planning and fertility: A review of major trends and issues." Pp. 211–227 in C. V. Kiser (ed.), *Research on Family Planning.* Princeton, N.J.: Princeton University Press.
Freedman, R., P. K. Whelpton, and A. A. Campbell
1959 *Family Planning, Sterility, and Population Growth.* New York: McGraw-Hill.
Goldberg, D.
1974 "Modernism." Occasional paper of the World Fertility Survey, No. 14.
Grabill, W. H., and L. J. Cho
1965 "Methodology for the measurement of current fertility from population data on young children." *Demography* 2: 50–73.
Grabill, W. H., C. V. Kiser, and P. K. Whelpton
1958 *The Fertility of American Women.* New York: John Wiley and Co.
Retherford, R. D., and L. J. Cho
1974 "Age-parity-specific fertility rates from census or survey data on own children." Paper presented at the annual meetings of the Population Association of America, New York.
Rindfuss, R. R.
1974 "Annual fertility rates from census data: method, assumptions and limitations." Center for Demography and Ecology Working Paper 74–21.
1975a "Recent trends in fertility differentials among educational groups." Center for Demography and Ecology Working Paper 75–11.
1975b "Minority status and recent fertility trends." Paper presented at the annual meetings of the American Sociological Association, San Francisco.
1975c "Trends and differentials in the timing of fertility: 1945–1965." Unpublished manuscript.
1978 "Changing Patterns of Fertility in the South: A Social-Demographic Examination." *Social Forces* 57(2).
Rindfuss, R. R., and J. A. Sweet
1975 "Rural fertility trends, United States: 1945–1973." Paper presented at the annual meetings of the Midwest Sociological Society, Chicago.
1977 *Postwar Fertility Trends and Differentials in the United States.* New York: Academic Press.
Ryder, N. B.
1969 "The emergence of a modern fertility pattern: United States, 1917–1966." Pp. 99–123 in S. J. Behrman, L. Corsa, Jr., and R. Freedman (eds.), *Fertility and Family Planning: A World View.* Ann Arbor: The University of Michigan.

Spilerman, S.
1975 "Forecasting social events." Pp. 381–404 in K. C. Land and S. Spilerman (eds.), *Social Indicator Models*. New York: Russell Sage Foundation.
Sweet, J. A.
1974a "Differentials in the rate of fertility decline: 1960–1970." *Family Planning Perspectives* 6(2): 103–107.
1974b "Recent fertility change among high fertility minorities in the United States." Center for Demography and Ecology Working Paper 74–11.
1974c "Trends and differentials in the fertility of the rural farm population." Paper presented at the annual meetings of the Rural Sociological Association, Montreal.
1975 "Recent marriage trends in the United States." Paper presented at the Sex Stratification Seminar, Chicago.
Teitelbaum, M. S.
1973 "U.S. population growth in international perspective." Pp. 69–84 in C. F. Westoff (ed.), *Toward the End of Growth*. Englewood Cliffs, N.J.: Prentice-Hall.
U.S. Bureau of the Census
1963a Census of Population: 1960, Subject Reports, Final Report PC(2)-1B, Spanish Surname Population. Washington, D.C.: U.S. Government Printing Office.
1963b Census of Population: 1960, Subject Reports, Final Report PC(2)-1C, Nonwhite Population by Race. Washington, D.C.: U.S. Government Printing Office.
1963c Census of Population: 1960, Subject Reports, Final Report PC(2)-1D, Puerto Ricans in the United States. Washington, D.C.: U.S. Government Printing Office.
1966 Census of Population: 1960, Subject Reports, Final Report PC(2)-4E, Marital Status. Washington, D.C.: U.S. Government Printing Office.
1972 Census of Population: 1970, Subject Reports, Final Report PC(2)-4C, Marital Status. Washington, D.C.: U.S. Government Printing Office.
1973a Census of Population: 1970, Subject Reports, Final Report PC(2)-1B, Nego Population. Washington, D.C.: U.S. Government Printing Office.
1973b Census of Population: 1970, Subject Reports, Final Report PC(2)-1C, Persons of Spanish Origin. Washington, D.C.: U.S. Government Printing Office.
1973c Census of Population: 1970, Subject Reports, Final Report PC(2)-1D, Persons of Spanish Surname. Washington, D.C.: U.S. Government Printing Office.
1973d Census of Population: 1970, Subject Reports, Final Report PC(2)-1E, Puerto Ricans in the United States. Washington, D.C.: U.S. Government Printing Office.
1973e Census of Population: 1970, Subject Reports, Final Report PC(2)-1F, American Indians. Washington, D.C.: U.S. Government Printing Office.
1973f Census of Population: 1970, Subject Reports, Final Report PC(2)-1G, Japanese, Chinese and Filipinos in the United States. Washington, D.C.: U.S. Government Printing Office.
1975 Current Population Reports, Special Studies, Series P-23, No. 51, Characteristics of American Youth: 1974. Washington, D.C.: U.S. Government Printing Office.
Westoff, C. F.
1974 "The populations of the developed countries." *Scientific American* 231(3): 109–120.

3

Age and the Sociology of Fertility: How Old Is Too Old?[1]

RONALD R. RINDFUSS and LARRY L. BUMPASS

Age has received rather little attention from the sociology of fertility even though it is a basic variable in the demography of that subject. The biological features of the age pattern of fertility are well known. After menarche, the ability to reproduce increases with age to a plateau in the twenties and then declines at an accelerating pace until menopause is reached. The level and shape of the schedules vary, but marked age variations in fertility are found in all populations, with the consequence that age is routinely taken into account in fertility analyses. Although age differences in marital fertility[2] are readily explained by differential fecundity in the absence of contraception, fecundity need not have a major effect in low fertility populations. Nevertheless, the common understand-

[1] The analysis reported here was supported in part by a NIH grant, No. HD07682, and by a CPR grant No. HD05876 to the Center for Demography and Ecology, as well as NIMH Grant No. MH-24807.
[2] Other factors such as age at marriage patterns and widow remarriage sometimes play an important role in the shape of total fertility schedules.

Social Demography

ing of differential fecundity by age may partly explain the relative neglect[3] of the social and psychological effects of age on fertility decisions.

This chapter focuses on age and the related demographic concept of elapsed time as salient variables in the decision to terminate childbearing (or conversely, the absence of a decision to continue). The basic proposition can be simply stated: later means fewer. The chapter is meant to be provocative, rather than definitive; the intent is to explore and illustrate a set of ideas, rather than to systematically test any particular hypothesis. We hope to examine some of these ideas more adequately in future work.

In addition to being important to the sociology of fertility, the issue of age is obviously relevant to the interpretation of period changes in fertility. The frequent debate over whether period reductions reflect changes in reproductive goals or "simply" represent delays in fertility may be answered by the assertion that delays may be expected to result in an ultimate reduction in the level of fertility desired even in the absence of an initial change in goals.

The first part of the chapter discusses ways in which age may affect fertility decisions. The remainder of the chapter explores the utility of this approach for understanding two concerns of students of fertility behavior: differential fertility by age at marriage and the effect of marital disruption on fertility.

The Sociological Component of the Age Effect on Fertility

Being "too old" is often reported as a reason for not having more children (Hoffman, 1975; Rainwater, 1965; Whelpton *et al.*, 1966). Age is an important consideration in a couple's decision with respect to the termination of fertility. While in its simplest form this proposition refers to a decision process about whether or not another child is desired, it also applies to other aspects that affect the probability of another birth such as choice of contraceptive method and the vigilance with which contraception is practiced. For example, age differentials in contraceptive failure among couples intending no more children (Ryder, 1973) may be interpreted as reflecting this component as well as differential fecundity. Another example would be the delay of a sterilization until an age beyond which a couple is certain they will not want another child.

---

[3] This is not to imply that the issue has been completely ignored in the literature. For example, Ryder (1973) has "speculate[d] that one factor in the decision to end childbearing is the respondent's age, quite apart from the number of children she has already borne [p. 136]." The point is that the proposition has not received the attention it should.

The social aspects of age may affect fertility decisions in a number of ways. First, the longer a woman[4] postpones bearing a child of a given birth order, the greater the likelihood is that she will get involved in other ego-involved activities that consume time and energy. These activities may take the form of a career, completion of education, volunteer work, or the pursuit of avocational interests. Whatever form they take, these activities compete with childbearing and rearing for the woman's time and attention. It should be noted that this competition need not pit the "traditional" roles of wife and mother against the "modern" role of a career woman. Indeed, time invested in activities in connection with children already born may compete with additional childbearing.

Second, because fertility tends to occur within a comparatively short time span, its postponement increases the likelihood that other members of the couple's cohort will have completed their childbearing. To give birth at a later age implies a set of constraints over an extended portion of the couple's married life during which they will be "out of phase" with their age peers. While the couple goes through the progression of child-rearing phases from intensive infant care to coping with teenagers, at each phase members of their birth cohort will be in successive phases. Thus couples contemplating a parity progression at a relatively late age face both a set of constraints not shared by their age peers and the loss of an important source of advice and support in the childrearing process. One aspect of this is likely to be a diminution with age of pronatalist influences from friends and acquaintances.

The effect of age on fertility decisions also has a social–biological component that is not related to fecundity. Rather, it derives from the concern that with increasing age, the partners may not have sufficient time and energy to cope with a child (or another child)—viewing time and energy either in absolute terms or as scarce and diminishing resources for which childbearing comes into increasing competition with other life goals.

Finally, there may be normative bounds prescribing the "proper" time for childbearing. There are a number of sources and manifestations of such a norm. One source may be concern over the onset of secondary sterility—reflected in part in the admonition to young couples to have (more) children "before it's too late." Similarly, there may be a general awareness through the popular press that bearing children at relatively later ages involves increased health risks for mother and child. In the ideal–typical life cycle represented in the popular culture by television and press, childbearing belongs to the early stages, and couples with

---

[4] Throughout, age of wife is being employed. However, age of husband is also likely to have an effect, particularly when there is disparity between age of wife and age of husband.

babies are *young* couples. That it is considered somehow less appropriate to bear children at later ages may be suggested in the ambivalence of friends over how to respond to a pregnancy announcement by a couple in their late thirties.

In a fledgling attempt to approach this issue, women in the 1970 National Fertility Study[5] were asked about the ideal age of a woman at the birth of her first and last children:

Q. 3:   What do you think is the ideal age for a woman to have her *first* child?

Q. 4:   And what is the ideal age for a woman to have her *last* child?

Although these questions are subject to all the potential hazards involved in questions dealing with the ideals (for example, see Blake, 1966; Bumpass and Westoff, 1970; Rindfuss, 1973; Ryder and Westoff, 1969) and some difficulties of their own as well, the uniqueness of the questions merits a brief discussion. The averages are 21.8 for the ideal age to have a first child and 30.8 for the ideal age to have a last child. Thus the ideal span of childbearing (9 years) is a comparatively small fraction of the biological potential and is not very dissimilar from the average actual time used for childbearing.

The distribution for the ideal age to have the last child is very uneven. Thirty-one percent of the respondents give 30 as the ideal age to terminate, and the next most frequent responses are 35 and 25. These preferred numbers are also evident within various subgroups. This pattern of heaping is identical to that found in the reporting of age in societies where age is not well known (Stockwell and Wicks, 1974), and may reflect a general absence of a considered opinion on the subject. However, there is another plausible interpretation. Ages 25, 30, and 35 represent significant years in a social sense. Age 30 is perhaps the best example—as immortalized by the radical slogan of the 1960s. These birthdays, more than adjacent birthdays, are regarded as significant milestones in the life cycle process.

A second age-related factor that is likely to have a sociological effect on fertility is age of youngest child or, as it is sometimes termed, length of open interval. This variable is obviously related to age of woman, particularly in that, unless another birth intervenes, both variables increase over time at the same rate. Probably the main effect of age of youngest child is related to the level of child care the woman is involved in—an effect imperfectly captured by the age of woman variable. Clearly, the amount of

---

[5] The 1970 National Fertility Study, directed by Norman B. Ryder and Charles F. Westoff, is a national probability sample of 6752 ever-married women under 45 years of age, residing in the continental United States.

time spent in child care varies with age of youngest child. It has been estimated that the amount of child care time required of the woman is three to four times as great if the youngest child is an infant than if the youngest child is age 2 through 5 (see Stone, 1972). Other things being equal, the further the woman is from the intensive care required by very young children, the less willing she may be to have another child and reenter these intensive care obligations.

Age of youngest child is also an indication of the likelihood that a woman will have developed nonfamilial interests that compete with childbearing and rearing. The implication here is similar to that which applies to age of woman: As time becomes available that is not required for child care, the probability that the woman will become involved in nonfamilial activities increases. Furthermore, there may be a consensus, if not a norm, regarding the maximum desirable interbirth interval (see Westoff *et al.,* 1963, p. 63).

Methodological Concerns

It is not without reason that the issues addressed here have received little attention: Their empirical exploration is fraught with methodological pitfalls. One such problem is the measurement of the biological component of the age effect on fertility. The primary assertion is that age has an effect on fertility greater than its simple biological component, and that the reasons for that effect are sociological. The most straightforward procedure would be to control for the biological effect and examine what is left. But although the biological effect is well known, the measurement of fecundity is highly problematic where contraception is widely practiced. (This is not to imply that fecundity is easy to measure in a noncontracepting population—but that alternative need not concern us here.) The problem arises because periods of contraceptive use cannot be assessed for fecundability and nonuse tends to be related to perceptions of fecundability. What is measurable is known or suspected sterility. The former is generally the result of explicit events (a sterilizing operation or menopause) and thus can be reported and dated comparatively accurately. The latter is generally based on intervals of nonuse of contraception, and, as such, the perception and dating process vary from individual to individual.

A second major difficulty is that the proposition "later means fewer" is concerned with individual changes over time, and, as such, its testing demands longitudinal data. The argument is that the longer an intended birth is postponed, the greater the likelihood is that a couple will revise its fertility goals downward. While there is some longitudinal support for this point (Freedman *et al.,* 1965), our present exploration is confined to cross-sectional data.

In the absence of prior measures of fertility intentions, it is only possible to illustrate patterns consistent with our hypothesis. To do so, data from the 1970 National Fertility Study are employed. Whenever possible, the same analyses have been routinely performed on data from the 1965 National Fertility Study and essentially the same results are obtained. This is, of course, gratifying, but it provides little comfort with respect to the longitudinal problem since both are cross-sectional studies.

Age and the Termination of Childbearing

In examining the cross-sectional relationship between age and fertility intentions, we are concerned with the decision to terminate childbearing, and the measure of the dependent variable used is whether or not the respondent intends to have more children.[6] The sample has been restricted to currently married women who are without known or suspected fecundity problems. The focus on presumably fecund women minimizes the biological effects of age on the differentials we observe, since by definition it eliminates from the analysis women who have unsuccessfully tried to become pregnant. For the consideration of age of youngest child, women who are either childless or pregnant are also excluded.

The relationship between age and the intention to have an additional child is shown in Table 3.1. As we would expect, for any given parity, the proportion intending to have more children is strongly and inversely related to age. Similarly, Table 3.2 shows the cross-sectional relationship between age of youngest child and childbearing intentions, controlling for parity. Also as expected, the proportion intending more children is strongly and inversely related to age of youngest child.

In order to see if the relationships found in Tables 3.1 and 3.2 persist

---

[6] Among presumably fecund, currently married women, future childbearing intentions were measured by one of three questions depending on the respondent's current status. Those who were currently pregnant were asked:

Q. 199:   Do you and your husband intend to have another child in addition to the one you are now expecting?

Those who were not currently pregnant and had had zero live births were asked:

Q. 205:   Do you and your husband intend to have any children?

Those who were not currently pregnant and had had one or more live births were asked:

Q. 212:   Do you and your husband intend to have another child?

TABLE 3.1

Proportion Intending More Children by Age of Respondent and Parity: 1970[a,b]

Age	Parity					
	0	1	2	3	4+	Total
	Proportion intending more children					
<20	99	96	*	*	*	94
20–24	97	90	49	33	37	77
25–29	85	77	34	27	19	45
30–34	55	56	18	15	15	23
35–39	*[c]	20	8	7	5	9
40–44	*	10	3	5	6	6
Total	90	75	27	16	11	40
	Number of women					
<20	79	97	15	1	—	192
20–24	295	363	271	68	27	1024
25–29	112	208	346	214	152	1032
30–34	36	96	237	194	224	787
35–39	19	59	172	168	239	657
40–44	16	48	146	135	211	556
Total	557	871	1187	780	853	4248

[a] The following respondents are excluded: women with reported fecundity impairments, currently pregnant women, and women who are currently widowed, divorced, or separated.

[b] The 1970 National Fertility Study oversampled black women. To adjust for this, a weighting system based on Current Population Reports was used in calculating statistics in this and subsequent tables. However, the number of women reported are unweighted.

[c] Asterisk denotes base less than 20.

when other fertility decision related variables are controlled, a dummy variable multiple regression analysis was performed in which the dependent variable was whether or not the couple intended more children. The independent variables, in addition to age, age of youngest child, and parity, include education, race, religion, age at marriage, and the length of the interval between marriage and the birth of the first child. In addition to the restrictions previously described, this analysis was limited to women aged 25–34. The results are shown in Table 3.3 As might be expected, the differentials by age or age of youngest child are diminished somewhat with all the other variables in the model controlled (compare the gross and adjusted columns). However, the effects of age and age of youngest child are still substantial. The proportion intending more is twice as large in the youngest age group as in the oldest. Similarly, the proportion intending more children is two-thirds greater among those who have infants than among those whose youngest child is 6 years old or older.

TABLE 3.2

Proportion Intending More Children by Age of Youngest Child and Parity: 1970[a]

Age of youngest child	Parity				
	1	2	3	4+	Total
Proportion intending more children					
<1	94	49	25	20	59
1–2	88	41	32	16	49
3–5	79	27	17	8	29
6+	26	9	6	8	10
Total	75	27	16	11	32
Number of women					
<1	247	178	89	110	624
1–2	281	290	155	204	930
3–5	156	246	203	222	827
6+	187	476	335	321	1319
Total	871	1190	782	857	3700

[a] The following respondents are excluded: women with reported fecundity impairments, currently pregnant women, women who are currently widowed, divorced, or separated, and women who do not have any children.

These analyses may seem to demonstrate what is intuitively obvious. Our purpose is to draw attention to the fact that the age effects require *sociological* attention focused on the role of age as a factor in the decision not to have more children. Again, we note that the underlying argument is necessarily longitudinal.

If we are correct that age and elapsed time are important dimensions in the fertility decision process, then they may be part of the explanation of two related differentials in fertility: those by age at marriage and marital history. This possibility will be addressed in the next two sections entitled "Age at First Marriage" and "Age at Second Marriage."

Age at First Marriage

The relationship of age at marriage and fertility is among the strongest and most pervasive in the literature. However, theoretical attention to this differential is scant—undoubtedly for reasons similar to those outlined in our initial discussion of age effects. There are a number of likely demographic explanations for the negative effect on fertility of age at marriage: (1) Premarital pregnancy may select women who are both more fecund and less effective contraceptors into early ages at marriage; (2) the

TABLE 3.3

Unadjusted and Adjusted Percentage Intending More Children by Age and Age of Youngest Child for Currently Married, Presumably Fecund, Not Currently Pregnant Women Aged 25–34 Who Have Had at Least One Live Birth: 1970

	Unadjusted percentage intending more	Adjusted percentage[a] intending more	Number of women
Age			
25–26	53	56	343
27–28	35	32	371
29–30	29	29	357
31–32	21	25	308
33–34	17	23	292
Total	31		1671
Age of youngest child			
<1	45	40	252
1–2	38	35	475
3–5	29	30	509
6+	19	24	435
Total	31		1671

[a] The following variables are in the model: age, age of youngest child, parity, education, race, religion, age at marriage, and the length of the interval between marriage and the birth of the first child.

later a woman marries, the shorter will be the length of time she is exposed to the risk of unwanted fertility after she has had all of the children she wants; (3) later age at marriage may result in greater risk of subfecundity before desired childbearing is completed; and (4) some of the fertility differentials by age at marriage may be spurious due to its correlation with other variables such as education and social background.

These relationships have been analyzed in detail for white, once married women in the 1965 and 1970 National Fertility Studies who were married 10–14 years (Bumpass and Mburugu, 1976). While multivariate controls reduce the observed differential somewhat, strong net differences persist that seem best understood in terms of the age effects under discussion here. In both data sets, about one-third of the difference in fertility by age at marriage can be explained by differentials in sterility and unwanted births.

The remaining difference is extremely important in light of the sociology of fertility and may be interpretable in terms of the sociological effects described earlier: the older the woman, the more likely she is to be involved in nonfamilial activities; the older the woman, the more likely that her age contemporaries have completed their childbearing; and the older the woman, the less support and urging she will receive from significant others to have children.

Age at Second Marriage

Similar processes ought to be associated with age in the fertility of second marriages. In addition, the sociological effect of age at remarriage also incorporates some of the effect of age of youngest child. To the extent that fertility does not occur during the disruption, then the disruption has the effect of lengthening the open interval—that is, of increasing the age of youngest child.

To explore these ideas, this section examines the effect of age at remarriage on *intended* fertility in the second marriage for a subsample of respondents from the 1970 National Fertility Study. This subsample consists of all twice-married, currently married women, with the exception of those who had a sterilizing operation (or whose current husband did) before the remarriage, and with the exception of those who think they are sterile even though they have not had a sterilizing operation. The dependent variable is intended fertility in the second marriage, which is the sum of the number of *wanted* children born in the second marriage plus the additional number of children intended. Thus this analysis is directed at factors affecting childbearing decisions after remarriage.

As before, a dummy variable multiple regression routine is employed to control for a number of potentially confounding variables. The number of children the woman had borne prior to the beginning of the second marriage is controlled. Unfortunately, similar information is not available for the current husband. Because orientations toward second marriage fertility may be different for divorced women than for widowed women, the reason for dissolution is included in the models. In addition, the following background variables are controlled: education of wife, education of current husband, race of wife, and religion of wife. Table 3.4 shows the results of this analysis.

The first column in Table 3.4 shows the unadjusted mean intended fertility in second marriage for each category of age at second marriage. As expected, mean fertility decreases as age at second marriage increases. The second column shows the adjusted mean fertility. Although the differentials among the various groups decline somewhat when potentially confounding factors are controlled, the effect of age at second marriage is still strong and inverse, and this relationship is orderly with the exception

TABLE 3.4

Unadjusted and Adjusted Mean Intended Fertility in Second Marriage for Twice-Married, Currently Married Women: 1970

Age at second marriage	Mean intended fertility in second marriage					Unweighted number of women
	Unadjusted	Net$_1$[a]	Net$_2$[b]	Net$_3$[c]	Net$_5$[d]	
<20	2.62	2.24	2.34	2.25	2.55	39
20–21	2.06	1.74	1.76	1.76	1.87	64
22–23	1.64	1.60	1.53	1.60	1.57	69
24–25	1.51	1.57	1.56	1.59	1.55	69
26–27	1.38	1.43	1.42	1.42	1.39	54
28–29	0.89	1.18	1.15	1.17	1.06	41
30–31	1.06	1.15	1.10	1.11	1.01	36
32–34	1.13	1.36	1.45	1.34	1.31	32
35 +	0.46	0.72	0.77	0.71	0.63	36
Total	1.49					

[a] Model includes: number of children born by second marriage, reason for dissolution, education of wife, education of current husband, race, and religion of wife.

[b] Model includes: the basic six control variables, plus length of first marriage and length of marital disuption.

[c] Model includes: the basic six control variables, plus age at first marriage and length of first marriage.

[d] Model includes: the basic six control variables plus age at first marriage and length of marital disruption.

of women who began their second marriage at ages 32–34. Women who began their second marriage at age 19 or younger have a preferred fertility in second marriage that is three times greater than those who began their second marriage at age 35 or greater; and this is the case controlling for the number of children born by the beginning of the second marriage. Furthermore, there is a difference of more than half a child between those who began their second marriage at age 20 or 21 and those who began their second marriage at age 30 or 31.

Age at beginning of second marriage is the sum of three variables that are important for fertility preferences: age at first marriage, length of first marriage, and length of marital disruption. While these three components and age at beginning of second marriage cannot be entered into the same equation, it is possible to use any pair of these components and age at beginning of second marriage in the model. This has been done for each of the three possible combinations, and the results are shown in Table 3.4. In each of the three cases, age at second marriage still has the same strong, inverse relationship to mean intended fertility in second marriage.

Conclusion

One of the major advances in the demography of fertility has been the separation of the timing and number components of movements in period fertility. However, acknowledging the analytical dividends of this decomposition, there are also theoretical links between timing and quantity. It is, of course, well known that the two components tend to respond to similar influences, so that what affects the tempo of fertility of younger cohorts may effect the quantity of fertility of older cohorts in the same period. The perspective taken here is that, in addition, changes (over time) or differences (within a period) in the timing of fertility are associated with differences in the ultimate amount of childbearing. The sociological meanings of age as they affect fertility decisions are seen as the critical link in this relationship.

Moreover, we want to emphasize that it is relative age[7] that is important. Since the significant considerations are sociological rather than biological, "How old is too old?" is a question about the relative childbearing pace of one's peers, internalized ideal life cycles, and the expectations of significant others.

We feel that the social definition of childbearing age is a critical issue that has received far too little attention in the sociology of fertility, and that this is especially unfortunate because of the potential theoretical power of this question for the interpretation of other fertility differentials. We note in conclusion that an example of this might be education. One effect that education has is to distribute women into various ages at parenthood.

We do not intend to imply that the usual interpretations attached to education differences are irrelevant. For example, less traditional orientations among high education women could result in longer delays after the completion of education before motherhood. We do wish to note, however, that a significant part of the education differences in fertility may be a consequence of the delay of fertility required for a given level of education to be completed. Such delays may reduce fertility in both its unwanted and wanted components. The latter is our major concern here. When we examine the effect of education on wanted fertility (as defined in Ryder and Westoff, 1972), the negative effect disappears or becomes curvilinear when age at first birth is controlled. For example, for currently married, white mothers married 10–15 years in 1970, the education means are:

---

[7] See Ryder (1973).

	Observed	Adjusted for age at first birth	Number of cases
0–8 years	3.2	3.0	43
9–11 years	3.1	2.9	121
12 years	2.7	2.8	411
College 1–3	2.9	2.9	136
College 4+	2.8	3.0	94

It is quite possible that a number of other variables typically found to affect fertility do so, to an extent, because of their effect on the timing of fertility.

ACKNOWLEDGMENTS

The assistance of Sue Anne Cochrane, Mary Ann Hanson, Cheryl Knobeloch, Margaret Knoll, and Barbara Witt is gratefully acknowledged.

References

Blake, J.
   1966   "Ideal family size among white Americans: A quarter of a century's evidence." *Demography* 3(1): 154–173.
Bumpass, L. L., and E. K. Mburugu
   1976   "The effect of age at marriage on fertility in the U.S." Center for Demography and Ecology Working Paper 76–22.
Bumpass, L. L., and C. F. Westoff
   1970   "The 'perfect contraceptive' population." *Science* 169: 1177–1182.
Freedman, R., L. C. Coombs, and L. Bumpass
   1965   "Stability and change in expectations about family size: A longitudinal study." *Demography* 2: 250–275.
Hoffman, L. W.
   1975   "The value of children to parents and the decrease in family size." Paper presented at the annual meeting of the American Philosophical Society, Philadelphia.
Rainwater, L.
   1965.   *Family Design: Marital Sexuality, Family Size, and Contraception.* Chicago: Aldine Publishing Co.
Rindfuss, R. R.
   1973   "Measurement of personal fertility preferences." Unpublished doctoral dissertation, Princeton University.
Ryder, N. B.
   1973   "Contraceptive failure in the United States." *Family Planning Perspectives* 5(3): 133–142.
Ryder, N. B., and C. F. Westoff
   1969   "Relationships among intended, expected, desired, and ideal family size: United States, 1965." Center for Population Research working paper (March).
   1972   "Wanted and unwanted fertility in the United States: 1965 and 1970." P. 471 in C. F. Westoff and R. Parke, Jr. (eds.), *Demographic and Social Aspects of Population Growth.* Research Reports of the U. S. Commission on Population Growth

and the American Future. Vol. I. Washington, D. C.: U. S. Government Printing Office.

Stockwell, E. G., and J. W. Wicks
  1974 "Age heaping in recent national censuses." *Social Biology* 21(2): 163–167.
Stone, P. J.
  1972 "Child care in twelve countries." Pp. 249–264 in A. Szalai (ed.), *The Use of Time*. The Hague: Mouton.
Westoff, C. F., R. G. Potter, and P. C. Sagi
  1963 *The Third Child: A Study in the Prediction of Fertility*. Princeton, N. J.: Princeton University Press.
Whelpton, P. K., A. A. Campbell, and J. E. Patterson
  1966 *Fertility and Family Planning in the United States*. Princeton, N. J.: Princeton University Press.

4

Couples' Decision-Making Processes Regarding Fertility[1]

LINDA J. BECKMAN

The major objective of this chapter is to elucidate a social–psychological model of fertility decision making in order to call increased attention to the role of psychological and motivational variables in the determination of fertility. Social–psychological theory and research that pertain to how individuals and marital dyads form preferences and make choices regarding childbearing will be reviewed. The focus will be on these processes as they occur in the United States and other developed countries, for one likely concomitant of modernization is increased importance of decision making in the determination of fertility.

Women in developed countries use contraception to reduce their fertility far below their biological ability. Many couples (or individuals) are making choices regarding the use of contraception and the limitation of fertility. The questions to be considered are *how* they "decide" to limit fertility and *what* determines their decisions.

Fertility-related decision processes recently have attracted the interest

[1] Preparation of this paper was supported, in part, by grant HD-52807 from Center for Population Research NICHD and by Career Development Award AA-00002 to the author.

of psychologists and social psychologists for the following reasons. First, with increasing utilization of the more effective means of fertility regulation, it seems likely that fertility "decision" processes are becoming more salient, and preferences regarding fertility may be increasingly in accord with actual fertility. Second, as sociodemographic differentials in fertility decrease (Ryder and Westoff, 1972; Turchi, 1975; U. S. Bureau of the Census, 1973, 1974; Westoff and Ryder, 1969), individual factors in decision making attain increasing explanatory power. While the decline of sociodemographic differentials in fertility may be a reflection of declining variance in desired and actual fertility in the United States, an alternative assumption is that subgroup normative influences have become less salient while individual instrumental values and preferences regarding fertility have gained in predictive power. Motivational preferences are less likely merely to reflect sociodemographic differences and may operate independently to influence fertility behavior.

Demography's Implicit Recognition of Motivational Influences

Demographers have postulated implicitly that fertility decision making occurs, but, because of their emphasis on aggregate data, have generally not explicitly examined or defined decision-making processes. Psychologists (Edwards, 1954; Fishbein, 1967; Janis and Mann, 1977; Jones and Gerard, 1967; Lee, 1974) have examined the decision-making process extensively, but in the past have rarely applied it to the area of fertility.

Most demographers postulate underlying subjective psychological variables, as in use of the concept *value of children,* to explain transitions from high fertility to low fertility during economic development. But in their reliance on data from censuses and large-scale national sample surveys, demographers largely have avoided problems of reliability and validity that plague researchers dealing with these "softer" variables. Even when they have used motivational variables, these have tended to be unidimensional variables such as desired, expected, or ideal family size. Thus although implicitly recognizing that some type of decision making or preference–crystallization process occurs, demographers have left the area of choices, preferences, and decisions regarding fertility to two divergent groups, economists and psychologists.

Despite demographers' reluctance to examine these microlevel variables, I believe that our models must be reductionistic and must attempt to examine individual preferences and decisions. If contraceptive use depends on a process of individual and family decision making, macromodels of sociological or demographic variables are not sufficient. Attention

must be given to the correspondence or interaction between sociodemographic and motivational variables, that is, how macrovariables are translated into microvariables. Even more important is the possibility that motivational variables can explain differences in fertility not accounted for
by demographic differentials (Beckman, 1974, 1976). Such an approach
has been criticized severely (Hauser and Duncan, 1959, pp. 96–102) for
the psychological reductionism or rationalization inherent in such accounts, lack of representativeness, reliability and validity, and inability to
deal with fertility in the aggregate or to measure trends over time. However, none of these difficulties, except for reductionism, is inherent in
psychological variables, and the alternative is to postulate (implicitly if
not explicitly) intervening processes or variables while refusing to examine them.

Social–Psychological Approaches to Fertility Decision Making

There are several possible existing paradigms or theoretical orientations to a social–psychological approach to fertility decision making (Davidson and Jaccard, 1975; Fishbein, 1972; Fishbein and Jaccard, 1973;
Hass, 1974; Terhune, 1973; Terhune and Kaufman, 1973; Townes et al.,
1974). Most social–psychological theories of fertility decision making
owe much to the economists, but consider psychological as well as economic costs and benefits of parenthood. They begin with the premise that
behavior is motivated and that motivation is governed by positive and
negative incentives (Smith, 1973). Usually the assumption is made that if
costs of an additional child outweigh the benefits, the person will choose
not to have an additional child. If benefits outweigh costs, the person will
desire an additional child (Beckman, 1974; Hass, 1974). These models are
defined as "rational" because, in effect, it is assumed that the individual
makes a choice, based on perceived benefits and costs, which maximizes
his or her psychic (that is, subjective expected) utility.

Almost all theorists and researchers of fertility decision making (with
notable exceptions, for example, Hass, 1974; Mellinger, 1974) have looked
at individual preferences and decisions rather than couples' decision
processes regarding fertility. In so doing, they have inadvertently eliminated one extremely important stage of the fertility decision process,
that is, how individual preferences or choices are combined to reach a
joint decision regarding fertility. The assessment of the impact of the decision process itself on fertility levels is of importance. Although it is true
that either member of a couple may alone make a decision to control fertility, in 1975 81% of married women in Los Angeles County reported that

both spouses shared equally in the decision of how many children to have (unpublished data from a study conducted among a representative sample of 583 married women aged 18–49; see Beckman, 1976).

A Social–Psychological Model of Couples' Fertility Decision-Making Processes

In societies where knowledge and practice of contraception are widespread, the assumption is often made (Thompson, 1974) that rational–instrumental models of individual decision making (such as the Fishbein model) are most appropriate. The conceptualization that I shall develop is perhaps best characterized as a rational-type model of fertility, although it does not ignore normative influences. The model assumes that a continuum exists from preference to individual decision to joint decision. A decision indicates a conscious choice whereas a preference indicates a subjective favorability or affect. In this conceptualization it is assumed that individuals and couples, in varying degrees, make decisions or choices regarding fertility, based at least partially on personal tastes or preferences, for varying long- or short-term time spans.

MOTIVATION FOR A/ANOTHER CHILD

Before discussing couples' decision making, it is desirable to consider individual decision making. This necessitates explication of a hypothetical construct called *motivation for parenthood*. This construct can be defined as the general strength of the tendency to have a first or an additional child. It represents a predisposition to act and serves to arouse, maintain, and direct behaviors toward or away from the goal of having a first or an additional child. The strength of motivation for or against a/another child depends on the perceived satisfactions and costs of having an *n*th child (the marginal utility of an *n*th child), as compared to various alternatives to children. Rewards and costs can be defined as *perceived* positive outcomes (satisfactions or benefits) and negative outcomes (costs) associated with having and interacting with an *n*th child.

For women, the perceived rewards and costs of parenthood and the perceived rewards and costs of major alternative sources of psychic satisfaction (such as employment or leisure) affect decisions whether and when to have an additional child, and therefore, affect fertility variables such as use of contraception and length of time between marriage and first birth (see Figure 4.1). Fertility decision making is conceptualized as a sequential process (Hass, 1974) in which the key decision probably is whether to have another child, rather than how many children to have.

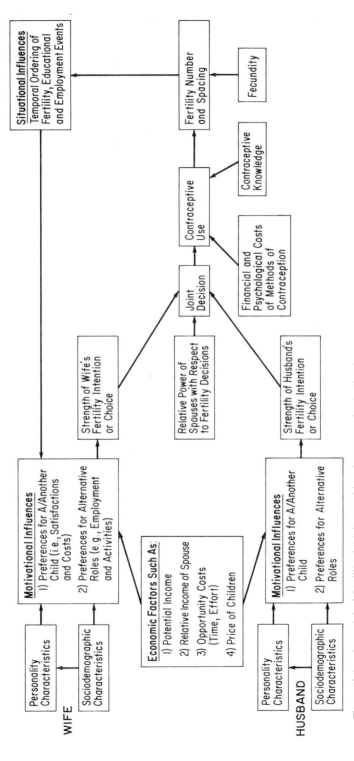

Figure 4.1. A model of fertility decision making (at one point in time).

The preference structures of individuals (that is, the perceived satisfactions and costs) may have built into them some preconscious satisfactions (that is, desiring a child because of an unconscious need to mother or an unconscious need to prove one's virility) or costs that are not easily measured and that may cause discrepancies between predicted motivation for parenthood and actual choices. Also it is possible that some satifactions or preferences serve as lexicographic events (Pope and Namboodiri, 1968), that is, they constitute normative or moral acts that, as ends in themselves, are not weighed against other alternatives as suggested in the general model. A normative or moral act (for instance, having at least two children) may be chosen automatically, whatever the disutility or opportunity costs involved; it is not bound by rational considerations. In such cases it is expected that situational and individual factors gain importance once minimal cultural norms have been met. For instance, the weighing of the salience of perceived advantages and disadvantages of parenthood for married couples may become more evident after the second child is born (Hass, 1974; Kammeyer, 1971). Before that point, for most people the weighing of positive and negative factors could determine the timing of the birth, but not the probability of occurrence of the birth. (Of course, the timing of early births is related to the probability of occurrence of later births.)

PROPOSED CAUSAL RELATIONSHIPS OF THE MODEL

Figure 4.1 shows the critical variables of interest in the present formulation. Underlying personality characteristics, sociodemographic characteristics, and situational determinants are thought to affect perceived satisfactions and costs, and thus motivation for parenthood. Sociodemographic variables may affect personality variables as well as directly influence the satisfactions and costs of a/another child. For instance, persons of lower socioeconomic status may evidence higher sex-role traditionalism than do persons of higher SES, and sex-role traditionalism may be one of several personality variables that mediate the association between demographic variables and preferences for children.

Factors such as race, urban–rural residence, education, or father's socioeconomic status may help to explain why, although two persons may have similar objective circumstances (for example, income, employment, standard of living), their *subjective* perceptions of the rewards and costs of having a child may greatly vary. However, it is not assumed that perceived satisfactions and costs of children are entirely dependent on such factors. When sociodemographic variables are controlled, it is predicted that some variation in preferences (arising from differences in other personality or situational characteristics) will remain. Data from both the Los Angeles County sample of married women (Beckman, 1976) and from a smaller pilot study of employed married women in the later years of child-bearing (Beckman, 1974) strongly support this contention.

In a similar way, normative influences that differ among demographic groups interact with situational determinants and personality factors to influence motivations for various alternatives to an additional child. The most prominent of these alternative roles for women is employment, and it is the alternative emphasized here. However, other socially acceptable alternatives, such as education, leisure activities, and volunteer work, are also relevant. Volunteer activities on a part-time basis may give women some of the same satisfactions (for example, self-esteem, a sense of making a social contribution) as does employment without many of the high costs involved (for instance, lack of time for children or housework).

The choice of additional motherhood or an alternative role does not represent an either–or decision for a woman. Allocation of time, energy, and money demands that a woman choose a certain amount of participation in each role (Turchi, 1975), and given limited resources (the economic factors in Figure 4.1), she will seek by her choice regarding amount of participation to maximize psychic utility, her sense of satisfaction. One manifestation of sex differences in factors affecting motivation for childbearing is that the issue of employment and parenthood as alternative roles rarely arises for men. Although it is possible that men may weigh parenthood against alternative material goods (a more expensive car) or alternative activities (foreign travel), it is assumed and accepted that a man will fulfill both roles. Even if the perceived positive benefits of children are identical for men and women, their respective desired and expected fertility may vary because women must make a trade-off between the two roles.

Contraceptive practices are directly affected by decision processes, contraceptive knowledge (including beliefs about susceptibility to conception), and perceived financial and psychological costs of use of various methods of contraception (Easterlin, 1969). In my model, an intention reflects an individual choice, while a joint decision implies couple communication. Obviously one member of a couple can make a unilateral decision regarding parenthood, but fertility regulation usually does not represent a unilateral choice. Individual intentions or choices lead to joint decisions, which in turn lead to the actual behavior of couples concerning birth planning practices. The decision outcome chosen in cases of disagreement depends on the relative power of the spouses, the relative ability of each person to influence the other. Contraceptive practices affect fertility outcomes such as number of children, interval between marriage and first birth, and other birth intervals.

OTHER CHARACTERISTICS OF FERTILITY DECISIONS

For decision making to take place, certain preconditions are necessary (Back, 1967). The person must be aware that a choice (in this case, the choice to limit conception) can be made, and he/she must have the means to implement it. The person must be motivated (and have the values) to make a definite choice. The person must have the environment that makes it possible to act on an intention, and the psychological makeup to act on it.

The fertility decision is important, irreversible after late pregnancy, and yet involves uncertain outcomes. A decision with these characteristics is likely to be delayed as long as possible (Janis and Mann, 1977). Individuals may actively avoid a fertility decision unless some action is forced on them. Whether this means delaying a decision to use contraception (that is, a decision to stop having children) or delaying a decision to discontinue the use of contraception (a decision to have a child) may depend on the personal dispositions and cultural norms of the individual decision maker or the couple.

Fertility decisions may follow various patterns. Many individuals cannot pinpoint a particular instance of having made a choice (for example, a definite decision to have an nth child). In some cases a series of minor choices leads to a slow drift into parenthood. Others may choose not to make a decision, which ultimately is itself a decision not to control one's fate. A decision to stop use of a contraceptive may be different than a decision for a nonuser to begin usage. The latter requires not only a choice to use fertility regulation but also a decision regarding what kind of contraception to use.

Fertility decisions may involve a long- or short-term time perspective. While some couples may plan their children several years in advance, many childless couples remain undecided about whether to have children and only gradually come to the realization that the wife is too old or they are too settled in a life style to desire children. Some persons may only make a decision not to have a child now, while others may decide that they want no more children. These different patterns of decision making are worthy of examination, because understanding the fertility decision-making process may help to predict future fertility behavior.

Because of the emphasis of the present chapter on decision processes, two components of Figure 4.1, motivational influences and the relative power of spouses in the joint decision, will be more extensively discussed.

Individual Preferences Regarding Children

My discussion of preference (motivation) for a/another child is primarily based on social exchange theory (Homans, 1961; Thibaut and Kelley, 1959). Social behavior may be explained in terms of the rewards and costs incurred in social interaction. The attractiveness of a present or future relationship (for example, a parent–child relationship) is a function of the reward–cost outcomes that persons experience or think they will experience in relation to some minimal level of expectation of what these outcomes should be. This minimal level is called the *comparison level* (CL) and is influenced by a person's past experience in the relationship, his past experience in comparable relationships (for example, with other children), his perception of what others like himself (for example, his sociodemographic group) are receiving, and his perception of the outcomes available in alternative relationships.

The comparison level is a standard against which a person evaluates the rewards and costs of a relationship in terms of what is felt to be deserved, that is, the minimum that a person thinks ought to be gained from the interaction. Usually it is not directly measured, but rather inferred from the level of a person's perceived satisfaction or dissatisfaction with the relationship. Thus the CL serves as a psychologically meaningful neutral point on a scale of outcomes (that is, satisfaction versus dissatisfaction). The value that a person places on an outcome or choice is not determined by the absolute amount of gain or loss that a person expects, but rather by the amount expected relative to a comparison level. A person receiving outcomes at comparison level would be neither satisfied nor dissatisfied with a relationship. To the degree that outcomes are above CL, the person would be attracted to and satisfied with a relationship. On the other hand, relationships entailing outcomes falling below CL would be relatively unattractive and unsatisfying (Thibaut and Kelley, 1959).

Individuals may remain in a relationship even though the outcomes they receive are below comparison level, because they perceive that in the alternatives available the costs are greater or the rewards are less. For example, in a loveless marriage the couple may stay together even if they are both unhappy. The wife may stay because she sees no chance for getting a better husband and no prospect for adequate support for her and her children except through her current marriage. A parent–child relationship also can become nonvoluntary, that is, the person is constrained in the relationship despite the fact that outcomes are below CL and better outcomes are available from other relationships, activities, or roles. Because of normative constraints the parent usually cannot or will not leave the relationship.

In my past research I have used an exchange theory approach to examine motivation for a first or an additional child versus motivation for the alternative role of employment. According to the theory, a person should want or intend to have a child (have high motivation for parenthood) when the rewards or advantages strongly outweigh the disadvantages. He or she should not want to have a child (have low motivation for parenthood) when the costs or disadvantages of parenthood outweigh the rewards. To determine if a person wants to have another child, it is necessary to delineate the perceived rewards and costs of an additional child and the salience of each. There should be a high correlation between a summary measure of rewards and costs and desires or behavioral intentions (Fishbein, 1967, 1972) regarding additional parenthood. Application of the theory requires specification of the type of cognitive algebra or psycho-logic to be used in deriving a summary index that combines the relative strength of these incentives. Many theorists have used a decision theory or subjective expected utility approach that assumes that likelihood of an outcome as well as its evaluative component must be taken into account. In most such formulations the value of an outcome is multiplied by its expectancy of occurrence, and then scores are summed (Davidson and Jaccard, 1975; Fishbein, 1967, 1972). A simpler additive approach that utilizes importance ratings may be just as effective. Salience or importance ratings may already include a person's internal assessment of likelihood (that is, an outcome would not be rated as important if the expectation that it would occur was very low). Because of measurement problems (that Townes *et al.*, 1974, may have adequately solved), I initially chose this simpler model.

Because an economic approach requires that the strength of preference for a child must be compared to the strength of preferences for possible alternatives, motivation for a/another child was compared to motivation for the alternative of employment or a career. Those women with greater preferences for the alternative of employment should have lower fertility and fertility intentions. It was predicted that women would choose their amount of interaction within each of these social situations (parenthood and employment) depending on the reward–cost outcomes (that is, ΣRewards $-$ ΣCosts) of additional participation in each situation and their combined outcomes. For instance, a woman would choose (or desire) to have a child or an additional child (and not to work) when the net reward–cost outcome of the motherhood role was considerably greater than the net reward–cost outcome of the work role, and the satisfactions of additional parenthood clearly outweighed the costs. Similarly, she would choose both roles if the rewards of both roles were high and the costs low.

Empirical Evidence Regarding Individual Preferences for Children

In my study of the motivation for parenthood of approximately 600 married women from Los Angeles County, respondents assessed the salience of a series of satisfactions and costs of an additional child and satisfactions and costs of employment on 7-point rating scales. Motivation for parenthood was defined as the sum of the importance ratings of the rewards of a/another child minus the sum of the importance ratings of the costs of a/another child. Motivation for employment was defined in an analogous manner. Then the relationship between these summary measures and desires regarding children and employment was examined. Respondents were divided into groups based on their scores (high or low) on motivation for a/another child and their scores (high or low) on motivation for employment. Of those with high motivation for a/another child, 83% wanted at least one additional child, while of those low in motivation, 10% wanted a child. Similarly, 85% of those with high motivation for employment intended to work in the next year, while only 27% of those with low motivation for employment intended to work.

As in other studies, employment appeared to influence fertility. Women with greater employment experience had produced fewer children, and currently employed women had lower motivation for a/another child than did unemployed women.

THE BIDIRECTIONALITY OF
THE EMPLOYMENT—FERTILITY RELATIONSHIP

My data suggest that one of the opportunity costs of a/another child that is more important to women who are currently employed is limitation of employment or a career. The perceived limitation of employment, that is, the degree of perceived role incompatability between parenthood and employment, appeared to be influencing employed women to have fewer children than women who were not employed. Causality also can operate in the reverse direction; women with smaller families have more time to work (Sweet, 1970). The existence of an inverse relationship between female employment and fertility is well documented (Blake, 1965; Hoffman, 1974; Nye and Hoffman, 1963; Siegel and Haas, 1963). Studies explicating the relationship have examined both the effects of work activity on fertility (Fortney, 1972; Freedman and Coombs, 1966; Groat et al., 1976) and the effects of fertility events (number of children, birth intervals, desired number of children) on female labor force participation (Stycos and Weller, 1967; Sweet, 1970; Weller, 1971; Whelpton et al., 1966). The best that can be said about the employment–fertility relationship at this point is that causality is most probably bidirectional, and the multiple causal paths involved are not clearly understood (Terry, 1975).

STABILITY OF REWARDS AND COSTS OF PARENTHOOD

The manner in which rewards and costs of parenthood change over time and the relationship between changes in rewards, costs, and changes in preferences for children have not been adequately examined. It may well be that some perceived satisfactions and costs of children (for example, motherhood as "woman's role") are established early in adolescence or even in childhood. These stable motives for or against having children may have been incorporated by the child during the process of identification with the same-sex parent. However, it can be argued that other satisfactions and costs of children are unstable and change systematically. If, as cognitive psychologists have postulated, thinking and reasoning precede decision and action, changes in desired or actual family size may be preceded or accompanied by changes in perceptions regarding the value of parenthood. Also, "naive" psychology tells us that the birth of a child (especially a first child) affects motivation for future childbearing. The process by which this occurs may be conceptualized as follows:

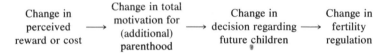

Before the child's birth, the parent may perceive the costs of parent—child interaction as relatively low and the rewards as great. Later on, for some parents the rewards may remain constant or become even greater, but the costs (changes in the form of husband—wife relations, anxiety over the child's development) also may rise drastically. Other persons may perceive the costs of children but not the high rewards of children until they are able to watch their own children grow and develop. For them, having children raises the level of satisfaction with the parenthood role and may increase their motivation for additional children. Cross-sectional studies that have compared the preference structures of persons of differing fertility have revealed some differences in the salience of various satisfactions or costs (Beckman, 1976; Townes et al., 1974; Vinokur-Kaplan, 1976). Although changes in rewards and costs as a result of a child's birth have been inferred from such cross-sectional research, adequate examination of these hypotheses awaits further results of longitudinal studies of family decision making, some of which are currently in progress.

Relative Power and Joint Decision Making of Couples

Social—psychological theories are most important when the members of the marital dyad initially do not have similar preferences or behavioral intentions regarding children. In such cases they do not agree about the importance of the perceived satisfactions and costs of children and as a consequence do not always concur about having a/another child, desired number of children, or spacing of children. In a pilot study of North Carolina couples married from 10 to 12 years, Mason (1974) observed that 28% disagreed as to the total number of children desired. Among newly married couples who have not yet settled initial disagreements, differences in fertility intentions might be even more evident.

The process by which couples decide whether or not to have an *n*th child or decide on an acceptable family size is incompletely understood. The manner in which such decisions are translated into fertility regulation has been relatively unexplored. Two streams of research bear on these processes, those of family sociology and social psychology. In comparison to social psychology, the family sociology literature has a large amount of empirical information available but is often weak on theory. The great advantage of the social psychology research is its base in several sophisticated social psychology theories. One of the common areas of application of these theories is the family or marital dyad. Particularly applicable to fertility decision making are studies of social power and influence (French and Raven, 1959; Raven and Kruglanski, 1970), conflict resolution (Deutsch, 1969; Rausch *et al.*, 1974), social exchange, and bargaining processes (Schelling, 1960; Siegel and Fouraker, 1960; Shubik, 1964; Thibaut and Kelley, 1959).

CONFLICT RESOLUTION

A theoretical model developed by Jourard (1971a, 1971b), Rausch *et al.* (1974), and others is concerned with the constructive resolution of conflict in intimate relationships. It is assumed that hostilities and conflicting needs, desires, and preferences are inevitable in any close relationship. It is proposed that conflicts cannot be resolved adequately unless they are expressed openly and managed constructively. Couples in our society often try to suppress hostile feelings and avoid overt conflicts that lead to resentment and dissatisfaction.

The model identifies three essential requirements in order to resolve conflict constructively:

1. Open communication
2. Accurate perceptions regarding the degree and nature of conflict
3. Constructive efforts to resolve conflict, which at minimum include each partner being willing to consider the other's point of view and alternative solutions, and to be willing to compromise if necessary

Breakdown of communication at any level can lead to defensiveness, self-doubt, confusion, and behavior perceived as inappropriate.

Mellinger (1974) has applied this theory to fertility decision making by suggesting that unsuccessful resolution of conflict may be an important factor in unwanted fertility. As long as overt decision making does not occur, conflict appears to be avoided, but covert decisions may be made to "take a chance" or to be careless in use of contraception. Such covert decisions may end the stress of internal conflict or avoid overt conflict with one's spouse.

EXCHANGE AND BARGAINING

Social exchange theory, which originated in economic analysis and game theory, already has been discussed in relation to individual preferences. Originally it was applied to social interaction in two-person groups and can be used to represent an exchange relationship between husband and wife under conditions of divergent interests. Game theory is a method for the study of decision making in situations of conflict. When two persons (in this case, the marital dyad) have different goals or objectives but their fates are intertwined, each person must consider how to achieve the most favorable outcome for self while taking into account the desires and strategies of the other person (Shubik, 1964). *Bargaining* typically refers to the processes by which parties attempt to reach a joint decision regarding what each shall obtain in some transaction between them (Raven and Rubin, 1976). Although generally applied to tangible outcomes such as a buyer and seller attempting to reach agreement on the price of a used car, it also could be applied to areas of family decision making such as where to go on vacation or when to have a next child. Although bargaining generally assumes that parties interact through a series of offers and counteroffers, it is possible to conceive of a bargaining process taking place in the marital dyad.

TYPES OF SOCIAL POWER

Once spouses realize that they hold divergent positions, each may attempt to convert the other to his/her own viewpoint. The outcome will depend upon several factors, two of the most important being the type of influence employed and the relative power of each spouse. The most well-known bases of power (that is, ability to influence) are reward power and coercive power. At least four additional bases of social influence can be defined: legitimacy (norms or accepted behavioral rules); reference (the desire to be similar to another person or group); expertness (superior knowledge); and informational (influence based on information communicated).

Among couples one or more of these forms of power may be operative in any situation. Measurement is complicated because the power sources operate in a somewhat nonadditive fashion and because of structural dissimilarities between some of the power bases and individual differences in susceptibility to the various power bases.

Various power bases may be negatively related to each other. For instance, if expertness is high, referent power may be reduced; by definition a person is dissimilar to another who has a different level of knowledge. If reference is high, expertness may be diminished.

A person susceptible to one power base may be relatively invulnerable to another. Persons who are highly authoritarian or sex-role traditional may be much more susceptible to legitimate or expert influence than to the other power bases. While in certain situations use of several power bases might be more effective than use of any one power base, in other situations the spouse's concomitant use of several power bases may be interpreted as "manipulation" and may increase the partner's resistance to influence attempts. Often a person has a choice regarding which power base to use. The husband may give rewards like affection to his wife for doing as he wants, or he may state that his demands are a legitimate part of his marital relationship. He may emphasize his greater experience in the world in certain areas, or he may try to move his wife to his point of view with more facts and new information. Which approach is more effective depends on the situation and the goals to be accomplished. If it were possible to determine which source of power would be more effective in different types of families with regard to fertility decision making (for example, sex-role traditional couples may be more susceptible to legitimate or expert influence) and which spouse tended to utilize each power base, predictions could be made regarding spouses' relative power when a discrepancy existed in a couple's preferences for children.

Reference, expert, and informational influence from sources external to the marital dyad may be of prime importance in determining what kind of contraception is used. Although my previous research (Beckman, 1974) suggests that on a conscious level the expectations of friends and relatives have little influence on decisions to use or not use contraception, friends (referent power) or the woman's physician (expert power) may have primary influence over the *method* of fertility control used. Because methods differ greatly in effectiveness, friends or physicians indirectly influence the rate at which unwanted pregnancies are likely to occur. In addition, since there may be a method–person interaction (that is, some type of persons have more success than others with certain methods), the judgment of the physician or friend regarding ability of a person to use a method becomes important.

OTHER SOCIAL–PSYCHOLOGICAL FACTORS AFFECTING COUPLES' FERTILITY DECISIONS

Other social–psychological factors such as openness of communication also are related to the success of fertility regulation. Many studies have found a relationship between aspects of marital interaction and contraceptive effectiveness (in the United States, Rainwater, 1960, 1965; in France, Michel, 1967; and in Puerto Rico, Hill *et al.,* 1959). Michel showed that in a French urban sample the amount of communication in the couple was more closely related to contraceptive success than was education or income. Thus it would appear that unwanted pregnancies were more characteristic of those who, because of lack of communication, did not coordinate fertility control efforts.

The resolution of discrepancies between marital partners with respect to strength of preferences or intentions for roles or material goods that compete with childbearing may indirectly affect fertility. We know that even when demographic factors such as education are controlled, women with full-time labor force participation have lower fertility rates than other women in the United States (Fortney, 1972; Ridley, 1969). If a wife desires to work full-time and the husband does not want her to work, does the woman acquiesce to her husband's wishes or assert her own will? Assuming employment affects fertility, the resolution of this disagreement may have indirect implications for that woman's completed fertility. To give another example, if a husband desires a lavish life style (a new car every year, a boat, an expensive vacation) that keeps him in debt and a wife prefers to save money, the resolution of these differences should have implications for fertility; couples have only so much money to allocate between children and alternative goods. The higher the couple's life style, given a constant amount of money, the lower the desire for children.

MEASUREMENT OF RELATIVE POWER IN THE MARITAL DYAD

A conflict or disagreement regarding fertility intentions or other factors affecting or interacting with fertility desires may be resolved in various ways. The key variable appears to be the relative *power,* that is, ability to influence, of each member of the couple. Power in the marital dyad is rarely equal. Changes in behaviors, values, or attitudes regarding fertility that occur through interaction or communication are more likely to converge on the high power person. Thus if a couple has divergent perceptions of children and motivation for an additional child, the less powerful member of the dyad may tend to adopt or at least behaviorally comply with the attitudes and values of the more powerful member. This formulation suggests that the more powerful person in the marital dyad will have more stable preferences regarding parenthood.

One problem that has plagued both the family sociology and social psychology literature is how best to measure power in the marital dyad. Although power is a multidimensional concept, too often decision making (which is assumed to be a measure of power) is defined only in terms of who "wins" or makes the final decision without regard to the process of decision making. We need to know not only who makes a decision, but who has the authority to make the decision and who controls who makes the decision (Safilios-Rothschild, 1970). Resistance to influence is also a variable. For example, the more publicly committed a person is to a belief, the more resistant it is to change (Deutsch and Gerard, 1955; Kiesler and Kiesler, 1969).

Unfortunately, in the subtle complex area of family interaction indirect nonobservable methods of influence between husband and wife abound. Some authors (Safilios-Rothschild, 1970) have attempted to describe these influence patterns and suggest nonobtrusive ways of measuring them. Survey questions, for example, can elicit reports of activities that cannot be recorded using observational techniques (Safilios-Rothschild, 1969, 1970), because of their intimate nature, because of the optimal timing required for their application (for example, "when he is in a good mood"), because influence is exercised through application of highly personal techniques ("cooking something he likes" or "buying the wife a gift I know she will like" as a use of reward power), or because it takes a long time (for example, "nagging" as a case of coercive power).

Blood and Wolfe's (1960) resource theory view of marital power suggests that each individual's relative power is determined by the relative resources each spouse brings to the marriage (in terms of education, occupation, income, and so on). The spouse with the greater amount of resources should be the most powerful. Safilios-Rothschild (1975) suggests expanding the acknowledged resources brought into the marriage to include the entire range of resources exchanged between spouses, such as love, sex, and companionship. These intrinsic resources can be extremely effective instruments of power manipulation. The most crucial hypothesis of her interpretation of marital power is the contention that the relative degree to which one spouse loves and needs the other spouse determines who can most effectively influence family decision making. This same principle was expounded by Waller and Hill (1951) as the "principle of least interest."

Recent formulations of equity theory (Walster, 1973) offer similar concepts, although here outcomes as well as inputs are considered. Heer's (1963) exchange theory also incorporates these outcomes by introducing the concept of marital alternatives. His assumption is that the person who has greater alternatives outside the marriage, for example, the person who could more easily find a spouse as desirable or more desirable than the one he/she currently has, also is more powerful. One problem with these formulations is that no one has adequately measured all important resources. How, for example, does one measure housekeeping ability or affection of each spouse? What these relative resource theories do suggest, which may be of importance, is the need for and some approaches to measuring relative power independent of decision-making outcomes. Relative power, if measured, could then be used as a proxy for ability to influence.

A methodological controversy in the study of family decision making is that between use of survey, in-depth interviewing, and observational techniques (Bahr, 1972; Olsen, 1969; Safilios-Rothschild, 1970; Turk and Bell, 1972). Because I doubt that social demographers are likely to begin using observational techniques or in-depth interviewing, my general approach here has been to discuss fertility decision making with the implicit assumption that any data collected will be survey data. Although a few brave souls (Lee, 1974) have tried, it is unlikely that fertility decision making can be effectively studied in the field or in the laboratory using observational techniques. It is possible, however, that researchers can observe couples' power, decision making, or communication style in general and that a variable identifying general style could be applied to specific decision-making situations.

The relationship between general measures of power and decision making and measures of decision making in a specific decision area such as fertility rarely has been addressed. The assumption is often made that there is a strong relationship between general and specific decision making. (I have assumed this myself in my earlier discussion.) However, attempts to relate global measures of power or decision making to decision making in specific areas where power may be completely delegated to one spouse may have questionable validity. In computation of indices of overall decision making, the total decision-making score depends on the particular decisions sampled (Centers *et al.*, 1971; Safilios-Rothschild, 1970). The relationship between general decision making and behavior specific decision making must be empirically studied, for it cannot safely be assumed.

Given that power can be operationalized and its relationship to fertility decision-making outcomes hypothesized, the picture still is cloudy. It can be predicted that, in general, the more powerful or dominant the husband is in the family, the more control he has over decisions regarding childbearing. However, the wife might bear primary responsibility for seeing that such decisions are effectively carried out through use of contraception. Findings regarding the specificity of dominance within task and decision domains (Blood and Wolfe, 1960; Centers *et al.*, 1971) suggest that "fertility control and regulation" is a domain that is traditionally considered feminine. Decisions or behaviors relating to fertility regulation (especially among lower SES groups) may be considered women's work. The husband's use of coercive or reward bases of social influence may not be effective in this situation, because the wife has the means to subvert his wishes through her effective or ineffective use of contraception, and her behavior may not be easily observable by the husband.

Theory and research on joint decision making in the marital dyad in cases of disagreement between spouses are sketchy and unclear. Much of the past research on family decision making can be faulted on methodological or conceptual grounds (Bahr, 1972; Olsen and Rabunsky, 1972; Safilios-Rothschild, 1970; Turk and Bell, 1972). Nevertheless, I believe there are a few general areas of social–psychological explanation—influence processes, bargaining processes, conflict resolution, and so on—that can usefully be applied to couples' decision making regarding fertility and that have the potential of helping us to make sense of this muddied area.

Conclusion

This chapter has been concerned primarily with explicating rather than with testing a model of fertility decision making. Because several other social–psychological models of fertility decision making also exist, more empirical evidence to distinguish between alternative models seems essential. A review of those aspects of the social–psychological approach outlined in this chapter that have been inadequately examined suggests future directions for our empirical efforts and for conceptual development.

Attention should be devoted both to individual preferences and to couples' joint decision-making processes. Although conceptualizations and research on individual intentions and decisions are fairly extensive, the value of this line of research is still questioned by many demographers. However, researchers have found relationships of significant magnitude between the various components of their models and fertility intentions, decisions, or behaviors. In general, these relationships have been with fertility intentions or past fertility rather than with actual future fertility.

Especially in research on psychological variables that are subject to rationalization and distortion, this is an obvious weakness, but it is a weakness
that future longitudinal designs can correct.

Research on individual intentions or choices may follow several directions. Primary are studies of how persons make fertility decisions, including examination of the formation of preferences and their changes over
time. Second, the issue of whether or not people make conscious fertility
decisions, that is, the rationality of fertility decision making, should be
examined. From the first two areas it follows that research is needed on
individual characteristics or personality traits that are related to whether
people make conscious decisions regarding fertility and how they make
these decisions. Such characteristics could include rationality, locus of
control, modernity, and competence. Finally, it is important that innova-
tive, reliable, and valid instruments be developed to measure individual
preferences and desires and that these be tested on national representative samples to determine the distribution of each psychological characteristic.

Studies of joint decision making regarding fertility are in one sense less
important than studies of individual decision making, for if initial intentions are congruent, a joint decision making or influence process is not
important. However, there are a large number of marriages or relationships in which couples do not agree regarding fertility desires. One
method of studying such couples is to select a sample in which we would
expect a high proportion of couples to have discrepant views because of
different cultural backgrounds, demographic characteristics, personality
characteristics, or situational contexts. While we would not have a representative sample of all disagreeing couples, any common features of the
decision-making process regarding fertility should be revealed.

In this chapter the importance of social–psychological theory in explanation of couples' decision making has been suggested. While primary
concentration has been on social power and influence and the relative
power of the spouses, conflict resolution and bargaining and exchange
processes also have been noted. The difficulties in measuring some of
these variables as they occur in the marital dyad are enormous, and the
question of the relationship between general decision making and fertility-
specific decision making remains to be answered. While survey data have
the potential of providing valuable information on couples' decision-making processes, diverse question formats and other methodologies must be
developed and tested. Methodologies such as in-depth interviewing and
laboratory observation probably will have to be utilized in order to provide a fuller multidimensional picture of couples' decision-making processes. While social demographers may not always feel comfortable with

these techniques, I do hope they will recognize their potential value in explaining fertility decision making, and that future research on fertility will incorporate the concepts and methodologies of a number of disciplines.

ACKNOWLEDGMENTS

I am grateful for the comments and suggestions of Larry Bumpass, Edward Conolley, and Betsy Bosak Houser.

References

Back, K. W.
   1967   "New frontiers in demography and social psychology."*Demography* 4: 90–97.
Bahr, S. J.
   1972   "Comment on the study of family power structure: A review 1960–1969." *Journal of Marriage and the Family* 34: 239–243.
Beckman, L. J.
   1974   "Relative costs and benefits of work and children to professional and non-professional women." Paper presented at the American Psychological Association meetings, New Orleans.
   1976   "Motivations, roles, and family planning of women." Final report prepared for Center for Population Research, NIH, Grant HD-07323.
Blake, J.
   1965   "Demographic science and the redirection of population policy." *Journal of Chronic Diseases* 18: 1181–1200.
Blood, R. O. and D. M. Wolfe
   1960   *Husbands and Wives.* New York: Free Press.
Centers, R., B. H. Raven, and A. Rodrigues
   1971   "Conjugal power structure: A reexamination." *American Sociological Review* 36: 264–278.
Davidson, A., and J. Jaccard
   1975   "Population psychology: A new look at an old problem." *Journal of Personality and Social Psychology* 31: 1073–1082.
Deutsch, M.
   1969   "Socially relevant science: Reflections on some studies of interpersonal conflict." *American Psychologist* 24: 1076–1092.
Deutsch, M., and H. G. Gerard
   1955   "A study of normative and informational social influence upon individual judgment." *Journal of Abnormal and Social Psychology* 51: 629–636.
Easterlin, R. A.
   1969   "Towards a socioeconomic theory of fertility: A survey of research on economic factors in American fertiity." Pp. 127–156 in S. J. Behrman, L. Corsa, and R. Freedman (eds.), *Fertility and Family Planning: A World View.* Ann Arbor: University of Michigan Press.
Edwards, W.
   1954   "The theory of decision making." *Psychological Bulletin* 51: 380–417.

Fishbein, M.
  1967   "Attitude and prediction of behavior." Pp. 477–492 in M. Fishbein (ed.), *Readings in Attitude Theory and Measurement*. New York: John Wiley and Sons.
  1972   "Toward an understanding of family planning behaviors." *Journal of Applied Social Psychology* 2: 214–227.
Fishbein, M., and J. Jaccard
  1973   "Theoretical and methodological considerations in the prediction of family planning intention and behavior." *Representative Research in Social Psychology* 4: 37–51.
Fortney, J. A.
  1972   "Achievement as an alternate source of emotional gratification to childbearing." Paper presented at the annual meeting of the Population Association of America, Toronto.
Freedman, R., and L. Coombs
  1966   "Economic consideration in family growth decisions." *Population Studies* 20: 217–221.
French, J. R. P., Jr., and B. H. Raven
  1959   "The bases of social power." Pp. 150–167 in D. Cartwright (ed.), *Studies in Social Power*. Ann Arbor: University of Michigan Press.
Groat, H. T., R. L. Workman, and A. G. Neal
  1976   "Labor force participation and family formation: A study of working mothers." *Demography* 13: 115–125.
Hass, P. H.
  1974   "Wanted and unwanted pregnancies: A fertility decision-making model." *Journal of Social Issues* 30: 125–165.
Hauser, P. M., and C. D. Duncan
  1959   "Demography as a body of knowlege." Pp. 76–105 in P. M. Hauser and C. D. Duncan (eds.), *The Study of Population*. Chicago: University of Chicago Press.
Heer, D. M.
  1963   "The measurement and bases of family power: An overview." *Marriage and Family Living* 25: 133–139.
Hill, R., J. M. Stycos, and K. W. Back
  1959   *The Family and Population Control: A Puerto Rican Experiment in Social Change*. Chapel Hill, N. C.: University of North Carolina Press.
Hoffman, L. W.
  1974   "The employment of women, education, and fertility." *Merrill-Palmer Quarterly* 20: 99–119.
Homans, G. C.
  1961   *Social Behavior: Its Elementary Forms*. New York: Harcourt, Brace.
Janis, I. L., and L. Mann
  1977   *Decision-Making: A Psychological Analysis of Conflict, Choice, and Commitment*. New York: Free Press.
Jones, E. E., and H. B. Gerard
  1967   *Foundations of Social Psychology*. New York: John Wiley and Sons.
Jourard, S. M.
  1971a   *The Transparent Self*. New York: Van Nostrand.
  1971b   *Self-Disclosure: An Experimental Analysis of the Transparent Self*. New York: John Wiley and Sons.
Kammeyer, K. C. W.
  1971   *An Introduction to Population*. San Francisco: Chandler.

Kiesler, C. A., and S. B. Kielser
  1969   *Conformity*. Reading, Mass.: Addison-Wesley.
Lee, J.
  1974   "Spousal decision making process: A study of families, planned and unplanned."
          Paper presented at NICHD Conference on Fertility Related Decision Making,
          Belmont, Maryland.
Mason, K.
  1974   "Women's labor force participation and fertility." Final Report to National Insti-
          tutes of Health.
Mellinger, G. D.
  1974   "Individual and couple fertility decisions as related to parity, marital stage, and
          education: A pilot study." Proposal submitted in response to RFPNICHD-BS-75-
          2.
Michel, A.
  1967   "Interaction and family planning in the French urban family." *Demography* 4:
          615–625.
Nye, F. I., and L. W. Hoffman Eds.
  1963   *The Employed Mother in America*. Chicago: Rand McNally.
Olsen, D. H.
  1969   "The measurement of family power by self-report and behavioral methods."
          Journal of Marriage and the Family 31: 545–550.
Olsen, D. H., and C. Rabunsky
  1972   "Validity of four measures of family power." *Journal of Marriage and the Family*
          34: 224–234.
Pope, H., and N. K. Namboodiri
  1968   "Decisions regarding family size: Moral norms and utility model of social
          choice." *Research Previews* 15: 6–17.
Rainwater, L.
  1960   *And the Poor Get Children*. Chicago: Quadrangle.
  1965   *Family Design: Marital Sexuality, Family Planning, and Family Limitations*. Chi-
          cago: Aldine Publishing Co.
Rausch, H. L., W. A. Barry, R. K. Hertel, and M. A. Swain
  1974   *Communication Conflict and Marriage*. San Francisco: Jossey-Bass.
Raven, B. H., and A. W. Kruglanski
  1970   "Conflict and power." Pp. 69–109 in P. G. Swingle (ed.), *The Structure of Con-
          flict*. New York: Academic Press.
Raven, B. H., and J. Z. Rubin
  1976   *Social Psychology: People in Groups*. New York: John Wiley and Sons.
Ridley, J. C.
  1969   "The changing position of American women: Education, labor force participa-
          tion, and fertility. Pp. 199–250 in *The Family in Transition*. Fogarty International
          Proceedings, Washington, D.C.: U. S. Government Printing Office.
Ryder, N. B., and C. F. Westoff
  1972   "Wanted and unwanted fertility in the United States: 1965 and 1970." Pp. 467–
          487 in C. F. Westoff and R. Parke, Jr. (eds.), *Demographic and Social Aspects of
          Population Growth*, vol. 1. (The Commission of Population Growth and The
          American Future Research Reports) Washington, D.C.: U. S. Government Print-
          ing Office.
Safilios-Rothschild, C.
  1969   "Family sociology or wives' family sociology? A cross-cultural examination of de-
          cision-making." *Journal of Marriage and the Family* 31: 290–301.

1970   "A study of family power structure: A review 1960–1969." *Journal of Marriage and the Family* 32: 539–552.

1975   "A macro- and micro-examination of family power and love: An exchange model." Paper presented at "Dynamics of Family Ecology" session of the ISS BD symposium, Surrey, England.

Schelling, T. C.
1960   *The Strategy of Conflict.* Cambridge, Mass.: Harvard University Press.

Shubik, M.
1964   "Game theory and the study of social behavior: An introductory exposition." Pp. 3–77 in M. Shubik (ed.), *Game Theory and Related Approaches to Social Behavior.* New York: John Wiley and Sons.

Siegel, S., and L. E. Fouraker
1960   *Bargaining and Group Decision Making.* New York: McGraw-Hill.

Siegel, A. E., and M. B. Haas
1963   "The working mother: A review of research." *Child Development* 34: 513–542.

Smith, M. B.
1973   "A social–psychological view of fertility." Pp 3–18 in J. T. Fawcett (ed.), *Psychological Perspectives on Population.* New York: Basic Books.

Stycos, J. M., and R. H. Weller
1967   "Female working roles and fertility." *Demography* 4: 210–217.

Sweet, J. A.
1970   "Family composition and the labor force activity of American wives." *Demography* 7: 195–209.

Terhune, K. W.
1973   "Fertility values: why people have children." Paper presented at American Psychological Association convention, Montreal, Canada.

Terhune, K. W., and Kaufman, S.
1973   "The family size utility function." *Demography* 10: 599–618.

Terry, G. B.
1975   "Rival explanations in the work-fertility relationship." *Population Studies* 29: 191–205.

Thibaut, J. W., and H. H. Kelley
1959   *The Social Psychology of Groups.* New York: John Wiley and Sons.

Thompson, V.
1974   "Family size: Implicity policies and assumed psychological outcomes." *Journal of Social Issues* 30: 93–124.

Townes, B. D., F. L. Campbell, L. R. Beach, and D. C. Martin
1974   "An application of decision theory to the study of birth planning." Paper presented at the American Psychological Association convention, New Orleans.

Turchi, B.
1975   *The Demand for Children: The Economics of Fertility in the U. S.* Cambridge, Mass.: Ballinger.

Turk, J. T., and N. W. Bell
1972   "Measuring power in families." *Journal of Marriage and the Family* 34: 215–222.

U. S. Bureau of the Census.
1973   Birth Expectations of American Wives: June, 1973. Current Population Reports. Series P-20, No. 254. Washington, D.C.: U. S. Government Printing Office.

1974   *Statistical Abstract of the |United States: 1974* (95th ed.). Washington, D.C.: U. S. Government Printing Office.

Vinokur-Kaplan, D.

1976   "Family planning decision-making: A comparison and analysis of parents' consideration." Unpublished manuscript.
Waller, W., and Hill, R.
1951   *The Family*. New York: Dryden Press.
Walster, E.
1973   "New directions in equity research." *Journal of Personality and Social Psychology* 25: 151–176.
Weller, R. H.
1971   "The impact of employment upon fertility." Pp. 154–166 in A. Michel (ed.), *Family Issues of Employed Women in Europe and America*. Leiden: E. J. Brill.
Westoff, C. F., and N. B. Ryder
1969   "Recent trends in attitudes toward fertility control and in the practice of contraception in the United States." Pp. 388–412 in S. J. Behrman, L. Corsa, and R. Freedman (eds.), *Fertility and Family Planning: A World View*. Ann Arbor: University of Michigan Press.
Whelpton, P. K., A. A. Campbell, and J. E. Patterson
1966   *Fertility and Family Planning in the United States*. Princeton, N. J.: Princeton University Press.

II
SPATIAL DISTRIBUTION

5

Spatial Aspects of Population: An Overview

AMOS H. HAWLEY

Population is, as a first approximation at least, an aggregate of finite things. As such it is an occupier of space. But the experience with space might not have occurred to man if (1) the circumstances and substances man uses were evenly distributed and (2) each individual were completely self-sufficient. Since neither of these conditions has ever obtained, space has always been one of man's major preoccupations. It enters into his thinking in numerous ways almost all of which can be expressed as some kind or degree of access.

A population's occupancy of space, in fact, invariably represents some kind of reconciliation of diverse accessibility requirements. On the one hand, the necessary interdependence among human beings generates a centripetal tendency. It tends to draw them into compact clusters where interindividual accessibility is maximized. On the other hand, the pursuit of sustenance exerts a centrifugal pressure, inasmuch as access to sustenance materials and conditions is no less important than is access to one's fellows. How these two classes of accessibility requirements are joined depends in large measure on the production technology employed and the

Social Demography

efficiency of transportation and communicative facilities possessed by a population.

Where production is labor intensive and confined for the most part to primary industry, specialization is not highly developed and accordingly interdependences are comparatively few. Accessibility to land takes precedence over accessibility to one's fellows. Population concentrations seldom attain large size. But where secondary and tertiary industries have gained ascendancy over primary industry, specializations are numerous and interdependences are extensively ramified. The location requirements of overriding importance for a great many activities are shifted from the land to the market, that is, to points of maximum interindividual accessibility. Thus large concentrations of populations can and do take form.

The contrast of types of economy implies also a significant difference in the facility for movement. The two cannot be readily separated. A labor-intensive, self-sufficient economy is a creature of primitive means for overcoming the friction of space. At the other extreme a highly differentiated, capital-intensive society can only occur where an efficient transportation and communication technology exists. Indeed, it is difficult to overestimate the importance of transportation and communication technology for the pattern and content of social life. Improvements in the facility for movement are probably the most critical of all technical acquisitions. They affect access to and the spread of new ideas and are thus instrumental in the initiation of cultures change. Space is a function of the time consumed in this movement from point to point; hence its meaning is determined by the efficiency of transportation and communication technology. That technology, then, regulates the diversity of occupations that can be joined in a division of labor and the variety and abundance of materials available at any one place. By the same token, it determines the scope of the market or, in ecological parlance, the scope of the ecosystem. It also regulates, by implication, the number of people who can live together and whether they must live in compact agglomerations or in more open settlement patterns. The extent of centralization—economic, political, or social—that is feasible is also contingent on the means at hand for movement. In short the effects of transportation and communication techniques pervade every aspect of social organization. Together they constitute one of the great necessary conditions for human collective life.

But the potentialities of that condition cannot be obtained from the tools alone or from the tools together with the knowledge required to make and employ them. They presuppose a standardization of the terms of discourses—weights and measures, monetary units, rules of the road, criteria of justice, and language. Standardization is the cultural counter-part of mobility. They also call for institutions of various kinds, such as postal systems, credit agencies and insurance firms, laws, police, courts, licensing and planing offices, hotels, restaurants, repair services, and various other administrative agencies. The relationship of population to space, in other words, is contingent upon the conjoint operation of organization and transportation and communication technology.

It is not clear, however, whether the actual history of man's ability to deal with the friction of space was necessary or accidental. Whatever may be the answer to that question, the fact is that the earliest developments were adapted to the long-haul carriage of bulk cargoes. Not until very late in the process of changes did significant improvements in the facilities for short-distance movements occur. Some tendency for this sequence to be repeated in developing countries is noticeable, though the causes are probably different. Whereas initially it was a matter of cumulative techno-logical change working its way slowly through a series of steps, the second or short-distance stage in the sequence seems now to be delayed not by nonavailability of the technology but by the inability of the masses of populations to afford automobiles, telephones, pipelines, and other items of equipment for the overcoming of distances. In any case, the spatial aspects of population have shifted radically as one technological stage has succeeded another, and more gradually, of course, as improvements have occurred within stages.

Given the changeability of the determinants of the spatial aspects of population, an understanding of the relationship is aided immeasurably if examined in historic perspective. Thus it will be seen that whether we approach the matter from the standpoint of density, scope of organization, or distribution of units there is no constant relationship to space.

Density

The simplest way of viewing population distribution is as the number of people per unit of space, or density. It is also one of the crudest of measures. As with all averages for highly skewed distributions, the density measure becomes more unstable as the size of the universe is increased. It is further subject to great variations as the size of areal unit employed in the denominator is altered (Day and Day, 1973). The crudeness of the measure becomes even more apparent when its interpretation is attempted. So many significant variables are excluded that all but one or two very rough inferences that might be made are unsupportable.

Yet density has a limited utility, at least in a preliminary way. As a relative value it offers some improvement over the absolute value of aggregate size. That is so because it provides an estimate of the extent of accessibility among the individuals comprising the aggregate, given the existing transportation and communication technology and organization of the population. A question of importance concerns how appropriate is the degree of accessibility. Because of unevenness in rates of change, density at one time may be too much or too little for the efficient operation of a system.

That is to say, in any given state of technology and organization there is conceivably an optimal density, a figure above which the frictions and collisions raise the costs of communication to prohibitive levels, and below which the costs again rise owing to the time and energy that must be spent in overcoming the distances separating members of the population. A plotting on a cost–density grid would inscribe a U-shaped curve. Where the technology and the organization are relatively primitive, the curve would be steep sided. But with each improvement in technology and organization, holding constant the size of the aggregate, the slopes of the curve would be more gradual and the U would be progressively flattened.

But in the great outpouring of research and commentary on density during the past decade, none of it deals with an optimum concept and very little touches upon insufficient density. On the latter point, the work of Barker *et al.,* (1962) at the individual level and of Bollinger (1972) at the institutional level are noteworthy. But apart from a few exceptions, virtually all of the work is devoted to the effects of excessive density. It explores the relation of density to the quality of life, to physical health, to vital processes, and to various pathologies such as mental disorder, delinquency and crime, and conflict (Choldin and McGinty, 1972). It ranges from rather casual inferences about cause and effect relations to a few careful studies employing multivariate models of analysis. Chapter 6 in this volume, by Galle and Gove, reviews that literature so thoroughly that a repetition is not needed here. This paper is also unique in its recognition of the opposite pole of a density continuum.

Positive findings on the relation of density to pathologies are rare. Most impressive on this score is the Galle *et al.* study (1972), which indicates that social structural variables, such as class and ethnicity, may operate through density (persons per room) in their association with pathologies. The increment added by density, however, is exceedingly small. It also might be questionable that these large "community areas" of Chicago, employed by the authors, are suitable as areal units; their mean values may conceal large ranges of variability. Incidentally, the measure of density found to have the highest explanatory value in this study is number of persons per room, or privacy, a property for which the conventional density measure is presumed to be a surrogate. But it should be noted that persons per room and persons per acre or per square mile have no necessary relationship.

The ground swell of interest in density as a cause of deviant behavior and its persistence in spite of unrewarding results is a phenomenon that in itself calls for explanation. If it represents a search for continuities from lower to higher forms of animal behavior, a great deal more attention to the establishment of parallels in research design is needed. If density studies are inspired by high rates of population growth and their future social implications, this would seem to be a miscalculation of the ultimate results of current growth trends. It is highly unlikely that densities the world over or within nations will reach levels that might threaten physiological or psychological functions. But the surge of interest comes at an odd time. For, as I have remarked elsewhere (Hawley, 1972), urban densities in the United States and in most of the Western world are in decline. And, pending the outcome of the present energy crisis, there is no reason to believe the trend will not continue.

In any event if I may repeat a point made earlier, the critical though neglected meaning of density would seem to lie in its bearing on the functioning of an organization.

Urban Expansion

One of the significant trends in population distribution has been the transition from the compact urban agglomeration developed during the nineteenth century to the more open, metropolitan scale unit of the present century. The shift from high to low density settlement patterns, though retarded by the inertia inherent in the physical structure of cities, has followed upon the great improvements in facilities for short-distance movements. A general centrifugal drift of population has been augmented by an accretion of new growth increments in the areas surrounding central cities. In the process, central cities declined at first relatively—as a proportion of the total dispersed agglomeration—and then absolutely.

Much more is involved, of course, than a redistribution of population. That is merely a symptom of fundamental changes at work in the organization of the urban unit. Urban expansion has been viewed as a species of the general process of cumulative social change. An accumulation of culture is associated with the growth of a system and that, in turn, requires an enlargement of territory from which to draw sustenance, and a development of an administrative capability at a center to provide coordination and integration of the system. Such a process obviously assumes improvements in transportation and communication. The applicability of the general expansion concept to the local area varies with the transportation regime, or more specifically with the degree of independence of the local system. If the local system is relatively self-contained, then most, if not all, of the elements of the general concept are present and the model is directly applicable. But when the local unit, the metropolitan area, is embedded in an extensive territorial network embracing many local units, the general concept has a rather limited applicability. This is the essential point of Franklin Wilson's argument, with which one must agree at least in part. The Kasarda paper (1972) with which Wilson takes issue is a correlation analysis of central city employment in selected professional and service occupations with size of central city, size of urbanized area population, and size of suburban area population, successively. From one point of view, Kasarda's work appears to be another attempt to determine the most appropriate measurement of population size for the prediction of central city characteristics. The SMSA does not contain the total area from which the center draws its sustenance, were it possible to isolate such a territory, and Kasarda's central city occupations are not clearly identified as metropolitan as distinct from urban services. Given these reservations, it still seems true, as the expansion concept holds, that a territorial dispersal of interrelated activities is associated with an increased amount of administrative function; that deconcentration of physical components and a centralization of integrative activities are counterpart trends.

Although longitudinal studies of an historico-descriptive character are well represented in the literature, there are none which examine the process under controlled conditions. Thus we have been unable to observe how external as well as internal relations change with the enlargement of an urban system. Cross-sectional studies provide us with an opaque picture of a functional hierarchy of urban places, but we are even less clear as to how such an ordering takes form. Nor do we know much about the repercussions for internal urban structures resulting from being relegated to different positions in a functional hierarchy.

Nor have the implications of the heightened mobility afforded by the conquest of intramural distance been very fully explored. We know that the average daily vehicular miles traveled by members of a household have increased more than five-fold in the past 50 years. With this has gone a departure of traditional functions from the household, a multiplication of specialized services, a decline of the local vicinage as a social unit, a reorganization of the uses of urban spaces, and a general regrouping of residents in urban areas. It seems very plausible, too, that the increased facility in daily trips has reduced the need for residence changes. A person can remain at a given place and enjoy access to a field of employment and other opportunity several times larger than was the case a short time ago. The one longitudinal series of annual data we have indicates that since 1947 there has been no significant change in the frequency of residence changes (U. S. Bureau of the Census, 1971). Those data show, incidentally, that intracounty residence changes have become relatively fewer. It is entirely probable that, if it were possible to sum all kinds of movement over space—rail and truck shipments, air passenger and freight miles, pipeline flows, mail deliveries, telephone calls, daily trips of persons, and residence changes—for a series of years, one would find that residence changes have been a declining proportion of all movements. Traffic densities are replacing residential densities.

Population Redistribution

Increased facility in daily movements and declining residential densities are features of the late phase of the redistribution of population that has characterized settlement in the United States from the beginning. Since early in the process of urban concentration, the zones of maximum population growth rates have tended to move outward from the inner core. At first that was due to the superior competitive powers of business and industrial activities for locations adjacent to central business districts. That influence had not yet spent itself when improvements in short-distance transportation and communication facilities appeared to carry forward the centrifugal drift of high growth rates. Before the first quarter of the present century was ended, the zone of highest growth was moving across central city corporation limits into adjacent rural territory, leaving behind a widening area of declining and negative growth rates. The emergence of the metropolitan area with the maturation of its suburban zone has not halted this movement of high growth rates; they have continued to drift deeper into outlying territory. Then with the tabulation of 1970 Census returns, we discovered that the most rapidly growing sector of the population during the preceding decade was the nonmetropolitan nonfarm population, and particularly that found in counties adjacent to the largest metropolitan areas (Campbell, 1975). Thus it seems that the concept of the SMSA as a definition of the effective urban unit is becoming inadequate just as did the city concept before it.

The fairly continuous long-term trend of peak growth rates to drift outward and away from the inner cores of metropolitan centers appears to have run its course by 1970. For as Chapter 8, by Beale and Fuguitt, indicates, a new trend in population distribution may have become unmistakable in the period between 1970 and 1973. While nonmetropolitan counties adjacent to metropolitan areas experienced the most rapid growth in that period, nonadjacent, nonmetropolitan counties grew more rapidly than metropolitan counties. That this began somewhat earlier is shown by the fact that in 1965 to 1970 in-migration rates were highest in urbanized nonmetropolitan counties which were not adjacent to metropolitan areas (Hines *et al.*, 1975). I can add little to Beale and Fuguitt's explanatory suggestions for the recent changes in distribution trends. It is noteworthy that, whereas departures from long-term distribution trends are usually led by special groups, the Beale and Fuguitt data show that virtually all categories of population are represented in the recent trend. In any case the new trend should be closely monitored over the ensuing years, for at this date we cannot be sure that we are not witnessing another short-term variation from a long-term trend.

This shift in trend, assuming it is that, is one of the many reminders that have forced themselves upon our attention of the historical particularity of much of our knowledge. Most of what we have learned over the years about population movements in the United States describes a society in transition from agrarian to industrial and perhaps to postindustrial phases. Consequently, one component after another in that body of knowledge has tended to become obsolete before it has been perfected. The rural to urban flows, for example, have all but dried up and interurban or intermetropolitan movements have loomed progressively larger. Furthermore, increased mobility allows the erstwhile farmer to remain in place and to travel to a nonagricultural job. Now, it seems, the drift may be turning from metropolitan to nonmetroplitan areas. But unlike the earlier movements from urban to rural areas, recent moves are not returns to the farm to escape occasional or cyclical urban unemployment; they are now moves to rural nonfarm and small city destinations, that is, to competing opportunities. Whereas until 1930 migration was the principal source of urban growth, it currently accounts for less than two-fifths of the population increments in urban areas. Patterns of selectivity in migration also are changing. To the selectivity of the young is now added the selectivity of persons in retirement ages. The narrowing of regional educational resources reduces the differences in educational attainment as between migrants and nonmigrants. The changing participation of women in the labor force is diminishing the tendency to sex selectivity. But the most conspicuous changes in selectivity have occurred in the intrametropolitan moves. While formerly the suburban-ward movement was domi-

nated by young white families with heads engaged in white-collar occupations, the movement now is much more representative of the total
population; single persons, broken families, and retired couples are prominent in the streams, blue-collar workers outnumber white-collar workers
in the movements in many areas, and blacks are becoming increasingly
numerous relatively as well as absolutely in the suburban drift (U. S. Bureau of the Census, 1975). Until quite recently, however, movement into
the suburban zones drew from the upper income levels of all occupational
and educational categories (Hawley and Zimmer, 1970). Whether that remaining selectivity has continued into the 1970s we do not know. Nor are
we adequately informed as yet on the patterns of selectivity of movements into nonmetropolitan counties. The Department of Agriculture report by Hines *et al.* (1975) compares various social and economic characteristics of metropolitan and nonmetropolitan residents and reveals
convergences in several respects, but it does not indicate how migration
might have affected the comparisons.

That the process of improvement in transportation and communication
techniques has brought about a progressive reduction of distances is an
observation so commonplace as to be trivial. What is not so obvious,
however, is where that trend is leading, for certainly it has not run its
course. If one were to imagine the extreme case in which the time and
cost of getting from point to point were reduced to zero, all locations in
space would be stripped of accessibility value and the spatial distributions
of people and of their activities could be completely random. Improbable
as that may be, there are some who argue we have advanced so far toward
that end that social organization need have no correlation in a spatial
order (Webber, 1963). Indeed, radio, television, satellite communication,
supersonic air travel, and the cheapening of toll telephone calls have all
but neutralized the immediate felt limitations of long distances. Of course,
although distance costs might seem to have disappeared as a result of
these technical improvements, many of the costs are merely translated
into advertising charges levied on consumer goods prices or into taxes to
provide government subsidies for the support of research and development, capital outlays for roads and for various services to transportation.
Short-distance movements have not yet had a second round of dramatic
improvements. But when they do occur, they may also involve a spreading of increased costs over a wider range of budget allocations. In short,
as long as there are costs of overcoming the frictions of space, a kind of
order in the spatial distribution of activities can be expected. That can be
radically different, however, from anything with which we are familiar.

References

Barker, R., with P. V. Gump and others
  1962 *Big School-Small School: High School Size and Student Behavior.* Stanford, Calif.: Stanford University Press.
Bollinger, W. L.
  1972 "The economic and social impact of the depopulation process upon four selected counties in Idaho." Pp. 561–596 in *Commission on Population Growth and the American Future, Research Reports,* Vol. V. Population Distribution and Policy. Washington, D. C.: U. S. Government Printing Office.
Campbell, R. R.
  1975 "Beyond the suburbs: The changing rural scene." Pp. 93–122 in A. H. Hawley and V. Rock (eds.), *Metropolitan America in Contemporary Perspective.* New York: John Wiley and Sons.
Choldin, H. M., and M. J. McGinty
  1972 "Bibliography: Population density, crowding and social relations." *Man–Environment Systems* 2(2)(May): 131–158.
Day, A. T., and L. E. Day
  1973 "Cross-national comparisons of population density." *Science* 181: 1016–1023.
Galle, O., W. R. Gove, and J. M. McPherson
  1972 "Population density and pathology: What are the relations for man." *Science* 176(April): 23–30.
Hawley, A. H.
  1972 "Population density and the city." *Demography* 9(4): 521–529.
Hawley, A. H., and B. Zimmer
  1970 *The Metropolitan Community: Its People and Government.* Beverly Hills, Calif. Sage Publications.
Hines, F. K., D. L. Brown, and J. M. Zimmer
  1975 "Social and economic characteristics of the population in metro and nonmetro counties, 1970." Agricultural Economic Report No. 272, Economic Research Service. Washington, D. C.: U. S. Department of Agriculture.
Kasarda, J.
  1972 "The theory of ecological expansion: An empirical test." *Social Forces* 51(2): 165–175.
U. S. Bureau of the Census
  1971 Current Population Reports, Series P-20, N:235, "Mobility of the population of the United States: March 1970 to March 1971." Washington, D. C.: U. S. Government Printing Office.
U. S. Bureau of the Census
  1975 Current Population Reports, Series P-23, N:54, "The social and economic status of the black population in the United States, 1974." Washington, D. C.: U. S. Government Printing Office.
Webber, M.
  1963 "Order in diversity: Community without propinquity." Pp. 23–54 in L. Wingo, Jr. (ed.), *City and Space: The Future Use of Urban Land.* Baltimore: Johns Hopkins Press.

6

Overcrowding, Isolation, and Human Behavior: Exploring the Extremes in Population Distribution[1]

OMER R. GALLE and WALTER R. GOVE

The existence of some optimal level of population size and density, above or below which a population may exhibit deleterious effects, has been an intriguing and recurring notion in both animal and human population studies. In the late nineteenth century Durkheim (1933) and Spencer (1879–1882) came to rather different conclusions about the structural and behavioral consequences of increasing size and density of human populations. Even before this, Verhulst (1845) had observed positive correlations between the death rate and the population density of specific populations. Sociologists (and others) also have been impressed by the severe effects of the other end of the population distribution continuum: extreme isolation (Davis, 1940; Spitz, 1945, 1946; Spitz and Wolfe, 1946). In this chapter we review the evidence on the behavioral consequences of the two extremes of population distribution—overcrowding and high population density on the one hand, and isolation on the other.

Our review has four sections. We start by reviewing evidence from various animal studies of the effects of overcrowding and isolation. As

---

[1] The research for this paper was supported by NICHHD Grant #R01 HD0671 1.

95

Copyright © 1978 by Academic Press, Inc.
All rights of reproduction in any form reserved.
ISBN 0-12-682650-1

most studies of the effects of high population density and/or overcrowding in human population settings have focused on urban settings, in the second section we briefly review research on the determinants of urban population densities. Third, we review evidence from ecological studies of the effects of high population density, overcrowding, and isolation on human behavior. Fourth, we examine recent survey research that has focused on the same areas of interest as the human ecological studies, but that utilizes data on individual households rather than the ecologist's customary areal data.

Animal Studies of Overcrowding and Isolation

Allee (1938) claimed that there are serious deleterious effects of both overcrowding and very low levels of population density for a wide variety of animal populations. Since then, a large body of evidence has accumulated that supports Allee's contention. Because the range of animals and behaviors studied is large, we focus here on three major topics that may have particular relevance to human studies: morbidity and mortality; reproductive behavior (including fecundity, sexual behavior, and maternal behavior); and aggression and other forms of aberrant social behavior.

MORBIDITY AND MORTALITY

As the density of many animal populations increases, so does mortality (Allee *et al.,* 1949; Petrusewicz, 1957; Thiessen and Rodgers, 1961). Prenatal mortality in confined populations of mice is related to increased population density (Christian and LeMunyan, 1958; see also Helmreich, 1960). Christian *et al.* (1960) released a small herd of deer on an island. When left free to breed, the deer reached a density of about one deer per acre, after which the mortality rate soared unaccountably even though food and water were abundant and there was no evidence of exogenous disease. Evidence of cyclical mortality increases in lemmings and snowshoe hares is reported by Deevey (1960). Crowding adversely affects the course of acute and chronic tuberculosis in mice (Tobach and Block, 1956). Increased levels of infant mortality were observed for Norwegian rats under high-density conditions (Calhoun, 1962), while high levels of density have been found to be related to juvenile mortality among herring gulls (Paynter, 1949) and among wild voles (Chitty, 1952). Among the Tribolium, or flour beetle, high levels of density appear to induce high levels of mortality from cannibalism (Chapman, 1928; Chapman and Baird, 1934; Crombie, 1943). Among a variety of animals growth is inhibited with increased density of growing populations, and adrenal weight typically is 'increased markedly in males and frequently increased in females (Christian, 1959, 1961; Van Wijngaarden, 1960). Similarly, in their studies of mammals, Christian and Davis (1964) found significant changes in body chemistry and a decrease in antibody formation and other related body defenses. The detrimental effect of crowding on health appears to be greatest for young growing organisms and least for dominant adult animals (Christian, 1959; Klepinger, 1968).

One special influence of overcrowding that may lead to death in certain species has been called *shock disease*. Seemingly healthy snowshoe hares may die when trapped or when chased, and elaborate studies of the incidence of disease show no obvious reason for mortality other than hypoglycemia (Deevey, 1972), which follows the general idea of Selye's "General Adaptation Syndrome" (1950).

At the other end of the continuum, a too small population may lead to excessive inbreeding and the possible fixation of deleterious genes with consequent weakening or extinction of the isolated population (Allee *et al.*, 1949). Certain kinds of survival behavior may not be possible with a small population. For example, when a group of 12 to 15 American pronghorn antelope are attacked by wolves, the antelope form a defensive band that presents a minimum of group surface and the bucks are able to fight off the attackers; when the population of pronghorns falls below this critical level, the animals stampede instead of grouping, thereby exposing themselves to the attackers and permitting the weaker bucks to be killed easily (Leopold, 1933; see also Sdobnikov, 1935). Other examples of the survival ability of a species being decreased under low population density conditions are goldfish (Allee and Bowen, 1932), flatworms (Oesting and Allee, 1935), and planarian worms (Allee and Wilder, 1938). Although exact data on the population size below which a species might undergo extinction are difficult to obtain, some evidence has been gathered on such levels for various insect populations (Smith *et al.*, 1933; Soper and Wilson, 1942).

REPRODUCTIVE BEHAVIOR

The evidence on the relationship between overcrowding and reproductive behavior among animals is quite substantial, generally indicating an inverse relationship. Reduced fertility has been observed with crowding among various types of rats and mice, either through a regression of the reproductive organs, decreased litter size, or failure of the litter to go full term before being aborted (Calhoun, 1962; Davis, 1964; Keeley, 1962; Schrag, 1972; Snyder, 1966a; 1966b; 1968; Terman, 1965). In addition, Calhoun (1962) and Louch (1956) report ineffectual maternal care, ranging from inadequate nest building to cannibalism of the young. Christian *et al.*

(1965) allowed an experimental population to reach a level of 51 animals in 5 months, after which 30 litters were born but no young survived. Decreased fertility as a reaction to high population density also has been found for birds (Perrins, 1965), elephants (Laws and Parker, 1968), rabbits (Lockley, 1961), wolves (Hoffman, 1958), deer (Christian *et al.*, 1960), and chickens (Hoffman and Tomhave, 1945; Pearl and Surface, 1909; Siegel, 1959).

In contrast to these findings of an inverse relation, certain studies have indicated either no relation between population density and reproductive activity or a positive one. No relationship obtains between mixed-sex crowding and depressed testes weight among gerbils, while a positive relationship obtains for the same-sex crowding (Syme, 1973). Fecundity in the drosophila (fruit fly) may be reduced by crowding, but only when there is a corresponding reduction in the food supply (Robertson and Sang, 1944, clarifying, to some extent, the earlier work of Pearl and Parker in 1922). In some protozoans the fission rate may actually increase as a result of crowding (Ludwig and Boost, 1939; Robertson, 1921).

The possibility that there is a minimum threshold of numbers necessary for producing offspring in birds has been suggested by several authors (Darling, 1938; Fauten, 1941; Fisher and Vevers, 1944; Fisher and Waterson, 1941). In many bird colonies, as the size of the colony decreases so does the reproductive success. Male birds reared in isolation may fail to mate because they show more fear than controls reared in groups (Fisher and Hale, 1956–1957; Hinde, 1959; Krujit, 1962). Social isolation in early rearing often influences sexual behavior (and thus reproduction) in a number of ways. Gruendel and Arnold (1969) compared isolated and mother-reared rats and found deficient mating behavior in almost all of the isolates. These results contradict earlier findings that male rats raised in isolation were more responsive to females and more likely to copulate than males group-raised with females (Beach, 1942, 1958; Kagan and Beach, 1953). Hamsters reared in isolation apparently show normal sexual responses at adulthood (Dieterlen, 1959; Eibl-Eibesfeldt, 1961; Thorpe, 1963), but the rearing of female guinea pigs in isolation is reported to have detrimental effects on sexual performance (Goy and Young, 1956–1957).

Abnormal sexual behavior has been widely reported in isolate-reared monkeys (Hansen, 1962; Harlow, 1961, 1962; Harlow and Harlow, 1962; Harlow *et al.*, 1966; Maple *et al.*, 1974; Mason, 1965). The importance of this abnormal sexual behavior for normal reproductive behavior is subject to some debate (Maple *et al.*, 1974). Other research on monkeys and chimpanzees has focused on the nature of social contacts, arguing for the importance of peer contacts (as opposed to just contact with the mother) in the development of adequate adult sexual development (Hansen, 1962; Harlow and Harlow, 1962; Mason, 1960; Nissen, 1954). Abnormal maternal behavior due to isolation during rearing ranges from poor nest building and neglect of the young for rats (Reiss, 1954; but see Eibl-Eibesfeldt, 1955) to an absence of typical maternal behavior in monkeys (Chappell and Meier, 1974; Harlow, 1962; Harlow *et al.*, 1966; Seay *et al.*, 1964).

AGGRESSIVE BEHAVIOR

Crowding animals in artificial cages or pens causes an increase in social stress that seems to induce fighting behavior (Petrusewicz, 1957). Greenberg (1972) studied the effects of floor area on aggressive behavior in aggressive and nonaggressive strains of mice. His results indicate that crowding causes more aggressive behavior in both strains of mice. Gregor *et al.* (1972) have replicated Petrusewicz's observations on increased fighting behavior as a direct result of crowding in cages or pens, and Fenderson and Carpenter (1971) report that salmon in high densities become more aggressive with time. A decrease in available space is accompanied by higher rates of aggression in pigeons (Willis, 1966) and in leghorns (Flickinger, 1966). Short-term acute crowding has led to increments of mild and severe aggression in captive monkey populations (Alexander and Roth, 1971; Southwick *et al.*, 1965).

Hemingway and Furumoto (1972) report that rats in moderately crowded groups fight more than those in overcrowded and uncrowded groups and suggest from these findings that population density up to a certain point encourages territorial defense (and drinking alcohol). After that point the decrease in fighting (and drinking) was accompanied by a transition from territorial to social rank behavior. After reviewing over 200 articles dealing with the effect of population density on rodent behavior, Archer (1970, p. 201) concludes, "the usual response to increased population density in natural populations is emigration. When the animals have no opportunity to emigrate, increased aggressive behavior, associated with changes in dispersion and social structure, is the primary consequence of increased density." Among mice, as among most other vertebrates when crowded, a dominance hierarchy (called the *pecking order* in chickens) is readily established as a consequence of fighting (Deevey, 1972). Snyder (1968) uses the term *dominance hierarchy* to indicate the social organization among animals involving one or two dominant individuals and several subordinates. Wynne-Edwards (1962) uses the hierarchy as an example of a typical group character and visualizes the dominance hierarchy as a mechanism for regulating population density.

The effects of isolation appear in some respects to be very similar to those of overcrowding, at least with regard to aggressive behavior. Monkeys living in partial isolation until adolescence were more aggressive than age-matched controls, perhaps because isolation hindered the development of mechanisms for the control of aggression (Mason, 1960, 1961). Similar results are reported by Chamove (1973) who found that aggression decreased as an increasing function of number of rearing partners. Similar results also have been found for rats (Ely and Henry, 1974), mice (Valzelli, 1969), and rabbits (Wolfe and Von Haxthausen, 1960). Isolated fox terriers were found to be deficient in fighting behavior when placed with other dogs, that is, the isolates continued to isolate themselves when put in groups (Fisher, 1955). Fuller (1964) confirmed this result, but he also found that if his puppies were removed from isolation as early as 7 weeks of age, they showed no abnormal effects and became normally socialized.

SUMMARY

Other harmful effects of either overcrowding or isolation have been noted in many animal studies, but this skimming of the substantial literature should suffice to give the flavor of the research findings. For many species high population density or overcrowding appears to increase mortality, decrease fertility, and lead to higher levels of aggression. The evidence on the isolation end of the density continuum is more mixed, although the general weight of the evidence suggests similar relationships between isolation and behavior—increased probability of high mortality (possibly even extinction), lowered fertility (possibly through inadequate sexual or maternal behavior), and increased aggression. These broad generalizations are based on studies of a limited number of species and do not hold for all studied species. Even in those species where the same general effect is observed (for example, increased mortality or decreased fertility), the specific mechanisms identified as involved in this changed behavior vary substantially among species and among different investigators.

HUMAN IMPLICATIONS

Animal studies have demonstrated the possibility of harmful effects for certain species under extremes of population distribution—high or low population density. The implications of these findings for the species Homo sapiens are still being debated and discussed with great vigor. The writers on this topic fall into three broad categories: (1) those who feel that what is true for other animals is equally true for humans (Ardry, 1970; Deevey, 1972; Hartley, 1972); (2) those who believe there is little connection between animal and human studies and generalizations about humans based on animal studies are virtually worthless (Hawley, 1972; Lawrence,

1974); and (3) those "middle-of-the-roaders" who believe that the various animal studies are suggestive and offer valuable insights for exploration of the effects of population distribution on human behavior, and that certain comparisons warrant exploration, albeit with great caution (Cassell, 1971).

We place ourselves in the third category, although we recognize the problems and dangers of simplistic and facile generalizations. Beyond the substantial problems of generalizing from one species to another, cultural factors enter into the picture in human populations. Hall (1966), for example, claimed that Japanese persons seem better able to endure high-density living arrangements than do German persons, and he pointed out the long period of time the Japanese have lived at high densities, allowing them to develop customs and cultural constraints for dealing with high-density situations.

Man lives under several different conditions of population density at the same time. This is an unstudied aspect of animal life and obviously an extremely important aspect of human life. Cities, for example, are built in such a way that some of an individual's time may be spent in areas of incredibly high density while other time is spent in very low-density surroundings. The movement back and forth may permit him to partake of the "good" or the "bad" in both areas. Man's technology of building construction permits him to build multistory high-density apartment buildings with great spaciousness within each dwelling unit, so that high intensity of land use need not lead to high levels of individual contact. Human population densities are complex and variable, much more so than the population densities of most other animals. Because most of the studies of human behavior and population density occur in an urban context, we believe it fruitful to consider the character of urban population densities before we proceed to our review of studies of the effects of densities on humans.

Determinants of Variations in Urban Population Densities

THE COMPONENTS OF POPULATION DENSITY

Gross density, population per unit area, may seem like a simple variable especially for most animal studies, but for humans in an urban setting it is actually a composite of several different measures of land use. A useful way of expressing this complex set of activities is the following equation:

$$P/A = (P/R)\ (R/D)\ (D/S)\ (S/N)\ (N/A)$$

where P equals population, A equals area, R equals the number of rooms in the area, D equals the number of dwellings in the area, S equals the number of residential structures in the area, and N equals the area in residences or the net residential area. Each term thus has a substantive interpretation: P/R is a measure of room crowding (persons per room), R/D is the average number of rooms per dwelling unit, D/S is the average number of dwelling units per structure, S/N is the number of structures per unit of land area devoted to residential use, and N/A is the proportion of the area which is used for residential purposes (Carnahan *et al.*, 1974b). By taking the logarithm of both sides, the equation just given may be transformed into an additive one, allowing the utilization of standard statistical techniques in analyzing variations between the several components.

In studies of urban density in the United States it has been found that gross density (P/A) is primarily a consequence of the components D/S, S/N, and N/A, while persons per room (P/R) and rooms per dwelling (R/D) have less effect (Duncan, 1966; Guest, 1970, 1972). The "minor" components, however, may be important at certain times or places. For example, in recent decades population densities have declined in many urban neighborhoods because of a declining number of persons per dwelling, not because of a declining number of dwelling units (Guest, 1972). In any case, two neighborhoods may have identical population densities but for very different reasons. One area may have a low population density because a large portion of the land is devoted to nonresidential uses (business or industrial) in conjunction with a few high-rise apartment buildings, while another area may have equally low population density because each single-family dwelling unit is surrounded by a large lawn.

THE DENSITY GRADIENT EQUATION

Density patterns in cities have been described by the formula

$$D_x = D_0 \, e^{-bx}$$

where D_x is the density of an area x units of distance away from the center of the city (usually the central business district, or CBD), D_0 is the extrapolated density of the city at its hypothetical center, and b equals the rate of change in density with each unit of distance from the CBD. The coefficient b may be interpreted as an indicator of the concentration of population around, or average distance of the population from, the CBD (Winsborough, 1963). A high value of b would indicate a high concentration of population around the CBD. D_0 is interpreted as a measure of congestion of population, because it indicates crowding at the city center. These two parameters—congestion and concentration—may vary independently.

Traditionally, human ecologists cite competition as the mechanism that results in the tendency toward congestion and concentration in most cities (Hawley, 1950, p. 280, pp. 382–404). Transportation facilities (especially harbor and rail) often converged in the CBD so that those producing and selling goods could reduce costs by proximity to transport facilities. The CBD was traditionally the most accessible point in the city to customers, allowing (with the concentration of business there) comparison shopping. Location within easy access to the CBD also was attractive to residents, for most jobs were in or near the CBD and costs of travel could be kept low by locating close to the city center.

Out of this competition for centrality came a sifting and sorting so that activities with the greatest need and economic power managed to occupy sites around the CBD. These generally included retailers, wholesalers, and some types of manufacturers who could afford high central city rents. Because residential activities were largely preempted at the center, population densities were often unusually low in the area right around the CBD. Nevertheless, some residences were found in this area, and the number of dwellings per structure and the number of structures per acre was often high because of the high land costs resulting from the competition. Residential density should decrease with distance from the CBD, primarily because the number of dwellings per structure and the number of structures per areal unit should also decrease with distance from the CBD.

TRANSPORTATION CHANGES

Changes in urban transportation in the United States have radically altered the competition for sites around the CBD, leading to a less centripetal pattern of population around the CBD and lower urban levels of congestion. Increased use of the truck and governmental highway construction have permitted establishment of transportation depots on the urban outskirts, reducing the utility of location near the CBD. The speed of the automobile and its wide-spread ownership have reduced the need of residents for close geographic centrality to place of work and of businesses to locate centrally for access to their customers. In a situation of reduced competition for the CBD, it appears that the metropolis is becoming organized around numerous subcentral transportation nodes, such as shopping centers and industrial parks.

DENSITY AS URBAN SPRAWL

Sociologists are notoriously inaccurate at predicting the future, yet, assuming that transportation systems continue to improve and given the further development of freeway–highway systems, there is every reason to believe that metropolitan areas will continue to decrease in their values of b and D_0 and that neighborhoods in cities will probably build up to very low levels of density. This seems a safe assumption as long as urban transportation has the necessary energy or fuel, and as long as automobile manufacturers can decrease levels of auto pollution or diminish public resistance to high pollution levels in cities. However, recent restrictions on speed and the changing government emphasis on the character of urban transportation may lead to a trend at least partially back toward the population patterns of the pre-automobile city.

In summary, urban population densities in the United States may be seen to be both (1) variable in their composition and (2) apparently moving toward a new pattern of less steep gradients from the central city. For our purposes here, it is most worthwhile to reiterate several points. The concept of density itself is a complex one when the reference is to urban human populations. From a conceptual point of view it may be useful to distinguish two major components of overall or gross population density (P/A). On the one hand, there is what might be called "structural density," or the way in which an area is built up (consisting primarily of D/S, S/N, and N/A). This has been the major factor in determining gross densities in urban areas. On the other hand, there is what might best be termed interpersonal crowding (primarily P/R, though it might also be encompassed partly by R/D). The fact that these two components of gross density may vary independently is important in distinguishing what precisely has been occurring in major urban areas. Over the last 30 years, for example, the percentage of the U. S. population living in urbanized or metropolitan areas has increased greatly. At the same time, however, levels of overcrowding have been reduced quite drastically. In 1940, 20% of all households in the U. S. averaged more than one person per room; by 1970, this percentage had declined to 8% (Carnahan *et al.*, 1974a). Along with this dramatic decrease in overcrowding, we have had a similar rise in the proportion of persons who live alone. Primary individuals (mainly one-person households) have increased from 11% of all households in 1950 to 19% of all households in 1970. In the United States, then, isolation may be becoming a more substantial problem for human populations in urban areas than overcrowding.

As this brief review suggests, density is a very complex variable involving many interacting components. Almost all of the research on density that has been done has treated these components separately. As a consequence, we have very little idea, for example, of how the aspects of the microenvironment—such as living in an overcrowded household or living alone—interact with structural density or gross density. Furthermore, as the characteristics and interactions of the components of density are clearly in a state of flux, relationships that are seemingly well established at one point in time may disappear or even be reversed at another. In addition there is always the possibility of a change over time in cultural adaptations to the various levels of density. As a consequence, research on the effects of density will necessarily be an ongoing process.

Ecological Studies of Overcrowding and Isolation in Human Populations

In our review of ecological studies of human populations, we begin with a review of the effects of high density and overcrowding; this is followed by a brief discussion of the effects of isolation. There are many more studies of the effects of high density and overcrowding than of isolation. We group high density and overcrowding together for, although we have specified the conceptual differences between the two concepts, this distinction is not always made in the literature.

HIGH DENSITY AND OVERCROWDING

Theoretical support for an effect of population density on social relationships rests on the notion that the number of social actors per unit of area affects the potential contacts, both for a given individual and within the aggregate. Frequencies of contact and communication are potentially multiplied exponentially as density increases. These contacts and communications create the possibility of increases in cooperation and/or conflict. On an aggregate level, high-density settlements and the large number of contacts each individual may make have been assumed to create a preponderance of secondary and segmental role relationships (Simmel, 1957; Wirth, 1938).

At the individual level, density may affect one's health and level of well-being. Most of the theoretical literature on the experience of crowding focuses on two analytically distinct but interrelated concepts: an excess of stimulation and a lack of privacy. For example, Desor (1972) defines crowding as "receiving excess of stimulation from social sources." Other investigators who have emphasized stimulus overload in the experience of crowding are Rapoport (1973), Galle *et al.* (1972), Wohlwill (1974), and Milgram (1970). Perhaps the best theoretical discussion of the effects of the environment on behavior is the book by Altman (1975). Altman, while recognizing the importance of stimulus overload, feels that the concept of privacy is the key to understanding crowding. We would note that there is a fairly extensive *conceptual* literature dealing with the nature and importance of privacy (for example, Altman, 1975, 1976; Bates, 1964;

Chermayeff and Alexander, 1965; Fischer, 1975; Jourard, 1966; Kelvin, 1973; Marmor, 1972; Pastalan, 1970; Pennock and Chapman, 1971; Schwartz, 1968; Shils, 1966), and that privacy is typically related to aspects of the physical environment, such as the number of persons per room in a household (for example, Chapin, 1951; Schwartz, 1968; Smith *et al.*, 1969). However, there has been virtually no empirical investigation of the effects of a lack of privacy (Altman, 1975, p. 6).

The National Academy of Sciences (1971) reports that crowding increases the incidence of infectious disease mainly through a greater opportunity for the spread of infection. The NAS report cites evidence that crowding also has other injurious health effects that occur primarily when the degree and extent of crowding are rapidly increasing. Thus the rapidity of growth and accompanying urbanization may be more deleterious to health than population density per se. The NAS report claims that animal experiments and experience with humans confirm that social stresses due to cowding produce physiological disturbances that in turn increase the susceptibility to disease. The relationship may be far more complex than this. Crowding under some circumstances appears to be clearly associated with poor health states, while under other circumstances it may be neutral or even beneficial (Taylor and Knowelden, 1957). Indeed microbial disease is not necessarily acquired through exposure. In many cases disease occurs as a result of factors that upset the balance between ubiquitous organisms and the host that harbors them (Dubos, 1965).

A number of the studies of the effects of crowding have utilized urban–residential neighborhoods as their units of analysis. A study of 42 census tracts in Honolulu for 1960 utilized five measures of population density: population per acre; proportion of dwellings with 1.5 or more persons per room; average household size; proportion of "doubled up" families; and proportion of dwelling units in structures with five or more units (Schmitt, 1966). These measures were then correlated with nine indicators of pathology: death rate, infant mortality rate, suicide rate, tuberculosis rate, and rates of venereal disease, admissions to mental hospitals, illegitimate births, juvenile delinquency, and adult crime. After controls for social class, persons per acre correlated much more strongly with the nine pathology measures than did any of the other component measures of density. Unfortunately, when Schmitt attempted to control for social class he dichotomized his variables (education and income) instead of treating them as continuous measures, which tended to weaken their effects and thus our faith in his results.

A negative relationship between gross density and general mortality was found across Chicago community areas for 1950, after controlling for socioeconomic status, quality of housing, and migration (Winsborough,

1970). Negative associations also were shown for public assistance rates and tuberculosis rates. However, a positive relationship obtained between gross density and the infant mortality rate (after controls). Winsborough's negative results, however, may be due to including the percentage of dwellings with 1.5 or more persons per room as one of his controls (a measure of housing quality). This measure is very closely related to persons per room, which was later shown to be more closely associated with pathology than the gross density measure Winsborough employed (Galle *et al.*, 1972).

In another analysis of data for Chicago community areas, this time for 1960, we (Galle *et al.*, 1972) attempted a roughly approximate rendition, in a natural human setting, of Calhoun's (1962) well-known study of population density and pathology in rats. A measure of gross density (persons per acre) was shown to be related slightly to five measures of "pathological behavior": standardized mortality rates, general fertility rates, juvenile delinquency rates, rates of admissions to mental hospitals, and rates of public assistance to persons under 18 years of age. Indices of social class and ethnicity were constructed in an attempt to take the complex human social structure into account. The density effects were reduced to insignificance when the controls for social class and ethnicity were introduced.

We then decomposed gross density into four component parts—persons per room, rooms per dwelling unit, dwelling units per structure, and structures per acre. On the basis of this decomposition we concluded that, after social class and ethnicity are controlled for, there appears to be a small but significant effect of overcrowding (persons per room) on rates of pathological behavior. However, the effects of density and social structure are so intertwined at the ecological level that it is extremely difficult to separate the two effects. For example, of the total variance in mortality, fertility, and juvenile delinquency explained by density and social structural measures taken together, over 90% is variance held in common by density and social structure, and it cannot be allocated independently to either density measures or social structural factors. This finding of high collinearity between measures of overcrowding and other relevant social structural controls appears in most of the ecological studies; unambiguous interpretation of any of these studies is inappropriate. However, the problem of collinearity has been lost in the debate over whether or not overcrowding is an important factor in the determination of behavior in human populations.

The complexity of the data and their interrelations also have caused a number of methodological questions to be raised about our Chicago study. The specific indices of social class and ethnicity have been questioned (Ward, 1975) along with the use of ratio measures for density (Schuessler, 1974). In addition, it has been suggested that the use of measures of central tendency (such as average persons per room) should have been replaced by measures of extremes of the distribution under examination (for example, percentage of housing units with more than one person per room (Ward, 1975). Finally, the cross-sectional, one-point-in-time nature of the analysis has been criticized (McPherson, 1973). In a more recent analysis (Galle and Gove, 1974) we considered each of these criticisms and examined each census period from 1940 through 1970 for Chicago. Extreme measures of each variable were used: Percentage of housing units with more than one person per room and percentage of housing units in structures with more than five housing units were our measures of overcrowding and structural density; percentage nonwhite, percentage of families with low incomes, percentage with less than 8 years of education, and percentage of labor force in lower blue-collar occupations were our measures of social structure. For all time periods between 1940 and 1970 and for all "pathologies" (mortality, fertility, juvenile delinquency, and marital instability) the two density variables are able to account for an average of 6.6% of variation independently. Social structure is able to account for slightly more—12.3%—of variation independently. The amount of explained variance held in common by the two sets of variables, however, is much larger—57.7% (Galle and Gove, 1974).

Several recent studies using cities as units of analysis have attempted to examine the effects of overcrowding on murder rates. A positive relationship between a set of density variables and homicide rates was found for 171 U. S. cities in both 1950 and 1970, although the relationship was greatly reduced after social class and racial controls were introduced (McCarthy et al., 1975). Using a larger sample of U. S. cities ($n = 389$) Gove et al. (1976a) found overcrowding and city size to be positively correlated to homicide. The relationship for overcrowding (but not city size) was reduced to insignificance after controls were introduced. Among an even larger set of U. S. cities ($n = 656$) Booth et al. (1976) found a small relationship between density and a variety of personal and property crimes. Density had more effect on large than on small cities. Their study, however, suffered from a severe methodological problem: They used census data from 1960 and crime data from 1967. The analysis by McPherson (1973) suggests the time lag was great enough to distort the relationship they found.

The effect of population density and crowding on health and social behavior was assessed among 145 economic–geographic regions in the Netherlands (Levy and Herzog, 1974). After economic status and population heterogeneity were controlled for, density was positively associated only with age-adjusted death rates. Weak or inverse relations were found between crowding (persons per room) and measures of age-adjusted male heart disease rate, admissions to general hospitals, admissions to mental hospitals, delinquency, illegitimate births, and divorce.

A study by Collette and Webb (1974) looked at the effects of density (persons per acre) and crowding (persons per room) in the 18 urban areas of New Zealand; unfortunately, no socioeconomic controls were used. However, New Zealand has a system of free public hospital care that greatly diminishes class-related differences in health care utilization. A fairly strong positive relationship was found between density and psychological disorder, but the relationship of density with physical disorder was negative. In general, weak and inconsistent relationships were found between crowding and the dependent variables.

In a study using census tracts in Edmonton, after controls for income and national origin, building type (that is, multiple unit dwellings) had a strong positive association with juvenile delinquency and social allowance (public assistance), but the relationships of those dependent variables with density and overcrowding were nonsignificant (Gillis, 1974).

A study of Peoria used city blocks rather than census tracts, controlled for a large set of other variables, and examined the relationship among measures of density and crime and mortality (Choldin and Roncek, 1976). Compared to the effect of some of their control variables, that of density was relatively weak; however, it was significantly related to child and infant mortality and the general crime rate and more strongly to the violent crime rate.

Booth and Welch (1974) looked at the relationship between areal density and civil disorder using 65 nations as their units of analysis. They found that "household crowding and, to a far less extent, areal density are linked to the emergence of civil strife [p. 153]." It is noteworthy that household overcrowding had a much greater explanatory power than did measures of industrialization, urbanization, and discrimination. Fischer *et al.* (1975, p. 416, footnote 10) refer to this study and a similar one by Factor and Waldron (1973) that use national averages of density, including countries composed largely of uninhabited territory, as "representing a *reductio ad absurdum,* so much so that one is tempted to suspect they are purposeful caricatures." In a subsequent study of cities in the United States Welch and Booth (1975) found a much weaker relationship between density and civil disorder; most of the variance in the civil disorder measure was accounted for by the size of the black population.

In sum, ecological studies of overcrowding, high population density, and various rates of "pathological" behavior show very mixed results.

Part of the difficulty of generalizing from these studies arises from confusion among the several aspects of high population density, particularly overcrowding versus structural density. Also contributing to the mixed results are the different ways of managing and interpreting the high degree of collinearity between density variables and control variables. Our summary assessment is a cautious affirmation of a positive relationship between crowding and some rates of "pathological" behavior. Although social structural factors are highly intercorrelated with high levels of structural density and interpersonal crowding, there does appear to be a small but significant amount of explained variance in certain rates of behavior, which can be attributed to density and/or overcrowding factors independently of other social-structural factors.

ISOLATION

There have been surprisingly few ecological studies of the relationship between isolation and behavior. In fact we know of only two studies, both of which are recent. One study is based on a survey of all pharmacists in the 45 New Zealand urban areas with populations of over 10,000 (Webb and Collette, 1975). Use of stress alleviative drugs (tranquilizers, antidepressants, and so on) was found to be very strongly related to living alone.

The second study is our own, and we shall review briefly our conceptualization as well as our findings (Gove *et al.*, 1976a). Those who live alone (our measure of isolation) are less likely to be firmly integrated into social networks. The literature on integration and isolation suggests the following premises. First, if one is integrated into a set of social networks one's life tends to take on meaning and value, whereas if one is isolated life tends to be meaningless and empty. Second, social control of behavior requires social interaction, and the individual who lives alone, lacking such control, will be free to act in deviant ways. Third, when one confronts a problem the social support and feedback of others put the problem into perspective and often suggest ways of handling it; isolated individuals tend to lack such support and feedback. Fourth, living alone is characterized by an environment that lacks the input and structure that tend to involve the individual in the daily affairs of life; individuals in such a situation may withdraw into a fantasy world and, if they are emotionally disturbed, this may lead them to brood about and thus magnify their problems. A fifth issue, which has received very little attention in the literature, is the fact that if others are present there is a high probability they will intervene (see, for example, Gove and Howell, 1974). In the case of suicidal behavior, for example, if others are present generally they will act to prevent the prospective suicide. All five of these factors suggest a positive relationship between the percentage of the population living alone in a given areal unit and the suicide rate.

A positive relationship also may be anticipated between the percentage of the population living alone and the death rate due to cirrhosis of the liver (a measure of alcoholism). This expectation is based on two factors that play a role in a person's drinking behavior. First, drinking is highly regulated by social norms (Bacon, 1957; Bales, 1946; Blacker, 1966; Larson and Abu-Laban; Patrick, 1952; Pittman, 1967; Pittman and Snyder, 1962; Roman and Trice, 1970; Skolnick, 1958; Snyder, 1962; Ullman, 1958; Whitehead and Harvey, 1974; Wilkinson, 1970). Second, many persons drink in reaction to a stressful situation that produces feelings of discomfort and distress (Alexander, 1963; Borowitz, 1964; Chafetz *et al.*, 1962; Greenberg, 1963; Pearlin and Radabaugh, 1975; Seely, 1959; Strauss, 1971; Trice, 1966; Washburne, 1955). Living alone would appear to be related to both of these factors, for many of the same reasons just cited linking isolation to suicide. Persons who live alone tend, almost by definition, to be largely removed from the social control of others. The environment associated with living alone may produce a desire for alcohol. And, for the problem drinker, living alone tends to prevent other persons from intervening or procuring help, thus increasing the probability of death from cirrhosis of the liver.

Utilizing a sample of all U. S. cities with populations of 50,000 or more in 1970, we have tested the relationships of suicide rate and death rate from cirrhosis of the liver with the percentage living alone, while controlling for a number of social-structural factors, namely, age, race, education, income, and unemployment. Percentage living alone was by far the most powerful predictor of both suicide and alcoholism.

In summary, the effect of residential isolation on humans has received relatively little attention in empirical research. However, the proportion of persons living alone is increasing in our society and the limited ecological evidence that is available suggests that this mode of residence has a number of undesirable effects.

Surveys on Overcrowding, Isolation, and Human Behavior

The studies reviewed in the preceding section took areas—census tracts, city blocks, entire cities, even nations—as the units of analysis. The measures of density and crowding as well as the measures of outcome behaviors and control variables all were calculated to describe populations of areas. This is a legitimate and useful research approach, but it has limitations when the conceptualization is based on individual behavior. This is because relationships that occur at the aggregate level are not necessarily the same ones that occur at the level of the individual (Hannan, 1971). Because individual inferences from aggregate data have inherent limits, to truly establish relations for individuals it is necessary to utilize data obtained from individuals. In the studies reviewed in this section, the outcome and control variables are typically measured for individuals, while the density measure may refer to an aggregate index (persons/area) or specifically to the individual living circumstances (persons/room, living alone).

In 1970 Marsella *et al.* published a study on the effect of dwelling density on the mental health of a small sample ($N = 99$) of Filipino men. They found that high levels of density were associated with poor mental health; however, their results are difficult to interpret because there were no controls on socioeconomic factors.

The following year Mitchell (1971) published the results of a large survey on overcrowding in Hong Kong. The degree of household crowding in Hong Kong is extremely high by American standards. Mitchell found that high levels of crowding were related strongly to complaints about lack of space and lack of privacy. These complaints were particularly common among those who shared their dwelling unit with another household. The level of general unhappiness and amount of worrying also were strongly related to crowding, but under controls for income these relationships were only maintained among the poor. Two indices of more serious psychiatric impairment, an indicator of emotional illness (generally composed of psycho-physiological symptoms) and an index of hostility, were unrelated to levels of overcrowding. The index of emotional illness was related positively to floor of residence when there were two or more households per unit; the index of hostility also was related to floor of residence, and the effects were compounded when there were two or more households per unit. Overcrowding was found to affect husband–wife communication and emotional happiness, but not quarrels. Respondents in overcrowded households were much less likely to know where their children were, and this relationship was not particularly affected by controls for the education of the respondent.

Booth and his associates conducted a major survey in Toronto in which they looked at the effects of overcrowding. These results are available in a series of papers (Booth, 1975a; 1975b; Booth and Cowell, 1976; Booth and Edwards, 1976; Booth and Johnson, 1975; Edwards and Booth, 1975; Johnson and Booth, 1975; Welch, 1975; Welch and Booth, 1975) and a book (Booth, 1976). Booth's data were obtained from a stratified multiple-stage probability sample of Toronto families. All of the 13 census tracts used in the Toronto study "were selected for their potential in yielding a large number of families residing in dwellings in which the number of people exceeded the number of rooms [Booth and Edwards, 1976, p. 310]." Furthermore, from those census tracts "nearly 17,000 screening interviews [were held which] yielded 862 eligible households. In 560 of these we were able to obtain interviews with one or both parents for a 65% completion rate [Booth and Edwards, 1976, p. 311]." Booth and Edwards (1976, p. 311) go on to state "the majority (80%) of the household heads were employed in blue-collar occupations, typically ones requiring only modest skills. Only 23% had completed high school; however, more than half had completed the eighth grade." Thus they had a very atypical sample and one that was very homogeneous on both crowding and social characteristics. As a consequence of this homogeneity, one would expect little variation on most variables and that the relationships found would be very modest.

In their analysis Booth and his associates controlled for age, education, occupational status, and ethnicity. In almost all their analyses these control variables were entered first and their crowding terms were entered as a second step. Thus they allocated any variance associated with their crowding variables that was collinear with their control variables to the control variables. This form of analysis "represents an extremely conservative test of crowding [Booth and Cowell, 1976, p. 211]." Throughout their analysis they used four measures of crowding, (1) objective neighborhood crowding, (2) subjective neighborhood crowding, (3) objective household crowding, and (4) subjective household crowding, and in addition they at times used a "rooms deficit" measure; in Booth and Edwards (1976) they also used persons per room and households per block.

The major focus of the Toronto study was on the relationship between crowding and physical health. The presence of communicable infections or stress disease was based on responses to a set of 42 symptomatic questions, information obtained from an interview and examination by a nurse and physician, and data based on tests of urine and blood samples taken at the time of the medical examination (Booth and Cowell, 1976). Unfortunately, between the initial interview and the subsequent medical examination there was a 49% attrition rate, and this attrition included a number of persons who were physically ill. In their analysis they looked at physiological indicators of stress, stress-related illnesses, communicable diseases, physical trauma (bruises), and reports of illness. On all five of these indices household crowding tended to be associated with poor physical health. However, the relationships were weak and most did not reach statistical significance. In general the relationships were stronger for objective household crowding than for subjective household crowding and they were stronger for men than for women. Physical health was generally unrelated to either measure of neighborhood crowding.

Crowding, by itself, explained only a very modest portion of the variance in sexual behavior (Edwards and Booth, 1975; Johnson and Booth, 1975). However, the data indicate that (1) subjective crowding was related to reports that lack of privacy prevented intercourse, and (2) under very special conditions crowding was related to high levels of marital intercourse. There was some very limited evidence that crowding was related to extramarital involvement and sexual deviation.

Booth and Edwards (1976) looked at the effect of crowding on marital relationships, relationships with children, and sibling relationships. With or without controls, the relationships with crowding were generally weak. Their view of the magnitude of their relationships is perhaps best captured in their discussion where they refer to "the minute effect of crowding revealed in our analysis [Booth and Edwards, 1976, p. 319]." Nevertheless, some of their relationships were statistically significant; for example, among wives subjective household crowding was related to a love decrement scale, arguments with spouses, and threats to leave spouses, while among men it was related to the love decrement scale and the physical striking of children.

Booth and Johnson (1975) found that crowded household conditions had a small adverse effect on the physical and intellectual development of children, with crowded children tending to be somewhat small for their age and slightly behind in school.

In summary, Booth and his associates found neighborhood crowding generally was unrelated to their dependent variables. Subjective household crowding was related slightly to poor family relations and to a variety of sexual experiences. Objective and, to a lesser extent, subjective household crowding were related weakly to poor physical health. Household crowding was related to retarded intellectual development and physical stature of children.

Booth (1976, p. 1) concludes that "perhaps the most important finding of this study, contrary to our expectation before we began the study, is that crowded conditions seldom have any consequences and even when they do their effects are very modest." However, such a conclusion should be viewed with a great deal of caution. As we have already noted, their sample is very atypical, which makes generalization a rather hazardous procedure. It is also very homogeneous, with the independent variables having relatively little variance, which decreases the likelihood of finding strong relationships. Furthermore, as Booth himself notes, their analysis tends to be very conservative. However, as is noted in detail in Gove *et al.* (1976b), not only is their analysis (generally) very conservative, but it also contains serious flaws. There are, for example, a number of problems with the scales they use. Perhaps the most serious problem is that throughout virtually all of the analysis when they are looking at the effects of a crowding variable, they not only control for various demographic variables but they also control for all of their other crowding variables. Thus to the extent that one measure of crowding relates to another (that is, they both measure crowding), they are actually controlling for the effects of the very variables they are looking at. After going over the Toronto study in great detail, looking especially at the zero order relationships, we (Gove *et al.*, 1976b) feel that "perhaps the most that can be concluded [from the data produced by the Toronto study] is that household crowding has at least as much effect as, and possibly more than, some of the traditional demographic variables considered by sociologists when looking at the dependent variables under consideration."

We have recently completed a survey of 2035 residents of Chicago (Gove *et al.*, 1976c). Approximately 25 interviews were gathered from each of 80 selected census tracts within the Chicago city limits. Equal numbers of tracts were selected from each of four different categories: (1) tracts with low levels of crowding and low levels of socioeconomic status, (2) tracts with high levels of crowding and low levels of socioeconomic status, (3) tracts with high socioeconomic status and low crowding, and (4) high socioeconomic status tracts that also had high levels of crowding. For each combination of crowding and socioeconomic status we selected 5 predominantly black tracts, 5 racially mixed tracts, and 10 predominantly white tracts. Households were randomly selected from each census tract, and a randomly selected adult was interviewed from each of the selected households.

Of the 2035 respondents interviewed, 453 or 22% were living alone. As we were initially screening by households and since the proportion of households in the United States where persons were living alone in 1970 was 19% and rising rapidly (Carnahan *et al.*, 1974, p. 70), this is about the proportion one would expect. As persons living alone cannot be crowded in their homes (using a measure of persons per room), we have excluded them from our analysis. An analysis of the data that include those who live alone shows that by excluding these persons from our analysis we are weighting the analysis against the overcrowding hypothesis.

The levels of crowding in our full sample are very similar to those of both the nation as a whole and central cities in 1970, and they are considerably less than those of the nation as a whole and central cities in 1950. As a consequence our results, unlike those of the Toronto study, have very broad generality for most persons living with others in the United States.

In the analysis we introduced controls for family income, education, race, sex, age, and marital status. Statistical significance was tested *after* these variables were controlled for.

The literature on crowding emphasizes the need to consider the subjective experience of crowding. While in the household the number of persons per room probably tends to be the key determinant of the experience of crowding in that setting, it is clear that other factors are imporant. First, due largely to cultural and experiential factors, there is wide variation in the extent to which persons experience a particular situation as crowded (for example, Altman, 1975; Booth, 1976; Hall, 1966; Mitchell, 1975). Second, the organization of activities in the home will vary greatly by household. As a consequence, in some households there may be a great deal of time spent in a crowded room, whereas in other households with the same ratio of persons per room, there may be very little time spent in a crowded room. Thus the indices of the experience of crowding may be, in some cases, a more accurate measure of the amount of actual crowding than the more objective measure, persons per room (Booth, 1976; Fischer, 1975).

In our analysis we introduced two measures: (1) a social demands scale, which measured an excess of social stimulation, and (2) a lack of privacy scale. These involve measures of the two key concepts that have been the theoretical bases for the explanation of the subjective experience of crowding. To our knowledge this is the first time there has been an attempt to measure these experiences in a household study. We woule note that the demands scale and lack of privacy scale are fairly strongly related to persons per room. Furthermore, when these measures are used as controls they tend to "interpret" or "explain" the relationships between persons per room and the various dependent variables.

MENTAL HEALTH

It would seem that, if overcrowding has adverse effects on the individual, it would almost have to be related to poor mental health.

After controls, the crowding variables are related to experiencing psychiatric symptoms, a lack of positive affect, having a nervous breakdown, manifest irritation, feeling alienated, having low self-esteem, and feeling unhappy. These relationships are statistically significant for all mental health items with all the crowding indices, except for the relationship between felt demands and positive affect. Taking an overall average shows that the crowding variables independently account for 40.4% of the total explained variance and the five control variables independently account for 41.3%, with 18.3% being collinear. Taken as a composite, these results provide strong support for the hypothesis that crowding has a substantial negative effect on a variety of aspects of mental health.

SOCIAL RELATIONS IN THE HOME

If overcrowding has an adverse effect on social relations, it would seem that this would be primarily manifested in the home. Our data on marital relations show that, after controls, the three indices of crowding are significantly related to a lack of positive marital relations, the presence of negative relations, a low score on the marital relations balance scale, and not feeling close to one's spouse. Regarding the respondents' relationships with (*a*) their children and (*b*) others living in the home, the data showed that persons per room is unrelated to, while lack of privacy and felt demands have significant adverse effects on, such relationships. Crowding also is significantly related to arguments and physical violence in the home.

Comparing the effects of crowding with those of the five control variables shows that crowding tends to explain more variance. On the average, the crowding variables independently account for 57.0% of the total explained variance and the control variables independently account for 34.6%, while 8.4% is collinear.

SOCIAL RELATIONS OUTSIDE THE HOME

It would seem that crowding in the home would have a relatively slight effect on social relationships outside the home, particularly in comparison to its effect on social relations in the home. However, if, as our data suggest, crowding has an effect on the mental state of the individual, we would expect it to have some effect on social relationships outside the home. In all cases at least some, and in some cases all three, of our crowding indices show a significant effect on the respondents' relationships with relatives and neighbors and on the number of close friends the respondents had. Some of the crowding variables are also positively related to arguments and physical violence outside the home. Overall, however, the data indicate that the effect of crowding on social relations outside the home is minor compared to that of the social structural variables.

PHYSICAL HEALTH

Our study did not focus on physical health and, lacking a physical examination, we have only a crude measure of the respondents' physical health. However, we had one innovation that allowed us to shed light on the relationship of crowding to physical health. The literature assumes that, if crowding is related to physical health, it is because persons in crowded households are physically run-down, more susceptible to infectious disease and, when sick, tend to be involved in the flow of activities, cannot get a good rest, and are not well cared for (for example, Galle *et al.,* 1972). In the interview we obtained information on all of these presumed relationships, and the data indicate crowding is strongly related to two of them. In contrast, the effect of crowding on the respondents' evaluation of their overall health is relatively minor, although significant.

FERTILITY

Data on fertility-related behavior were collected only from married respondents. They indicate that (1) crowded respondents had more children than they wanted, (2) crowding has a slight relationship with ineffectual family planning, (3) crowding at least occasionally inhibits sexual intercourse, and (4) crowding is not related to hypersexuality. Support for one of the recurrent themes in the literature, that crowding is related to fetal mortality, is provided by the data that show that crowding is related to having a pregnancy end in stillbirth, miscarriage, or abortion.

CARE OF CHILDREN

Our data show a mixed pattern in the effect of crowding on parental care. Crowded parents feel hassled by their children, and they are relived when the children are out of the house, tend not to get along well with their children, and do not like the way their children behave. Furthermore, they tend not to know their children's friends or the parents of their children's friends. However, crowding is relatively unrelated to parents' supportive or punitive behavior toward their children, and it is unrelated to juvenile delinquency.

To date we have made only a very preliminary analysis of the effects of structural density (primarily the number of housing units per structure) and the effects of living alone. This analysis suggests (with a few important exceptions) that these variables are not nearly as imporant as overcrowding. The number of housing units per structure has a strong negative relationship with one's being satisfied with where he or she lives. Increase in housing units per structure, particularly the shift from single unit to multiple unit structure, is significantly associated with three indicators of poor mental health: unhappiness, symptoms, and alienation. In general, housing units per structure appears to be largely unrelated to social relations inside the home, physical health, and fertility-related behavior. Consistent with the finding by Gillis (1974), the number of housing units per structure is significantly related to juvenile delinquency. Among residents in multiple-unit structures, there is a strong association between juvenile delinquency and floor of residence: If the floor of residence is the first floor the rate of delinquency is low; if it is other than the first floor the rate of delinquency is high.

Now let us briefly look at the respondents who live alone and compare them to respondents who live with others. The respondents who live alone do not differ significantly from the other respondents in their satisfaction with their living arrangements or on any of the indicators of mental health. They are less likely to act overtly aggressive, probably due to the fact that there is no one at home to act aggressively toward. They do tend to report better physical health than the other responents. Our ecological analysis of cities over 50,000 suggested that persons who live alone were likely to have a drinking problem. This relationship held up in the survey. Respondents who live alone are much more likely to drink heavily and to manifest problems associated with drinking.

With the Chicago survey data we looked at the interactive effects of number of persons per room, number of housing units per structure, and floor of residence. Persons who live in households with more than one person per room and in structures with more than 40 housing units are particularly likely (1) to be dissatisfied with their living arrangements, (2) to be in poor mental health, (3) to be in poor physical health, and (4) to have children who have participated in delinquent activities. Similarly, persons who live in homes with more than one person per room and who live above the fifth floor (our upper category for floor of residence) are particularly likely to be (1) dissatisfied with their living arrangements, (2) in poor mental health, (3) in poor physical health, and (4) aggressive. A tentative finding is that women are more reactive to crowding than are men, which is consistent with the fact that women typically spend a greater proportion of their time at home than do men.

Concluding Remarks

We have been exploring the idea that either end of the population distribution continuum—either very high or very low density—may have deleterious effects on the behavior of human populations. Evidence from various animal studies suggests that overcrowding and isolation have negative effects on a variety of species, although the specific effect and the mechanisms bringing about that effect vary across species. Evidence from studies of human populations, including both ecological analyses and survey data, is not as rich, but several general themes emerged in our review. First, the concepts of high population density and overcrowding are substantially more complex for human than for animal populations, but this fact has been sometimes obscured in the studies reviewed. Future studies ought, at least, to distinguish between structural density—the way an area is built up—and interpersonal crowding, for many studies indicate that these two aspects of density have somewhat different relationships to behavior. The same might be said for the other end of the population distribution continuum. The percentage of the population living alone is a measure of isolation, but those persons who are living alone in urban settings are in fact living in the midst of many other humans. In this case human contacts are not obviated by living alone, but the frequency and character of contacts are probably quite different from those of persons living with others. Similarly, those living alone in an isolated environment probably have very different social relationships from those of persons living alone in a city.

Our review of the literature on density suggests that it probably has some effect on "pathology," but that such an effect has not been conclusively demonstrated, and it appears unlikely that with further research density will emerge as a variable of major substantive importance. Most of the studies that have looked at the relationship between overcrowding and human behavior have relied on ecological data. There is some problem in interpreting the results, for the studies are essentially concerned with individual experiences and behavior, while the items of analysis are usually large aggregate units. Furthermore, crowding tends to be highly related to class and race, and collinearity cannot be avoided in such studies. Taken in toto the areal aggregate studies indicate that crowding probably is related positively to "pathological" behavior but that the strength of the relationship is unclear.

The three major surveys also show a mixed pattern. We take Mitchell's study in Hong Kong as suggesting crowding has a very discernible but not a huge effect. However, in part because of the mode of analysis and measures used, but primarily because the study involves such a very different culture, it is not clear what implications this study has for Western society.

The general conclusion reached by those involved in the Toronto study is that crowding has very little effect. However, as we have noted here and discussed at greater length elsewhere (Gove *et al.*, 1976b), the sample is so atypical and homogeneous and the measurement and analysis so flawed that it is difficult to draw any conclusions about the effect of crowding. (There is, of course, the possibility that our perspective leads us to a biased interpretation, and we recommend the reader look at the works by Booth and his associates—keeping our comments in mind.)

The only other survey is the one we did in Chicago. We managed to avoid the problem of collinearity between class, race, and crowding, and our levels of crowding are very similar to those in the United States as a whole. We used one objective measure of crowding (persons per room) and two subjective measures (a social demands scale and a lack of privacy scale) that tap the two concepts that the theoretical literature has linked to the subjective experience of crowding. We found crowding to be related strongly to poor mental health of the respondents and to poor social relationships in the home. It also is related strongly to certain aspects of physical health, fertility-related behavior, and child care. It has only a weak relationship with social relationships outside the home. We take our results as indicating that crowding in the home is a major variable that has a substantial impact on a varied set of behaviors. Of course, one should not consider the issue settled on the basis of one study. There has been a striking lack of studies of social isolation. What little research there is on social isolation (as indicated by living alone) suggests it may be an important variable, and it is clear that it deserves more attention than it has received.

ACKNOWLEDGMENTS

We would like to thank Gail Hyfantis, Lisa Heinrich, and Karl Taeuber for comments on an earlier draft.

References

Alexander, B. F., and E. M. Roth
1971   "The effects of acute crowding on aggressive behavior of Japanese monkeys."
          Behavior 39: 73–90.
Alexander, F.
1963   "Alcohol and behavior disorder." In S. Lucia (ed.), *Alcohol and civilization.*
          New York: McGraw-Hill.
Allee, W. C.
1938   *The Social Life of Animals.* Boston: Beacon Press.
Allee, W. C., and E. Bowen
1932   "Studies in animal aggregations: Mass protection against colloidal silver among
          goldfishes." *Journal of Experimental Zoology* 61: 185–207.
Allee, W. C., O. Park, A. Emerson, T. Park, and K. Schmidt
1949   *Principles of Animal Ecology.* Philadelphia: W. B. Saunders Co.
Allee, W. C., and J. Wilder
1938   "Group protection for Euplanaria dorotocephala from ultra-violet radiation."
          Physiological Zoology 12: 110–35.
Altman, I.
1975   *The Environment and Social Behavior.* Monterey, Calif.: Brooks/Cole.
1976   "Privacy: A conceptual analysis." *Environment and Behavior* 8 (March): 7–29.

Archer, J.
1970   "Effects of population density on behavior in rodents." In J. H. Crook (ed.), *Social Behavior in Birds and Mammals*. New York: Academic Press.

Ardrey, R.
1970   *The Social Contract*. New York: Atheneum.

Bacon, S.
1957   "Social settings conducive to alcoholism." *Journal of the American Medical Association* 164 (May): 177–181.

Bales, R. F.
1946   "Cultural differences in rates of alcoholism." *Quarterly Journal of Studies of Alcohol* 6 (March): 480–499.

Bates, A.
1964   "Privacy—A useful concept?" *Social Forces* 42 (May): 429–434.

Beach, F. A.
1942   "Comparison of copulatory behavior of male rats raised in isolation cohabitation, and segregation." *Journal of Genetic Psychology* 60: 121–136.
1958   "Normal sexual behavior in male rats isolated at 14 days of age." *Journal of Comprehensive Psychology* 51: 37–38.

Blacker, E.
1966   "Sociocultural factors in alcoholism." *International Psychiatry Clinics* 3 (Summer): 51–80.

Booth, A.
1975a   "Crowding and social participation." Unpublished manuscript.
1975b   Final report submitted to Department of Urban Affairs, Ottowa, Canada.
1976   *Urban Crowding and Its Consequences*. New York: Praeger.

Booth, A., and J. Cowell
1976   "The effects of crowding upon health." *Journal of Health and Social Behavior* 17 (September): 204–220.

Booth, A., and J. N. Edwards
1976   "Crowding and family relations." *American Sociological Review* 41 (April): 308–321.

Booth, A., and D. R. Johnson
1975   "The effect of crowding on child health and developments." *American Behavioral Scientist* (July–August): 736–749.

Booth, A., and S. Welch
1974   "Crowding and urban crime rates." Paper presented at the Annual Meetings of the Midwest Sociological Association, Omaha, Nebraska.

Booth, A., S. Welch, and D. R. Johnson
1976   "Crowding and urban crime rates." *Urban Affairs Quarterly* 2 (March): 291–307.

Borowitz, G. H.
1964   "Some ego aspects of alcoholism." *British Journal of Medical Psychology* 37: 257–263.

Calhoun, J. B.
1962   "Population density and social pathology." *Scientific American* 206 (February): 139–148.

Carnahan, D. L., W. Gove, and O. Galle
1974a   "Urbanization, population density and overcrowding." *Social Forces* 53 (September): 62–72.

Carnahan, D., A. Guest, and O. Galle
1974b   "Congestion, concentration and behavior: Research in the study of urban density." *Sociological Quarterly* 15 (Autumn): 488–506.
Cassell, J.
1971   "Health consequences of population density and crowding." Pp. 462–478 in National Academy of Sciences, *Rapid Population Growth*. Baltimore: Johns Hopkins Press.
Chafetz, M. E., H. W. Demone, Jr., and H. Soloman
1962   *Alcoholism and Society*. New York: Oxford University Press.
Chamove, A. S.
1973   "Rearing infant rhesus together." *Behavior* 47: 48–66.
Chapin, S. F.
1951   "Some housing factors related to mental hygiene." *Journal of Social Issues* 7: 164–171.
Chapman, R. N.
1928   "The quantitative analysis of environmental factors." *Ecology* 9: 111–122.
Chapman, R. N., and L. Baird
1934   "The biotic constants of tribolium coafusum Duval." *Journal of Experimental Zoology* 68: 293–304.
Chappell, P. F., and G. W. Meier
1974   "Behavior modification in a mother-reared dyad." *Developmental Psychobiology* 7(July): 296.
Chermayeff, S., and C. Alexander
1965   *Community and Privacy: Toward a New Architecture of Humanism*. New York: Doubleday.
Chitty, D.
1952   "Mortality among voles (*Microtus agresitis*) at Lake Vyrnwy, Montgomeryshire in 1936–1939." *Philosophical Transactions of the Royal Society of London* B236: 505–552.
Choldin, H., and D. Roncek
1976   "Density, population potential and pathology: A block level analysis." *Public Data Use* 4(July): 19–30.
Christian, J. J.
1959   "The roles of endocrine and behavioral factors in the growth of mammalian population." In A. Gorbman (ed.), *Comparative Endocrinology*. New York: John Wiley and Sons.
1961   "Phenomena associated with population density." *Proceedings of the National Academy of Science* 47: 428.
Christian, J. J., and D. E. Davis
1964   "Endocrines, behavior and population." *Science* 146: 1550–1560.
Christian, J. J., V. Flyger, and D. Davis
1960   "Factors in the mass mortality of a herd of sika deer (cervus nippon)." *Chesapeake Science* 1: 79–95.
Christian, J. J., and C. D. LeMunyan
1958   "Adverse effects of crowding on reproduction and lactation of mice and two generations of their progeny." *Endocrinology* 63: 517–529.
Christian, J. J., J. A. Lloyd, and D. E. Davis
1965   "The role of endocrines in the self-regulation of mammalian populations." *Recent Progress in Hormone Research* 21: 501–578.

Collette, J., and S. Webb
1974   "Urban density, crowding, and stress reactions." Paper presented at the meet-
          ing of the Pacific Sociological Association, San Jose, California.
Crombie, A. C.
1943   "The effect of crowding upon the natality of grain-infesting insects." *Proceed-
          ings of Zoological Society,* London, S. A., 113: 77–98.
Darling, F. F.
1938   *Bird Flocks and the Breeding Cycle: A Contribution to the Study of Avian So-
          ciality.* Cambridge: Cambridge University Press.
Davis, D. E.
1964   "The physiological analysis of aggressive behavior." Pp. 53–74 in W. Etkin
          (ed.), *Social Behavior and Organization Among Vertebrates.* Chicago: Univer-
          sity of Chicago Press.
Davis, K.
1940   "Extreme social isolation of a child." *American Journal of Sociology* 45 (Jan-
          uary): 554–565.
Deevey, E. S.
1960   "The hare and the haruspex: A cautionary tale." *The Yale Review* 49: 161–179.
1972   "The equilibrium population." Pp. 2–16 in W. Petersen (ed.), *Readings in Pop-
          ulation.* New York: MacMillan.
Desor, J. A.
1972   "Toward a psychological theory of crowding." *Journal of Personality and So-
          cial Psychology* 21: 79–83.
Dieterlen, F.
1959   "Das verhalten des syrischen goldhamsters (Mesocricetus auratus Water
          House)." *Zeitschrift Für Tierpsychologie* 16: 47–103.
Dubos, R.
1965   *Man Adapting.* New Haven: Yale University Press.
Duncan, O. D.
1966   "Path analysis: Sociological examples." *American Journal of Sociology* 72: 1–
          16.
Durkheim, E.
1933   *The Division of Labor in Society.* Translated with an introduction by George
          Simpson. New York: MacMillan Company.
Edwards, J., and A. Booth
1975   "Crowding and human sexual behavior." Unpublished paper.
Eibl-Eibesfeldt, I.
1955   "Angeborens und Erworbenes im Nestbauverhalten der Wanderratte." *Natur-
          wissenschaften* 42: 633–634.
1961   "The fighting behavior of animals." *Scientific American* 205 (December): 112–
          122.
Ely, D. L., and J. P. Henry
1974   "Effects of prolonged social deprivation of murine behavior patterns, blood
          pressure and adrenal weight." *Journal of Comparative and Physiological Psy-
          chology* 87 (October): 733–740.
Factor, R., and I. Waldron
1973   "Contemporary population densities and human health." *Nature* 243: 381–384.
Fauten, R. W.
1941   "Development of nestling yellow-headed blackbirds." *Auk* 58: 215–232.

Fenderson, O. C., and M. R. Carpenter
1971 "Effects of crowding on the behavior of juvenile hatchery and wild landlocked Atlantic salmon (salmo salar L.)." *Animal Behavior* 19 (August): 430–447.
Fischer, C., M. Baldassare, and R. Ofshe
1975 "Crowding studies and urban life: A critical review." *Journal of the American Institute of Planners* 41 (November).
Fischer, C. T.
1975 "Privacy as a profile of authentic consciousness." *Humanitas* II (February): 27–43.
Fischer, A. E.
1955 "The effects of differential early treatment on the social and exploratory behavior of puppies." Unpublished doctoral dissertation, Pennsylvania State University.
Fisher, A. E., and E. B. Hale
1956–1957 "Stimulus determinants of sexual and aggressive behaviour in male domestic fowl." *Behaviour* 10: 309–323.
Fisher, J., and H. Vevers
1944 "The changes in the world numbers of the gannet in a century." *Journal of Animal Ecology* 13: 49–62.
Fisher, J., and G. Waterson
1941 "The breeding distribution, history and population of the fulmar in the British Isles." *Journal of Animal Ecology* 10: 204–276.
Flickinger, G. L.
1966 "Response of the testes to social interaction among grouped chickens." *General Comparative Endocrinology* 6: 89–98.
Fuller, J. L.
1964 "Effects of experimental deprivation upon behavior in animals." *Proceedings, World Congress Psychiatry* (Montreal) 3: 223–227.
Galle, O., and W. Gove
1974 "Crowding and behavior in Chicago, 1940–1970." Unpublished paper.
Galle, O., W. Gove, and J. McPherson
1972 "Population density and pathology: What are the relationships for man." *Science* 176 (April): 23–30.
Gillis, A. R.
1974 "Population density and social pathology: The case of building type, social allowance and juvenile delinquency." *Social Forces* 53 (December): 306–314.
Gove, W., O. Galle, J. McCarthy, and M. Hughes
1976a "Living circumstances and social pathology: The effect of population density, overcrowding and isolation on suicide, homicide and alcoholism." Unpublished paper.
Gove, W., and P. Howell
1974 "Individual resources and mental hospitalization: A comparison and evaluation of the societal reaction and psychiatric perspectives." *American Sociological Review* 39 (February): 86–100.
Gove, W., M. Hughes, and O. Galle
1976b "Some comments on the Toronto study." Unpublished paper.
1976c "Overcrowding in the home: An empirical investigation of its possible consequences." Paper presented at the meeting of the American Public Health Association, Miami.

Goy, R. W., and W. C. Young
1956–1957   "Strain differences in the behavioral responses of female guineapigs to alpha-estradoil benzoate and progesterone." *Behavior* 10: 340–354.
Greenberg, G.
1972   "The effects of ambient temperature and population density on aggression in two inbred strains of mice, Mus musculus." *Behavior* 42: 119–130.
Greenberg, L. A.
1963   "Alcohol and emotional behavior." Pp. 109–121 in S. Lucia (ed.), *Alcohol and Civilization*. New York: McGraw-Hill.
Gregor, G. L., R. Smith, L. Simons, and H. Parker
1972   "Behavioral consequences of crowding in the deermouse (Permyscus maniculatus)." *Journal of Comparative and Physiological Psychology* 79 (June): 488–493.
Gruendel, A., and W. Arnold
1969   "Effects of early social deprivation on reproductive behavior of male rats." *Journal of Comparative and Physiological Psychology* 67: 123–128.
Guest, A. M.
1970   "Families and housing in cities." Unpublished doctoral dissertation, University of Wisconsin—Madison.
1972   "Patterns of family location." *Demography* 9: 159–171.
Hall, E.
1966   *The Hidden Dimension*. New York: Doubleday.
Hannan, M.
1971   *Aggregation and Disaggregation in Sociology*. Lexington, Mass.: Lexington Books.
Hansen, E. W.
1962   "The development of maternal and infant behavior in the rhesus monkey." Unpublished doctoral dissertation, University of Wisconsin—Madison.
Harlow, H. F.
1961   "The development of affectional patterns in infant monkeys." In B. M. Foss (ed.), *Determinants of Infant Behavior*. New York: John Wiley and Sons.
1962   "Development of affection in primates." Pp. 157–166 in E. L. Bliss (ed.), *Roots of Behavior*. New York: Harper and Row.
Harlow, H. F., and M. Harlow
1962   "The affectional systems." Pp. 287–334 in A. M. Schrier, H. Harlow, and F. Stolnitz (eds.), *Behavior of Nonhuman Primates* (Vol. 2). New York: Academic Press.
Harlow, H. F., W. D. Joslyn, M. Senko
1966   "Behavioral aspects of reproduction in primates." *Journal of Animal Science* 25: 45–67.
Hartley, S. F.
1972   *Population: Quantity vs. Quality*. Englewood Cliffs, N.J.: Prentice-Hall.
Hawley, A. H.
1950   *Human Ecology: A Theory of Community Structure*. New York: Ronald Press.
1972   "Population density and the city." *Demography* 9 (November): 521–529.
Helmrich, R. L.
1960   "Regulation of reproductive rate by intrauterine mortality in the deer mouse." *Science* 132: 417.
Hemingway, D. A., and L. Furumoto

1972   "Population density and alcohol consumption in the rat." *Quarterly Journal of Studies on Alcohol* 33 (September): 794–799.

Hinde, R. A.
1959   "Some factors influencing sexual and aggressive behavior in male chaffinches." *Bird Study* 6: 112–122.

Hoffman, E., and A. E. Tomhave
1945   "A relationship of square feet of floor space per bird and egg production." *Poultry Science* 24: 89–90.

Hoffman, R. S.
1958   "The role of reproduction and mortality in population fluctuations of wolves (Microtus)." *Ecological Monographs* 28: 79–109.

Hoover, E. M., and R. Vernon
1962   *Anatomy of a Metropolis.* Garden City, N.Y.: Doubleday.

Johnson, D. R., and A. Booth
1975   "Crowding and human reproduction." Unpublished paper.

Jourard, S. M.
1966   "Some psychological aspects of privacy." *Law and Contemporary Problems* 31 (Spring): 307–318.

Kagan, J., and F. A. Beach
1953   "Effects of early experience on mating behavior in male rats." *Journal of Comprehensive and Physiological Psychology* 46: 204–208.

Keeley, K.
1962   "Prenatal influence on behavior of offspring of crowded mice." *Science* 135: 44.

Kelvin, P.
1973   "A social-psychological examination of privacy." *British Journal of Social and Clinical Psychology* 12 (September): 248–261.

Klepinger, B. D.
1968   "Population size: Its effects on behavior and stress-responsive physiological systems." *Dissertation Abstracts,* Order No. 69-4769. Doctoral dissertation, Indiana University.

Kruijit, J. P.
1962   "Imprinting in relation to drive interactions in Burmese Red Junglefowl." *Symposium of the Zoological Society of London* 8: 219–226.

Larson, D., and B. Abu-Laban
1968   "Norm qualities and deviant drinking behavior." *Social Problems* 15 (Spring): 441–450.

Lawrence, J. E. S.
1974   "Science and sentiment: Overview of research on crowding and human behavior." *Psychological Bulletin* 81: 712–720.

Laws, R., and I. Parker
1968   In *Symposium of the Zoological Society.* Vol. 21: 319–359. London: Academic Press.

Leopold, A.
1933   *Game Management.* New York: Scribner.

Levy, L., and A. Herzog
1974   "Effects of population density and crowding on health and social adaptation in the Netherlands." *Journal of Health and Social Behavior* 15 (September): 228–240.

Lockley, R. M.
1961   "Social structure and stress in the rabbit warren." *The Journal of Animal Ecology* 30: 385–423.

Louch, C. D.
1956   "Adrenocortical activity in relation to the density and dynamics of three confined populations of Microtus." *Ecology* 37: 701–713.

Ludwig, W., and C. Boost
1939   "Uber das wachstum von protistenpopulationen und den allelokatalytischen effekt." *Archiv Protistenkunde* 92: 453–484.

McCarthy, J., O. Galle, and W. Zimmern
1975   "Population density, social structure and interpersonal violence: An intermetropolitan test of competing models." *American Behavioral Scientist* (July–August): 771–791.

McPherson, J. M.
1973   "A question of causality: A study in the application of regression techniques to sociological analysis." Doctoral dissertation, Vanderbilt University.

Maple, T., J. E., and G. Mitchell
1974   "Sexually aroused self-aggression in a socialized adult male monkey." *Archives of Sexual Behavior* 3 (September): 471–475.

Marmor, J.
1972   "Mental health and overpopulation." In S. T. Reid and D. L. Lyon (eds.), *Population Crisis: An Interdisciplinary Perspective.* Glenview, Ill.: Scott, Foresman.

Marsella, A., M. Escudero, and P. Gordon
1970   "The effects of dwelling density on mental disorders in Filipino men." *Journal of Health and Social Behavior* 11 (December): 288–294.

Mason, W. A.
1960   "Effects of social restriction on the behavior of rhesus monkeys: I. Free social behavior." *Journal of Comprehensive and Physiological Psychology* 53: 582–589.

1961   "Effects of social restriction on the behavior of rhesus monkeys: II. Test of gregariousness." *Journal of Comprehensive and Physiological Psychology* 54: 287–290.

1965   "The social development of monkeys and apes." In I. DeVore (ed.), *Primate Behavior.* New York: Holt, Rinehart, and Winston.

Milgram, S.
1970   "The experience of living in cities." *Science* 167: 1461–1468.

Mitchell, R.
1971   "Some social implications of high density." *American Sociological Review* 36 (February): 18–29.

Mitchell, R. E.
1975   "Ethnographic and historical perspectives on relationships between physical and socio-spatial environments." *Sociological Symposium* 14 (Fall): 25–40.

National Academy of Sciences
1971   *Rapid Population Growth.* Baltimore: Johns Hopkins Press.

Nissen, H. W.
1954   Unpublished manuscript.

Oesting, R., and W. C. Allee
1935   "Further analysis of the protective value of biologically conditioned fresh

water for the marine turbellarian, Procerodes wheatlandi. IV." *Biological Bulletin* 68: 314–326.

Pastalan, L. A.
1970   "Privacy as an expression of human territoriality." In L. A. Pastalan and D. H. Carson (eds.), *Spatial Behavior of Older People*. Ann Arbor: University of Michigan Press.

Patrick, C.
1952   *Alcohol, Culture and Society*. Durham: Duke University Press.

Paynter, R. A.
1949   "Clutch-size and the egg and chick mortality of Kent Island Herring Gulls." *Ecology* 30: 146–166.

Pearl, R., and S. L. Parker
1922   "Experimental studies on the duration of life. IV. Data on the influence of density of population on the duration of life in the Drosophila." *American Naturalist* 56: 312–321.

Pearl, R., and F. M. Surface
1909   "A biometrical study of egg production in domestic fowl. 1. Variation in annual egg reproduction." Department of Agriculture, *Animal Industries Bulletin* 110: 1–80.

Pearlin, L., and C. Radabaugh
1975   "Economic strains and the coping function of alcohol." Unpublished manuscript.

Pennock, J. R., and J. W. Chapman Eds.
1971   *Privacy*. New York: Atherton Press.

Perrins, C. M.
1965   "Population fluctuations and clutch size in the great tit." *Journal of Animal Ecology* 34: 601–647.

Petrusewicz, K.
1957   "Investigation of experimentally induced population growth," *Ekologija Polska* 5: 281–309.

Pittman, D. J.
1967   *Alcoholism*. New York: Harper and Row.

Pittman, D. J., and C. Snyder
1962   *Society, Culture and Drinking Patterns*. New York: John Wiley and Sons.

Rapoport, A.
1973   "An approach to the construction of man-environment theory." Pp. 124–136 in W. F. E. Preiser (ed.), *Environmental Design Research* (Vol. 2). Stroudsburg, Penn.: Dowden, Hutchinson and Ross.

Reiss, B. F.
1954   "The effect of altered environment and of age in mother–young relationships among animals." *Annals of the New York Academy of Sciences* 57: 606–610.

Robertson, F. W., and J. H. Sang
1944   "The ecological determinants of population growth in a drosophila culture. I. Fecundity of adult flies." *Proceedings of Royal Society,* London,s.B.,132:258–277.

Robertson, T. B.
1921   "Experimental studies on cellular multiplication. II. The influence of mutual contiguity upon reproductive rate and the part played therein by the 'X-substance' in bacterized infusions which stimulate the multiplication of infusoria." *Biochemical Journal* 15: 612–619.

Roman, P., and H. Trice
  1970   "The development of deviant drinking behavior: Occupational risk factors."
          Archives of Environmental Health 20 (March): 424–433.
Schmitt, R.
  1966   "Density, health and social disorganization." *Journal of the American Institute
          of Planners* 32 (January): 37–40.
Schrag, H. L.
  1972   "Effects of density, nesting material and sibling-non-sibling matings upon re-
          production in the deer mouse *peromyscus maniculatus gambelli.*" Unpub-
          lished doctoral dissertation, Washington State University.
Schuessler, K.
  1974   "Analysis of ratio variables: Opportunities and pitfalls." *American Journal of
          Sociology* 80 (September): 379–396.
Schwartz, B.
  1968   "The social psychiatry of privacy." *American Journal of Sociology* 73 (May):
          741–752.
Sdobnikov, W.
  1935   Relations between the reindeer and animal life of the tundra and forest." *Trans.
          Arctic Institute* 24: 5–66.
Seay, B., B. A., and H. F. Harlow
  1964   "Maternal behavior of socially deprived rhesus monkeys." *Journal of Abnor-
          mal and Social Psychology* 69: 345–354.
Seely, John R.
  1959   "The W. H. O. definition of alcoholism." *Quarterly Journal of Studies on Alco-
          hol* 20 (June): 352–358.
Selye, Hans
  1950   *The Physiology and Pathology of Exposure to Stress.* Montreal: Acta.
Siegel, H. S.
  1959   "Egg-production characteristics and adrenal function in White Leghorns con-
          fined at different floor space levels." *Poultry Science* 38: 893–898.
Shils, E.
  1966   "Privacy: Its constitution and vicissitudes." *Law and Contemporary Problems*
          31 (Spring): 281–306.
Simmel, G.
  1957   "The metropolis and mental life." Pp. 635–646 in P. K. Hatt and A. J. Reiss,
          Jr. (eds.), *Cities and Societies: The Revised Reader in Urban Sociology.* New
          York: Free Press.
Skolnick, J. R.
  1958   "Religious affiliation and drinking behavior." *Quarterly Journal of Studies on
          Alcohol* 19 (September): 452–470.
Smith, H. W., *et al.*
  1933   "The efficiency and economic effects of plant quarantines in California." *Bulle-
          tin of the University of California College of Agriculture* 555: 1–276.
Smith, R. H., D. B. Downer, M. T. Lynch, and M. Winter
  1969   "Privacy and interaction within the family as related to dwelling space." *Jour-
          nal of Marriage and the Family* 31 (August): 559–566.
Snyder, C.
  1962   "Culture and Jewish sobriety." Pp. 616–628 in D. J. Pittman and C. Snyder
          (eds.), *Society, Culture and Drinking Patterns.* New York: John Wiley and
          Sons.

Snyder, R. L.
  1966a   "Fertility and reproductive performance in grouped male mice." In K. Ben-
           irschke (ed.), *Symposium on Comparative Aspects of Reproductive Failure*.
           Berlin: Springer.
  1966b   "Collection of mouse semen by electroejaculation." *The Anatomical Record*
           155: 11–14.
  1968   "Reproduction and population pressures." In E. Stellar and J. M. Sprague
           (eds.), *Progress in Physiological Psychology* (Vol. 2). New York: Academic
           Press.
Soper, F. L., and D. M. Wilson
  1942   "Species eradication: A practical goal of species reduction in the control of
           mosquito-borne disease." *Journal National Malaria Society* 1: 5–24.
Southwick, C. H., M. A. Beg, and M. R. Siddiqi
  1965   "Rhesus monkeys in north India." Pp. 111–159 in I. DeVore (ed.), *Primate
           Behavior: Field Studies of Monkeys and Apes*. New York: Holt, Rinehart, and
           Winston.
Spencer, H.
  1879–1882 *Principles of Sociology*. New York: Appleton.
Spitz, R. A.
  1945   "Hospitalism: An inquiry into the genesis of psychiatric conditions in early
           childhood." *The Psychoanalytic Study of the Child*. New York: International
           Universities Press.
  1946   "Hospitalism: A follow-up report." Pp. 113–117 in *The Psychoanalytic Study
           of the Child*. New York: International Universities Press.
Spitz, R. A., and K. M. Wolfe
  1946   "Anaclitic depression: An inquiry into the genesis of psychiatric conditions in
           early childhood." Pp. 313–342 in *The Psychoanalytic Study of the Child*. New
           York: International Universities Press.
Strauss, R.
  1971   "Alcohol." Pp. 236–280 in R. Merton and R. Nisbet (eds.), *Contemporary So-
           cial Problems* 3rd ed. New York: Harcourt Brace Jovanovich.
Syme, L. A.
  1973   "Social isolation at weaning: Some effects on two measures of activity." *Ani-
           mal Learning and Behavior* 1 (August): 161–163.
Taylor, I., and J. Knowelden
  1957   *Principles of Epidemiology*. Boston: Little, Brown.
Terman, C. R.
  1965   "A study of population growth and control exhibited in the laboratory by prai-
           rie deermice." *Ecology* 46: 890–895.
Thiessen, D. D., and D. A. Rodgers
  1961   "Population density and endocrine function." *Psychological Bulletin* 58: 441–
           451.
Thorpe, W. H.
  1963   *Learning and Instinct in Animals*. Cambridge: Harvard University Press.
Tobach, E., and H. Block
  1956   "Effect of stress by crowding prior to and following tuberculosis infection."
           American Journal of Physiology 187: 399.
Trice, H.
  1966   *Alcoholism in America*. New York: McGraw-Hill.
Ullman, A. D.

1958   "Sociocultural backgrounds of alcoholism." *Annals* 315 (January): 48–54.
Valzelli, L.
1969   "Aggressive behaviour induced by isolation." In S. Garattini and E. Sigg
            (eds.), *Aggressive Behaviour*. New York: John Wiley and Sons.
Van Wijingaarden, A.
1960   "The population dynamics of four combined populations of the continental
            vole (Microtus arvalis (Pallas))." *Vers. Landbouwk Onderz* No. 66–22. Wagen-
            ingen, pp. 1–28.
Verhulst, P. E.
1845   "Reserches mathém. sur la loi d'accroissement de la population." *Nouveaux
            memoires de l'Academia R. des Sciences de Bruxelles*. 18: 1–38.
Ward, S. K.
1975   "Methodological considerations in the study of population density and social
            pathology." *Journal of Human Ecology* 3,4: 275–286.
Washburne, C.
1955   "Alcohol, self and group." *Quarterly Journal of Studies on Alcohol* 17
            (March): 108–123.
Webb, S. , and J. Collette
1975   "Urban ecological and household correlates of stress-alleviating drug use."
            American Behavioral Scientist (July/August): 750–770.
Welch, S., and A. Booth
1975   "Crowding as a factor in political aggression: Theoretical aspect and an analy-
            sis of some cross-national data." *Social Science Information* 13 (4/5): 151–162.
Whitehead, P., and C. Harvey
1974   "Explaining alcoholism: An empirical test and reformulation." *Journal of
            Health and Social Behavior* 15 (March): 57–65.
Wilkinson, R.
1970   *The Prevention of Drinking Problems: Alcohol Control and Cultural Influ-
            ences*. New York: Oxford University Press.
Willis, F. N.
1966   "Fighting in pigeons relative to available space." *Psychonometric Science* 4:
            315–316.
Winsborough, H. H.
1963   "An ecological approach to the theory of suburbanization." *American Journal
            of Sociology* 68: 565–570.
1970   "The social consequences of high population density." Pp. 84–90 in T. R. Ford
            and G. F. DeJong (eds.), *Social Demography*. Englewood Cliffs, N.J.: Pren-
            tice-Hall.
Wirth, L.
1938   "Urbanism as a way of life." *American Journal of Sociology* 44 (July): 1–24.
Wohlwill, J. F.
1974   "Human adaptation to levels of environmental stimulation." *Human Ecology*
            2: 127–147.
Wolf, A., and E. F. Von Haxthausen
1960   "Toward the analysis of the effects of some centrally-acting sedative sub-
            stances." *Arzneimittel-Forschung* 10: 50.
Wynne-Edwards, V. C.
1962   *Animal Dispersion in Relation to Social Behavior*. New York: Hafner.

7

The Organizational Components
of Expanding Metropolitan Systems

FRANKLIN D. WILSON

The most important aspect of man's evolution is the expansion of his niche in the world ecosystem.

This expansion has involved (1) increase in numbers sustained by (2) increasing human resourcefulness in extracting the requisite supplies of energy and materials from the environment and (3) an elaboration of the patterns of organization of the human collective efforts involved in this activity [Duncan, 1964, p. 40].

Urban communities, as territorially based systems of adaptation, constitute a form of social organization that has been at the center of the expansion process (Adams, 1966, 1974; Childe, 1950; Cohen, 1974; Hammond, 1972). Historically, urban communities have functioned as the locus of decision units whose activities include production and distribution of goods and services, control and coordination of the activities of other units, technological innovation, and information storage. Although the nature of the units with which such functions are vested has ranged from religious and military to political and economic, urban communities always have been in a position of dominance with respect to ecological expansion.

Social Demography

Copyright © 1978 by Academic Press, Inc.
All rights of reproduction in any form reserved.
ISBN 0-12-682650-1

This chapter focuses on a hypothesis derived from the theory of ecological expansion: As a territorial system expands both in size and land
area, there occurs at its center an increase in those units that perform the
functions of coordination and integration for the system as a whole. The
theoretical and empirical basis of this hypothesis will be summarized and
criticized, followed by an empirical test of its plausibility as it relates to
recent trends in U. S. metropolitan communities.

The Theory of Ecological Expansion

In one of the first empirical studies of metropolitan communities,
McKenzie (1933) observed that every metropolitan community is organized around a focal point of dominance, which, because of its location
and economic structure, is able to attract to it those units that mediate and
control the activities and relations that are carried on within the boundaries of the system. As the territorial scope of the activities of the community expands, the morphological structure of the community becomes
more differentiated with respect to the location of land usages and specialization of activities. There is "a progressive absorption of more or less
unrelated populations and land areas into a single organization [Hawley,
1950, p. 348]." At the center of settlement there occurs an increase in
those units whose basic functions consist of coordinating and integrating
the expanding system and mediating the relations that units within the settlement have with external units.

Thus expansion or growth of a territorial system involves (1) the growth
of a center of activity from which dominance is exercised, and (2) an enlargement of the scope of the center's influence:

> The process [expansion] entails the absorption and redistribution of the functions for-
> merly carried on in outlying areas, a centralization of mediating and control functions,
> an increase in the number and variety of territorially extended relationships, a growth of
> population to man a more elaborate set of activities, and an accumulation of culture
> together with a levelling of cultural differences over the expanding domain. [Hawley,
> 1968, p. 335].

The expansion process is based upon an increase in productivity of
what Hawley calls the "key function," which mediates the relations of
the system to its external environment. Productivity of the key function is
the primary factor that determines the degree to which a system can be
elaborated, the size of the population that can be sustained in the system,
and the territorial scope of the system. Two secondary factors that limit
expansion are the maximum distance over which dominance can be effec-

tively exercised and the functional boundaries of other territorial systems (Hawley, 1968, p. 332).

Expansion of the community usually begins at its nucleus and proceeds outward with extension and improvement of transportation and communication facilities. Accessibility of the center of settlement to outlying areas provides an opportunity for expansion by stimulating the the development of mediating and control functions. Because the center usually sits astride major routes of transportation and communication, technological innovations and the diffusion of information from other settlements are more likely to occur there.

Much of the evidence in support of this model of ecological expansion is historical in nature (Hawley, 1950, 1971; McKenzie, 1933). This model provides an excellent chronicle of the metropolitanization of American society. The model has been applied to the urbanization process in North American and other western nations, and also to the process in developing countries (Berry, 1972; Berry and Horton, 1970; Hawley, 1971, pp. 290–336).

THE ORGANIZATIONAL COMPONENTS OF METROPOLITAN EXPANSION

Relations between metropolis and hinterland form a topic to which the frame of reference of human ecology has been applied most effectively, although such varying concepts have been used as "metropolitanism" (Duncan *et al.,* 1960; Hawley, 1971; Duncan and Lieberson, 1970), "metropolitan dominance" (Duncan *et al.,* 1960; Schnore, 1963; Vance and Smith, 1954), "metropolitan decentralization" (Schnore, 1965), and the "urban hierarchy" (Berry, 1972). Most uses of these concepts portray the influence of metropolitan communities through a concern with structure at a single time, whereas the concept of metropolitan expansion points to the origin of that influence and its changes over time in form and structure.

The metropolitan community is a highly organized, multinucleated territorial system, with each territorial component performing some specialized role. The division of labor renders the components necessarily interdependent. At the center of the system stands an urban core that specializes in the coordinating functions of administration, exchange (of information and goods), and control. As the system extends its activities over a broader territory, it faces a problem encountered by all organizations: It must increase its administrative apparatus in order to maintain control and ensure efficient coordination of its activities.

It does not necessarily follow that the increase in control and coordinating activities will take place at the center of the expanding system. A metropolitan community is not a corporation with a formally organized structure, and therefore it is not capable of effecting a unified response to outside disturbances. The influence of a metropolitan area is simply a composite of the totality of influences exerted by decision units that are located within its boundaries. Thus if an increase is taking place in activities related to control and coordination, it is probably because those corporate units located within the boundaries of metropolitan systems are expanding their activities. It is logical but not automatic that such units will seek to augment their administrative apparatus at their existing centrally located bases, and that new key-functional units also will locate at the core.

Units whose activities are of particular relevance to the expansion model are (1) the headquarters units of local, regional, national, and multinational corporations and voluntary associations; (2) governmental units, particularly those at the state and federal levels; and (3) units whose activities involve the flow of information, people, and goods across the boundaries of territorially based systems of social organization, for example, such units as transportation and communication agencies, advertising, banking, and other financial intermediaries, law firms, public relation firms, management consultants, data-processing services, and research and development operations. These types of units are disproportionately concentrated in metropolitan areas, because of the greater accessibility afforded for carrying out extended hinterland relationships and the relative ease with which interorganizational personal contracts can be established when quick decisions have to be made. In addition, a large metropolitan area possesses a socioeconomic infrastructure that provides time- and cost-reducing externalities that are critical to these types of units for conducting their daily activities (Pred, 1974; Quante, 1976).

A recent test of the hypothesis that the organizational component of expanding metropolitan systems concentrates in the nucleus of the system used data on metropolitan areas in the United States during the 1960–1970 decade:

> The results presented in this study . . . provide empirical support for the theory that increases in the peripheral areas of territorially based systems will be matched with a development of organizational functions in its center to ensure integration and coordination of activities and relationships throughout the expanded system. Categoric and multivariate analysis indicate that central cities are far more developed in coordinative and integrative functions than their suburban ring. In fact, the size of the outer locus has substantially greater direct effects on organizational development within the central city than does either size of the central city, age of the SMSA, per capita income of central city residents, percentage nonwhite in the central city, or distance between metropolitan centers [Kasarda, 1972, pp. 174–175].

Although Kasarda's results appear to be consistent with the hypothesis that expansion of a metropolitan system results in an increase in organizational functions localized in its nucleus, there are a number of theoretical and methodological deficiencies inherent in his analysis that render the results suspect and the conclusion uncertain.[1] I have undertaken a separate analysis of the U. S. metropolitan experience during the 1960–1970 decade, seeking to avoid some of these problems, and have reached rather different conclusions that cast doubt on the ability of the hypothesis derived from historic experience to serve as a guide to recent and future trends.

[1] Kasarda's analysis is not a test of the theory of ecological expansion; he attempted only to test one important hypothesis associated with the theory. An adequate test of the hypothesis would require relating measures of expansion to measures of change in the spatial concentration of organizational activities. Kasarda treats size of the population outside the central city as if it were an indicator of expansion. This is simply faulty logic, unless it were the case that size is perfectly correlated with change in size. A test of the hypothesis requires data that permit one to associate changes in the critical variables in the model with each other.

Kasarda's measure of the organizational component of metropolitan systems is not a pure measure of the spatial concentration of industries. This can be seen by inspecting the components of the index used to measure this variable:

$$I = \frac{O_c/P_c}{O_m/P_m} \qquad (1)$$
$$(2)$$

or

$$I = \frac{O_s/P_s}{O_m/P_m} \qquad (3)$$
$$(4)$$

where O_c and O_s are the number of SMSA residents performing a given organizational function within the central city or suburban ring, respectively; P_c and P_s are the population size of the central city and the suburban ring, respectively; O_m is the total number of SMSA residents performing the same organizational function within all SMSAs; and P_m is the total population of all SMSAs. Components (2) and (4) are identical and are constant. Differences in the measure of spatial concentration of any one of the organizational functions are due to variations in the city or ring concentration of the Os or Ps or both. Kasarda's index is an expected measure of the spatial concentration of industries relative to the dispersion of population. For example, Kasarda (1972, p. 171) reports that the mean index of organizational development with respect to professional, technical, and kindred workers is 1.215 for central cities and .631 for suburbs. From these values, among others, he concludes that "central cities are far more developed in coordinative and integrative functions than their suburban rings." But this is not a correct interpretation of these index values. The correct interpretation would be that relative to the dispersion of population, central cities are far more developed in coordinative and integrative functions and their suburban ring. This difference in interpretation is important for a test of the expansion model, because not one of the scholars responsible for the development of the model indicates that the centralization of coordinative and control functions is to be assessed relative to the population size of either the inner or outer locus of the expanding system.

Methodology

SOME METHODOLOGICAL ISSUES

Empirical evaluation of hypotheses derived from the theory of ecological expansion requires the resolution of two important issues: (1) operationalization of the concept of the center of an expanding system and (2) sorting out the flow of influence between the expansion of territorial systems and changes in the concentration of activities associated with coordination and integration.

The definition of the center of an expanding territorial system should depend on the scope of influence exerted by that system. McKenzie (1933, p. 84) suggests two approaches that can be used to delineate the influence of metropolitan areas. The first approach defines community influence in terms of the commutation area in which the "daily economic and social activities of the local population are carried on through a common system of local institutions." The delineation of Standard Metropolitan Statistical Areas (SMSAs) by the Office of Management and Budget is an attempt to operationalize this concept. The appropriateness of the SMSA delineation of the large urban agglomerations characteristic of American Society has been questioned by Berry (1973). Essentially, Berry suggests that the economic regions, which he terms Daily Urban Systems (DUSs), developed by the Bureau of Economic Analysis of the U. S. Department of Commerce provide a better approximation to urban agglomerations than the SMSA concept. In the following analyses, measures based on both the SMSA and DUS concepts are employed.

The center of a SMSA or DUS may be taken as either the central business district or the central city, depending upon their size and the extent to which structural differentiation and the redistribution of land use activities have occurred. McKenzie (1933, pp. 70–71) explicitly recognized the importance of the central business district:

> Every region is organized around a central city or focal point of dominance in which are located the institutions and services that cater to the region as a whole and integrate it with other regions. . . . Certain functions, notably communications, finance, management, and the more specialized commercial and professional services, are becoming more highly concentrated in or near the center of the dominant city.

The second type of community influence identified by McKenzie is the "trade area," which "is defined as the surrounding geographic territory economically tributary to a city and for which such city provides the chief market and financial center." The trade area approach has been used extensively by human ecologists (Duncan and Lieberson, 1970; Duncan *et al.*, 1960; Schnore, 1967). The important implication to note here is that the center of this type of large-scale system is perhaps best taken to be the whole metropolitan or commutation area rather than simply the central urban core.

The appropriate definition of which activities are to be regarded as "integrating and coordinating" depends on whether community influence is being assessed from the metropolitan district or the trade area approach. In applying a trade area approach, Duncan *et al.* (1960) sought to identify industries oriented toward providing goods and services to areas outside the physical boundaries of the metropolitan area. Similarly, when using the metropolitan district approach care must be taken to exclude activities that are not metropolitan in scope. For example, industries that provide goods and services at the neighborhood level should be omitted, such as local retail and grocery stores, personal service establishments, and non-specialized medical services.[2]

Empirical assessment of the size and location of units that perform the functions of coordination and integration typically relies on employment and workplace data for selected industries and/or occupations. Such a methodological procedure is based on a connecting assumption, stipulating that the number of persons employed in the selected industry categories is proportional to the degree of organizational activities engaged in by units whose functions are those of control, coordination, and integration of the activities of all other units in the territorial unit.

The use of either the SMSA or the DUS as basic units for measuring expansion is not without its problems. Changes in the coordinating and integrating functions of a metropolitan area that are oriented primarily toward activities carried on within the boundaries of its commutation area are not independent of changes in similar functions performed for its trade area. Given sufficient development in the technology of communication and transportation, the major factor that tends to stimulate growth in the commutation area of a metropolitan community is the extent to which it is capable of broadening its exporting activities, or increasing and broadening the relations it has with other territorial units. The lack of a precise match between changes in organizational activities and changes in the size of the territorial unit responsible for producing that change creates a serious accountability problem. Part of the change in the concentration of organizational activities that our procedure attributes to change in the size of an SMSA or DUS may, in fact, reflect change in the size and scope of the extended trade area. The data bases available for this re-

---

[2] Along similar lines, the use of white-collar occupations as measures of organizational functions has one serious deficiency. The occupational distribution of a metropolitan area is not independent of its size nor its industrial structure (Winsborough, 1960, pp. 894–897). The results reported by Kasarda (1972) suffer from this deficiency. White-collar occupations make up a substantial part of the labor force of a number of the industry categories for which he reports results.

search do not permit proper differentiation between the metropolitan district and trade area approaches.

DATA

Most of the data for these analyses were obtained from decennial census information for 1960 and 1970. Some of the information was taken from published reports; other information was taken from the 1% Public Use Samples. Because not all of the data desired were available, two distinct metropolitan universes were used.

For the first analysis (Tables 7.1–7.4), data for the dependent variable were taken from the 1% Public Use Sample for states. This data file does not permit identification of central city and suburban workplace for the metropolitan population of states having fewer than two large SMSAs. The necessary data were available for 24 states (Alabama, California, Connecticut, Florida, Georgia, Illinois, Indiana, Kansas, Kentucky, Louisiana, Massachusetts, Michigan, Minnesota, Missouri, New Jersey, New York, Ohio, Oregon, Pennsylvania, Tennessee, Texas, Virginia, Washington, and Wisconsin). These states include most of the nation's metropolitan population.

In the first analysis, the organizational component of metropolitan systems is identified with a classification scheme based on one used by Duncan et al. (1960, pp. 199–209). "Extralocal" industries are treated as one category; included are wholesale trade, interurban transportation, banking, finance, advertising, and state and federal public administration. "Metropolitanwide" industries are those that provide goods and services for the total resident population of the SMSA; included are intraurban transportation systems, TV and radio broadcasting, motor vehicle dealers, detective and protective series, hospitals, museum, art galleries, local public administration, zoos, and real estate. All other industries were placed in a residual category ("Others"), including local community services and extractive and manufacturing industries.

In the analysis of the determinants of change (Tables 7.5–7.7), the organizational component of metropolitan systems is defined as employment in the following industries: transportation, communications, and utilities; wholesale and retail trade; finance, insurance, and real estate; business and repair services; professional and related services; and public administration. The universe for this analysis is 85 monocentered metropolitan areas that had a population in 1960 greater than 250,000.

Employment information for 1960 was obtained from the journey to work volume of the 1960 Census. Employment data for 1970 were obtained from a 1% Public Use Sample tape for county groups. This data set has several advantages over the use of the published census volumes (and the fourth count summary tapes for SMSAs). The information on labor force activities is provided for persons in households, which can be aggregated to obtain detailed information for subareas such as the central business district, the central city, and the remainder of the SMSA. Because the information is for persons, the data can be subjected to more extensive manipulation with respect to measuring organizational functions. Once the data are aggregated to the SMSA level, the records for SMSAs can be matched with published data to obtain additional information. Employment information from the sample tapes was inflated by a factor of 100 to approximate total labor force figures for 1970 (U. S. Bureau of the Census, 1972). This procedure has the shortcoming that the estimates of employment in industries by place of work for each SMSA are less reliable than those produced by the Bureau of the Census for its published reports that use a larger sample and a more complex weighting procedure.

Employment figures are for the resident population of SMSAs, which excludes persons who live outside but work inside the SMSAs included in our universe. For some SMSAs, this is a serious deficiency causing an underestimate of the number of persons employed in certain industries.

The data on population, land area, and age of central city (date central city reached 50,000 population) for SMSAs were obtained from the United States Census of Population Summary Reports for 1960 and 1970. Data for DUSs (population 1960 and 1970 and percentage of total earnings in 1967 from federal government or residentiary industries) were obtained from Berry (1973, pp. 18–28). "Functional distance" is defined as the road map distance of each SMSA to the nearest SMSA that occupies a higher position in the urban hierarchy as defined by Duncan *et al.* (1960, p. 271). The SMSAs nested under national metropolis, regional metropolis, diversified manufacturing with metropolitan functions, and regional capitals were used as reference points. A measure of industrial structure is derived from Kass (1973, pp. 427–446), and from Duncan *et al.* (1960), for areas for which Kass indicated that he could find no unique cluster. From these sources, a dummy variable was created in which a value of 1 is assigned to an SMSA if its industrial structure is defined as wholesale, retail, public administration, finance, education, or any combination of these.

Findings for U. S. Metropolitan Systems, 1960 to 1970

TRENDS IN THE CONCENTRATION OF EMPLOYMENT

The first step in analysis is a description of change from 1960 to 1970 in the concentration of organizational activities in central city and suburban components of SMSAs. The description will include specification by industry, region, occupation, and various combinations thereof. The character of the data base is illustrated in summary form by Table 7.1. The census data on place of work are arranged to show numbers employed in the central city and in the suburbs in 1960 and in 1970 for each of the designated industry categories, occupations, and regions. The full data base is a complete cross-classification of these variables.

Goodman's (1972) log linear model for the analysis of multidimensional contingency tables is employed to reduce the information to a set of meaningful parameters. The model evaluates for each specified attribute or combination of attributes the odds (probability) that a person possessing those attributes works in the central city (rather than in the suburbs). The general model being evaluated can be estimated with the following equation, in which the dependent variable is the logarithm of the odds of working in the central city:

$$\text{Log}_e \, E = \mu_E + \lambda_A + \lambda_B + \lambda_C + \lambda_D + \lambda_{AB}$$
$$+ \lambda_{AC} + \lambda_{AD} + \lambda_{BC} + \lambda_{BD} + _{CD} \tag{1}$$

$\text{Log}_e E$ is the natural log of the odds of working in the central city; μ_E is the grand mean effect, for example, the average cell value of E when variables A through D are zero; the parameters λ_A through λ_D represent the effects that industry, occupation, geographic regions, and time periods (1960 versus 1970) respectively have on the odds of working in the central city; and the parameters λ_{AB} through λ_{CD} represent two-way interaction effects. The general model expressed in equation (1) is hierarchial; each parameter is added sequentially to a baseline model.

The top panel of Table 7.2 reports the chi-square values associated with the general model. The values reported in the bottom panel of Table 7.2 were obtained by nesting occupation within industry groupings.

The log linear chi-square values associated with the "Total" rows provide a test of the hypothesis that the odds of a metropolitan resident working in the central city do not vary by industry, occupation, region, or year. The very large chi-square value (37,379) indicates that this hypothesis cannot be accepted. The other chi-square values in both panels of the table were generated to evaluate the relative importance of the sequential addition of each variable (or variable combination) to the baseline model. The full model (if the three-way and four-way interactions also were shown) will, by definition, completely explain the observed cell frequencies. Hence the log likelihood chi-square statistic reduces to zero. The percentage reduction in chi-square due to the addition of a new parameter to the model indicates the relative ability of the parameter to explain the total variation observed in the dependent variable.

TABLE 7.1

Employment in Central City and Suburbs Cross-Classified with Industry, Occupation, and Region. Metropolitan Population in Selected States in the U. S., 1960 and 1970

	1960		1970[a]	
Variables	Central city	Suburbs	Central city	Suburbs
Industry				
Extralocal				
Transportation– communications	1,262,200	438,200	1,228,400	647,000
Wholesale trade	1,017,500	284,200	1,124,100	638,100
Finance, insurance investments	1,065,400	265,000	1,327,300	475,600
Business services	388,900	137,300	544,900	307,900
Hotels–motels	229,200	74,500	199,300	120,900
Public administration	511,800	293,600	598,200	361,600
Metropolitanwide				
Transportation, utilities	529,400	195,300	502,900	264,700
Real estate	283,100	119,600	301,500	190,100
Auto repairs	286,700	141,600	284,900	215,600
Entertainment	176,600	109,200	174,100	144,400
Professional services	2,536,400	1,454,000	3,928,500	2,816,000
Public administration	640,900	274,600	763,200	404,600
Others				
Local community level	4,349,300	2,279,400	4,041,800	3,431,700
Agriculture–mining	93,300	149,300	134,400	166,300
Construction	1,024,900	751,500	948,900	911,700
Durable manufacturing	3,328,000	2,549,500	2,934,600	3,244,000
Nondurable manufacturing	2,773,600	1,228,500	2,207,800	1,453,500
Not reported	210,600	95,100	420,100	323,300
Occupation				
Professionals	2,516,400	1,512,200	3,451,800	2,642,700
Managers	1,916,600	927,300	1,827,600	1,242,000
Clerical	4,108,800	1,611,500	4,866,300	2,881,700
Sales	1,775,200	807,700	1,702,500	1,309,000
Others	10,390,800	5,981,700	9,816,700	8,041,600
Region				
West	2,518,500	2,093,300	2,951,500	2,056,700
North central	6,756,200	2,944,000	6,713,000	5,222,500
East	6,750,600	4,104,900	6,178,000	5,182,600
South	4,682,500	1,698,200	5,822,400	2,755,200
Totals	20,707,800	10,840,400	21,664,900	16,117,000

[a] Industry and occupational categories for 1970 were recoded to conform to these reported for 1960.

TABLE 7.2

Associated Chi Squares Derived from Two Hierarchical Models Predicting the Log Odds of Working in the Central City

Variables	Log linear chi square	DF	Percentage reduction in chi square
Total	37379	719	96.43
Industry	24246	702	35.13
Occupation	23569	698	1.81
Region	13419	695	27.15
1960	7423	694	16.04
Industry (×) occupation	4769	626	7.10
Industry (×) region	2940	575	4.89
Industry (×) 1960	2269	558	1.80
Occupation (×) region	2158	546	0.30
Occupation (×) 1960	2083	542	0.20
Region (×) 1960	1330	539	2.01
Total	37379	719	98.65
Industry–occupation	20914	630	44.05
Region	10817	627	27.01
1960	4769	626	16.18
Industry–occupation (×) region	2203	359	6.86
Industry–occupation (×) 1960	1261	270	2.52
Region (×) 1960	504	267	2.03

The percentage reduction values reported in the third column of the top panel of Table 7.2 indicate that the workplace structure of metropolitan areas is influenced very heavily by industry. The almost negligible reduction in chi-square value occasioned by the addition of occupation clearly implies that central cities and suburbs are differentiated primarily with respect to industry structure. Note, however, that the interaction of industry and occupation has a distinct effect on workplace location. This evidence of industry-specific variations in the spatial concentration of occupational groups is the reason we altered the general model slightly, as shown in the bottom panel.

The 27% reduction in chi square resulting from the addition of region to the model probably reflects the influence of two factors. First, the four major regions of the country, developed economically in different historical periods, can be expected to differ with respect to the spatial distribution of employment. Second, as I have shown elsewhere (Wilson, 1976), much of the effect attributed to region actually reflects regional variations in the size distribution of metropolitan area. Metropolitan areas with populations of 1 million or more are likely to have highly decentralized economic structures, whatever region they are in.

The 16% reduction in chi-square associated with time period attests to the pervasive decline that occurred between 1960 and 1970 in the location of employment activities in central cities. Although it is often asserted that this decline primarily reflects shifts in the location of manufacturing industries with predominant blue-collar occupational structures, results reported elsewhere suggest otherwise (Wilson, 1976). Indeed, Kasarda (1976) found that the volume of growth of white-collar employment in suburban districts was significantly greater than that for blue-collar employment.

While the chi-square values reported in Table 7.2 indicate the magnitude of the effect exerted by the variables considered, they do not describe the pattern of variation that exists within levels of these variables. To analyze patterns, another set of statistics generated from Goodman's log linear model is employed. The log probabilities or the log odds of having a given characteristic may be expressed as deviations from the average cell mean. Table 7.3 presents the log odds coefficients associated with the region, time, and region–time interaction portions of the hierarchial models reported in Table 7.2. These coefficients may be added to the

TABLE 7.3

Log Linear Additive Coefficients Indicating the Odds of Working in the Central City: Region of the Country and Time Period

Variables	Log odds of working in the central city (additive coefficients)
Regions	
West	− .1638
North central	.0638
East	− .0648
South	.1648
Time	
1960	.1004
Regions (×) 1960	
West	− .0379
North central	.0580
East	− .0022
South	− .0180
Grand mean effect	4.7179
Intercept value	.3504

grand mean effect to obtain the log odds of working in the central city for a person with the specified attribute (or combination of attributes), holding constant all other attributes (including industry and occupation). Thus the coefficient of + .1004 for the year 1960 indicates that the log odds of working in the central city are 4.7179 + .1004 for 1960 as compared to 4.7179 for 1970. A central city workplace was more likely in 1960 than in 1970, net of the other variables in the model.

Discussion of the log odds coefficients will focus on the nested industry and occupation classification that was used in the version of the general model reported in the bottom panel of Table 7.2. The coefficients for this portion of the model are presented in Table 7.4. The grand mean effect and intercept value given in Table 7.3 still apply, and the coefficients are net of the region and time effects. (The last two rows and two columns [totals] of Table 7.4 report the separate occupation and industry effects that correspond to the first version—top panel of Table 7.2—of the general model.)

The coefficients reported under the columns headed "Odds wk. cent. city" are the deviations from the grand mean of the log odds of working in the central city, net of region and time period. Positive values indicate that the odds of working in the central city are greater for a person in this industry–occupation group than for the average person. The coefficients reported in the column headed "Odds wk. cent. city (+) 1960" are the sum of the additive effect of (time = 1960) plus the interactional effect of (time = 1960) and industry–occupation. (For example, the value of (.1218) reported for professional workers in transportation and communications is the sum of the general additive effect of time [.1004] plus the specific interactional effect of time with this industry and occupation [.0214].) Positive values indicate that the odds of working in the central city were greater in 1960 than in 1970, and thus indicate a recent *decline* in the likelihood that persons employed in that industry–occupation group work in the central city.

The hypothesis concerning concentration of the organizational component of expanding metropolitan systems permits us to specify three patterns that should be discernible among the coefficients reported in Table 7.4. First, the locus of employment of persons in white-collar occupations should be in the central city. Second, changes in the concentration of organizational activities should be in the direction of increases in central cities. Third, the central city concentration of employment for white-collar occupations in extralocal industries should be especially high and increasing, for the organizational units in these industries serve very broad hinterlands.

The first pattern expected from the hypothesis is observed very weakly

TABLE 7.4

Log Linear Additive Coefficients Indicating the Odds of Working in the Central City: Industry–Occupation and Time Period[a]

Industry	Professionals		Managers		Clerical		Sales		Others		Total, all occupations	
	Odds wk. cent. city	Odds wk. cent. city (+) 1960	Odds wk. cent. city	Odds wk. cent city (+) 1960	Odds wk. cent. city	Odds wk. cent. city (+) 1960	Odds wk. cent. city	Odds wk. cent. city (+) 1960	Odds wk. cent. city	Odds wk. cent city (+) 1960	Odds wk. cent. city	Odds wk. cent. city (+) 1960
Extralocal												
Transportation, communications	.1584	.1218	.0975	.0592	.1769	.1134	.3449	.1588	-.0174	.1023	.1800	.1990
Wholesale trade	.0829	.2785	.1232	.1686	.1774	.2122	.1283	.2025	.0297	.1310	.1253	.1764
Finance, insurance, investments	.5572	.0933	.2040	.0575	.2696	.1042	.1349	.0666	.4643	.0921	.3631	.0799
Business services	-.0808	.0646	.1372	.1444	.1230	.1401	.0923	.1942	.0601	.1141	.0929	.1204
Hotels–motels	-.0015	.2062	-.2292	.1492	.2141	.1266	1.2620*	.0364	.0617	.1667	.0356	.1652
Public administration	-.0392	.0743	-.0205	.0299	.0501	.0182	-.0048	.0265	-.3824	-.0281	-.0430	.0206
Metropolitanwide												
Transportation, utilities	.2087	.0381	-.0758	.0582	.1492	.0786	.0706	.1183	.0139	.0970	.1167	.0933
Real estate	.1637	.1854	.0480	.0957	-.0077	.0861	-.2647	.1095	.1888	.1093	.0545	.0974
Auto repairs	-.0973	.1146	-.0780	.0535	.0127	.1003	.0063	.0238	.1190	.1196	-.0263	.1194
Entertainment	-.0318	.1308	-.2158	.0354	-.0291	.0881	.1068	.2488	-.2946	.0659	-.0706	.0366
Professional services	-.1614	.0514	-.0043	-.1015	.0010	.0838	.1485	.1197	-.1610	.0565	-.0056	.0614
Public administration	.1135	.0975	-.1454	.0010	.0405	.0730	1.4456*	-.0293	.0255	.0330	.0860	.0523
Others												
Local community level	-.0439	.0709	-.1481	.0962	-.0853	.1276	-.1618	.1274	-.1750	.1226	-.0933	.1211
Agriculture–mining	-.3282	.0137	-.4704	-.0092	-.2283	.0060	-.5944	.1027	-.7939	-.0693	-.4184	-.0408
Construction	.0766	.0769	-.3380	.0892	-.1132	.1030	.0884	.2886	-.3030	.0680	-.1156	.0830
Durable manufacturing	-.4316	.0899	-.2722	.0936	-.3057	.0900	-.0857	.2410	-.3129	.0775	-.2520	.0905
Nondurable manufacturing	-.1265	.0550	.0363	.1247	.0377	.1280	-.0594	.1505	-.0746	.0858	-.0156	.0849
Not reported	-.1932	.0916	-.0047	.2518	.0314	.1671	.2579	.2750	-.1096	.1218	-.0137	.0482
Total, all industries												
Odds wk. cent. city	.0155		.0429		.0557		.0443		-.0725			
Odds wk. cent. city (+) 1960		.0856		.0782		.1064		.1129		.0830		

[a] An asterisk indicates a cell frequency of less than 25.

147

and inconsistently. For each of the four white-collar occupation groups, the total effect (for all industries) is positive but barely above zero. For many specific combinations of industry and white-collar occupation, the coefficients are negative, indicating a greater than average likelihood of working outside the central city.

The second pattern expected from the hypothesis is contradicted by the data in Table 7.4. Of the 72 combinations of industry with a white-collar occupation, for only 3 did central city workplace become more likely in 1970 than in 1960.

The third pattern is partially discernible in the data. For the extralocal industries, several of the coefficients (odds wk. cent. city) for white-collar occupations are distinctly positive. However, the positive and frequently large coefficients in the second column for these industry–occupation groups indicate a pronounced decentralization, 1960–1970. The central city concentration of white-collar employment in extralocal industries may be reinterpreted as a residue of historical experience rather than an indication of current organizational necessity.

The coefficients derived from the log linear model document that the shift in location of employment from central cities to suburbs has been characteristic of most industry–occupation groups, and that those activities most indicative of the metropolitan key function have not been exempt from the trend. This finding is presented in simpler form in Table 7.5, where the analytical virtues and complexity of the earlier analysis are replaced by simple percentages. For each specified industry (except public administration) the percentage of employment located in the central city decreased between 1960 and 1970. Although these industries exhibited increasing central city employment, their aggregate rate of growth in the total metropolis was even greater (except for public administration). Of the total metropolitan increase in employment in these industries, only for finance, insurance, and so on, did the central cities capture more than half of the increase. The majority of employment growth, even in many industries that presumably perform key organizational functions for metropolitan areas, has occurred outside the central cities.

DETERMINANTS OF CHANGES IN CONCENTRATION

The major objective of this analysis is a test of the hypothesis that as a territorial system expands both in size and land area, there occurs at its center an increase in those organizational units that perform the functions of coordination, integration, and control for the system as a whole. Although McKenzie (1933) and Hawley (1950, 1968) were not explicit on this point, the hypothesis implies not simply an increase in the number or size of centrally located units engaged in activities related to coordina-

TABLE 7.5

Change in the Concentration of Employment in the Central Cities of 85 Selected Metropolitan Areas, for Selected Industries, 1960 to 1970[a]

Industry categories	Percentage in central city 1960	1970	Percentage increase in central city	Percentage increase in SMSA	Increase in central city relative to increase in SMSA (percentage)
Transportation, etc.	58.0	53.2	17.5	28.0	24.1
Wholesale and retail	57.2	45.8	21.9	52.1	26.7
Finance, insurance, etc.	63.1	59.9	46.1	53.8	55.3
Business services	58.1	48.4	46.8	76.2	36.5
Professional services	54.3	47.4	74.3	99.9	42.3
Public administration	53.3	54.2	43.4	30.2	45.3
Total employment	52.3	50.1	23.6	29.1	42.4

[a] Measures are calculated for the aggregate labor force in all 85 metropolitan areas.

tion, integration, and control, but a greater increase at the center than in the periphery. In our application of the hypothesis to recent U. S. metropolitan trends, the expectation is that central cities should have experienced a net increase in the designated organizational units. Such a net increase can occur in two ways: (1) The majority of the new growth in organizational units occurs in central cities; and (2) more organizational units shift their location from the suburbs to central cities than the reverse. The results presented in the previous section clearly demonstrate that suburban areas have captured the largest share of the increase in organizational activities. Although these results cast doubts on the plausibility of the expansion hypothesis, they do not suffice as a direct test of that hypothesis. Measures of change in the locus of organizational activities must be related to measures of metropolitan expansion.

For a direct test of the expansion hypothesis, three measures of the expansion of metropolitan communities are employed. The first is change in the size of the population resident in DUSs, SMSAs, and the two major components of SMSAs. The second is change in the amount of land area in SMSAs, central cities, and suburbs. The third measure is gross density, the number of persons per square mile of land area. Density is included for completeness, although it is felt that this variable is more an indicator of deconcentration than of expansion (see Winsborough, 1963, pp. 565–

TABLE 7.6

Population, Land Area, and Density for 85 Selected Metropolitan Areas, 1960 to 1970

Measure	Size		Percentage of total SMSA population		Absolute change (percentage)	Relative change (percentage)
	1960	1970	1960	1970		
Central cities						
Population	353,176	372,882	45.9	41.5	5.6	15.3
Land area (sq. mi.)[a]	69	90	3.5	4.4	29.3	20.3
Density[a]	6,519	5,606			−14.0	
Suburbs						
Population	417,176	526,412	54.1	58.5	26.2	84.7
Land area (sq. mi.)[a]	1,890	1,970	96.5	95.6	4.2	79.7
Density[a]	497	484			− 2.6	
SMSAs						
Population	770,352	899,294	100.0	100.0	16.7	
Land area (sq. mi.)[a]	1,959	2,060	100.0	100.0	5.1	
Density[a]	393	437			−11.1	
DUSs						
Population	1,327,529	1,531,529			15.4	

[a] The mean value of these variables among the 85 areas is reported.

570). An aggregate summary of changes in these three measures between 1960 and 1970 is reported in Table 7.6. During this decade metropolitan areas expanded in both population and land area, with suburbs capturing most of the growth in each.

For a test of the relation between changes in the central city concentration of key organizational activities and changes in the size of metropolitan communities, separate regression equations were fitted for each of six selected industry groupings. These industry groupings are identified in the column headings to Table 7.7. Employment in each industry grouping is an index of the size of a key organizational activity. The dependent variable, relative change in the concentration of an organizational activity in the central city, is the increase in central city employment in an activity, taken as a percentage of the total metropolitan employment increase for that activity. A relative measure of change is used as the dependent variable because the theory of ecological expansion clearly implies that the nucleus of the expanding system will be the locus of the majority of net growth that occurs in organizational activities. The hypothesis under evaluation specifies that changes in organizational concentration should be positively (and significantly) related to percentage change in metropolitan population and relative changes in suburban population and land area.

In Table 7.6, the first five measures listed in the stub are the basic independent variables, measures of metropolitan expansion. The remaining independent variables are city or metropolitan characteristics at a particular time, and most of them are not expected to change much during the decade. Each was included because of a presumed or possible relation to metropolitan structure or expansion.

The 5 variables indexing metropolitan expansion, taken together with the 13 control variables, do a poor job of predicting or specifying the change in the concentration of organizational activities within the metropolis. For three of the six regression equations, the fit is quite poor, as indicated by explained variance under 5%. Among 30 standardized regression coefficients relating the 5 principal independent variables to the 6 dependent variables, only 1 is large enough to reach statistical significance at the 5% level. The results reported in Table 7.6 are strongly inconsistent with the predictions derived from the theory of ecological expansion. An alternative analysis using measures of absolute rather than relative change as dependent variables yielded essentially similar results.

Discussion

I can suggest two major reasons why the results reported here lead to a disconfirmation of the hypothesis that as a metropolitan system expands

TABLE 7.7

Determinants of Relative Change in the Concentration of Organizational Activities in Central Cities, for 85 Selected Metropolitan Areas, 1960 to 1970 (Standardized Regression Coefficients)[a,b]

Independent variables	Transportation, and so on	Wholesale and retail	Finance, and so on	Business services	Professional services	Public administration
Relative change in suburban population	.3792	.0515	.0356	.1041	−.0956	.2530
Percentage of change in suburban density	−.1278	−.3459	.1845	.0168	−.1522	−.2905
Relative change in suburban land	.1166	.2955	−.0281	.1616	.0882	.4947*
Percentage of change DUS population, 1960–1970	−.1857	.1657	.0213	.0108	−.2390	.0165
Percentage of change in SMSA population	−.0045	.1492	.2408	.0590	.2348	.1163
Log central city population, 1960	−.3224	.9074	1.4735*	1.5718*	.0976	1.9500*
Percentage of SMSA Population in central city	.0637	−.3629	−.5640	−.6664*	.2143	−.9985
Ratio of central city to SMSA density	.0651	−.0166	−.1085	.0681	.0763	−.2032
Percentage of SMSA land in central city	.0327	.0584	−.0319	.1127	.1447	−.0503
Percentage of DUS population in SMSA	.3045	−.2109	−.1159	−.0955	−.3634	−.7538*
Log DUS population, 1960	.3049	−.3386	.0816	−.3493	−.3473	−1.3128*
Rank of SMSA	.2994	.4609	1.1215*	1.1215*	−.1938	.4743
Age of central city	.3693	−.1888	−.2292	−.1276	.0752	−.0958
Distance to other SMSA	.2457	.1494	.0076	−.0014	.1690	.0766
Per capita income	−.3186	−.3288*	−.1992	−.1446	−.3099*	−.2099
Percentage of earnings federal government	.0371	.0311	.0228	.0115	.1427	.2291
Percentage of earnings residentiary	.3247	.1604	.0082	−.0186	.1854	.0351
Industrial structure	.0817	−.0467	−.1154	.1599	.1376	.1404
Means	.4886	.3105	.6196	.4506	.4643	.4902
R² (corrected)	.0401	.1047	.0129	.0000	.2797	.3114

[a] Relative change in concentration of an organizational activity is defined as: $O_i^{T+n} - O_i^T / O_K^{T+n} - O_K^T$ where O is an organizational activity, i refers to central city, K refers to SMSA, and T refers to time period.

[b] An asterisk indicates statistical significance at the .05 level by the customary F test.

in size and land area, there occurs at its center an increase in those organizational units that perform the functions of coordination, integration, and control for the system as a whole. First, the assumption that SMSAs and DUSs are contained systems, not subject to influences from outside units, may have been violated. Although an attempt was made to satisfy this assumption through the use of monocentered territorial units, the boundaries of these units still may provide only crude approximations to the territorial scope of the activities such units carry on with extended hinterlands. Some effort should be directed toward developing measures of ecological expansion that reflect growth in both the commutation and trade areas of metropolitan communities.

The second explanation for the disconfirmation of the hypothesis under test is more fundamental. The spatial structures of metropolitan areas are still in the process of evolving. Practically every new development in the technology of transportation and communication, building designs and operation, marketing techniques, and organizational forms tends to be reflected in the manner in which activities are spatially distributed and redistributed within metropolitan areas. Improvements in transportation and communication technologies appear to have reduced the need for spatial clustering and centralization of key organizational activities.

Historically, the centralization of employment activities in the core parts of metropolitan areas was very much influenced by the centralization of the interurban transporation network, the difficulty of moving goods and people efficiently within the boundaries of urban areas themselves, and the existence of an urban socioeconomic infrastructure that provided cost-reducing externalities. The continual reduction of locational constraints on peripheral locations, the emergence of large negative externalities associated with congested central locations, the spread of traditional central city amenities over the urban landscape, the rapid residential decentralization of the labor force, and the changing ethnic composition of central areas are all leading to increased decentralization of industries.

Berry and Cohen (1973) suggested that although manufacturing and retailing activities have been shifting from center to peripheral locations, headquarters, and main office functions, as well as financial and marketing activities, still occupy central locations and will probably continue to do so. Indeed, this was one of the major conclusions reached by Kasarda (1972, p. 175):

> If the present centrifugal drift of population, manufacturing activity, and establishments providing standardized goods and services continues, we may expect to find the central cities becoming even more territorially specialized in coordinative and integrative functions in future years.

Our results suggest a different conclusion. While central cities traditionally have been the major recipients of growth in coordinative and integrative activities, much of this growth is now occurring in peripheral areas. During the 1960–1970 decade, the majority of the increases in the key organizational activities of expanding metropolitan systems occurred away from the center of the commutation area. If this trend continues, coordinative and integrative activities rapidly will become diffused throughout metropolitan areas.

Gold (1972, p. 463) noted that during the 1960s even the central offices and administrative activities of corporations and other organizations began to respond to the forces of decentralization as manufacturing had earlier. His interpretation of the shift in location is suggestive (1972, p. 464):

> For many corporations, the desire of top executives to move closer to their residences in the suburbs appears to be the principal motive for relocating headquarters facilities out of the urban core. The negative factors expelling corporate executives from the central city . . . include racial unrest, decline in the skill level of the central-city labor force, extensive and costly commutation patterns, the proliferation of commuter income taxes, and the general tensions that result from doing business in a crowded and impacted environment.

When these negative externalities of central location are combined with the positive attractions of the suburbs, the balance is currently in favor of continued suburbanization of office employment. More importantly, as Gold suggests, the trend may be accelerating as many of the business establishments that provide auxiliary services to corporations that have shifted their locations will themselves be induced to relocate as well (see also Quante, 1976).

Although the evidence presented in this chapter reveals that some of the most important functions traditionally performed by central cities are being diffused throughout metropolitan areas via the decentralization process, the recency of this shift prompts caution in making long-run forecasts. It is still true that large metropolitan areas exert considerable influence over extended territorial areas. What seems likely to change in the next several decades is that this influence may no longer be localized in the center of metropolitan areas.

References

Adams, R. McC.
1966 *The Evolution of Urban Society*. Chicago: University of Chicago Press.

1974   "The study of ancient Mesopotamian settlement patterns and the problem of urban orgins." Pp. 490–500 in Y. Cohen (ed.), *Man in Adaptation: The Biosocial Background*. Chicago: Aldine Publishing Company.

Berry, B. J. L., and F. E. Horton
   1970   *Geographic Perspectives in Urban Systems*. Englewood Cliffs, N. J.: Prentice-Hall.

Berry, B. J. L.
   1972   "Latent structure of the American urban system, with international comparisons." Pp. 11–60 in B. J. L. Berry (ed.), *City Classification Handbook*. New York: John Wiley and Sons.
   1973   *Growth Centers in the American Urban System*. Cambridge, Mass.: Ballinger Publishing Company.

Berry, B. J. L., and Y. S. Cohen
   1973   "Decentralization of commerce and industry: The restructuring of metropolitan America." Pp. 431–456 in L. H. Masotti and J. K. Hadden (eds.), *The Urbanization of the Suburbs*. Berverly Hills, Calif.: Sage Publications.

Childe, V. G.
   1950   "The urban revolution." *Town Planning Review* 21: 3–17.

Cohen, Y. A.
   1974   "The concept of culture: Evolution and adaptation." Pp. 9–18 in Y. A. Cohen (ed.), *Man in Adaptation: The Cultural Present*. Chicago: Aldine Publishing Company.

Duncan, B., and S. Lieberson
   1970   *Metropolis and Region in Transition*. Beverly Hills, Calif.: Sage Publications.

Duncan, O. D., W. R. Scott, S. Lieberson, B. Duncan, and H. H. Winsborough
   1960   *Metropolis and Region*. Baltimore: The Johns Hopkins Press.

Duncan, O. D.
   1964   "Social organization and the ecosystem." Pp. 36–82 in R. E. L. Faris (ed.), *Handbook of Modern Sociology*. Chicago: Rand McNally.

Gold, N. N.
   1972   "The mismatch of jobs and low-income people in metropolitan areas and its implications for the central city poor." Pp. 441–488 U. S. Commission on Population Growth and the American Future, Population Distribution and Policy, Sara Mills Mazie (ed.), Volume V of *Commission Research Reports*. Washington, D. C.: Government Printing Office.

Goodman, L. A.
   1972   "A modified multiple regression approach to the analysis of dichotomus variables." *American Sociological Review 37(February)*: 28–46.

Hammond, M.
   1972   *The City in the Ancient World*. Cambridge, Mass.: Harvard University Press.

Hawley, A.
   1950   *Human Ecology: A Theory of Community Structure*. New York: Roland Press.
   1968   "Human ecology." *The International Encyclopedia of the Social Sciences* 4: 328–337.
   1971   *Urban Society: An Ecological Approach*. New York: Roland Press.

Kasarda, J. D.
   1972   "The theory of ecological expansion." *Social Forces* 51 (December): 165–175.
   1976   "The changing occupational structure of the American metropolis: Apropos the urban problem." Pp. 113–136 in B. Schwartz (ed.), *The Changing Face of the Suburbs*. Chicago: The University of Chicago Press.

Kass, R.
1973 "A functional classification of metropolitan communities." *Demography* 10(August): 427–446.

McKenzie, R. D.
1933 *The Metropolitan Community*. New York: McGraw-Hill.

Pred, A. R.
1974 Major Job-Providing Organizations and Systems of Cities. Commission on College Geography Resource Paper No. 27. Washington, D. C.: Association of American Geographers.

Quante, W.
1976 *The Exodus of Corporate Headquarters from New York City*. New York: Praeger Publishers.

Schnore, L. F.
1963 "Urban form: The case of the metropolitan community." Pp. 167–197 in Werner Z. Hirsch (ed.), *Urban Life and Form*. New York: Holt, Rinehart and Winston.
1965 *The Urban Scene*. New York: The Free Press.

U. S. Bureau of the Census
1972 Public Use Samples of Basic Records from the 1970 Census: Description and Technical Documentation. Washington, D. C.-U. S. Government Printing Office.

Vance, R. B., and S. Smith
1954 "Metropolitan dominance and integration." Pp. 120–137 in R. B. Vance and N. J. Demerath (eds.), *The Urban South*. Chapel Hill, N. C.: University of North Carolina Press.

Wilson, F. D.
1976 Residential Consumption, Economic Opportunities, and Race. Unpublished manuscript. Department of Sociology, University of Wisconsin–Madison.

Winsborough, H. H.
1960 "Occupational composition and the urban hierarchy." *American Sociological Review* 25(December): 894–897.
1963 "An ecological approach to the theory of suburbanization." *American Journal of Sociology* 68(March): 565–570.

Yeates, M. H., and B. J. Garner
1971 *The North American Society*. New York: Harper and Row.

8

The New Pattern
of Nonmetropolitan
Population Change[1]

CALVIN L. BEALE and GLENN V. FUGUITT

The increasing concentration of people in and around large cities always has been a major dimension of population redistribution in the United States. Most of those concerned with population trends have assumed that this process would continue into the future, as an almost inevitable concomitant of economic development and increasing organizational complexity. There is recent evidence, however, of a new trend in which remote areas are growing more rapidly and gaining net migrants at a higher rate than is the metropolitan territory. In this chapter we examine the new pattern of redistribution by comparing population changes according to residence in metropolitan and nonmetropolitan areas for three periods between 1950 and 1974. We take into consideration specific resi-

[1] This work has been supported by the Economic Development Division, Economic Research Service, U. S. Department of Agriculture, and by the College of Agricultural and Life Sciences, University of Wisconsin–Madison, through a Cooperative Agreement. Analysis was aided by a "Center for Population Research" grant, No. HD05876, to the Center for Demography and Ecology, University of Wisconsin–Madison, from the Center for Population Research of the National Institute of Child Health and Human Development.

dence subgroups, geographic subregions, and selected factors associated with differential growth and migration.

In the 1960s the United States passed through a time of acute consciousness of the movement of people from rural and small town areas into the metropolitan cities. Concern about rural–urban migration as a potential problem was heightened by the ghetto riots of the time, although suppositions about the rural origins of rioters proved largely unfounded. There also came a growing awareness of increasing urban problems of poverty, pollution, crime, congestion, and other real or suspected effects of large-scale massing of people.

It is ironic that this concern came after the peak of rural-to-urban movement already had passed. Rapid rural outmovement had been occurring since the beginning of World War II. It continued in the 1950s as farms consolidated, and much farm labor became redundant through the continued mechanization of agriculture. From 1940 to 1960 a net average of more than 1 million people left the farms annually, although not all moved to metropolitan cities. By 1965, when alarm over rural-to-urban migration reached the highest political levels, the economy of the nonmetropolitan areas and the social outlook and affluence of metropolitan residents already were changing in ways that would soon lead to a halt in the net rural outflow. Since 1970, changes in rural and urban population flows have occurred so rapidly that nonmetropolitan areas are not only retaining people but are receiving an actual net inmigration as well. Most of our attention here is directed toward this unanticipated event.

Data and Procedures

The basic units in our inquiry are 3100 counties and county equivalents that include the entire population of the nation.[2] We have used a current metropolitan definition, treating as nonmetropolitan only those counties not in Standard Metropolitan Statistical Areas as of September, 1974. (County equivalents for SMSAs were used in New England.) Further residential refinement is obtained through a classification of nonmetropolitan counties as "adjacent" and "not adjacent" to an SMSA. In addition to geographic contiguity, counties to be classed as adjacent had at least 1% of their labor force commuting to the metropolitan central county for work in 1970 (Hines *et al.,* 1975, p. 3).

[2] Alaska is represented by 24 election districts for which comparable census data could be obtained over the time period. The Independent Cities of Virginia were combined with adjacent counties.

We recorded the number of inhabitants in each county for 1950, 1960, and 1970 from published census sources. The amount of net migration for 1950–1960 was taken from data for each county published by the U. S. Bureau of the Census (1962), and comparable data for 1960–1970 were obtained from a computer tape furnished by the bureau.

For the period since the Census of 1970, the best source of population data is the Bureau of the Census Federal–State cooperative series of county estimates, published annually (U. S. Bureau of the Census, 1975a, 1975b). Accurate local population estimates are not easy to make. Nevertheless, the estimates of the bureau for 1966 (the only complete county series in the 1960s) caught clearly the nonmetropolitan turnarounds of that period in the Ozarks, Tennessee Valley, Texas hill country, and Upper Great Lakes cutover lands, although mistaking the direction of trend in the Mississippi Delta. Subsequent improvement of the techniques, corroboration by employment and retirement data, and the strength of the demographic changes now occurring bolster confidence in the current series. Census Bureau staff members also have confirmed the general results of the Federal–State Cooperative series by comparing them with two almost wholly independent sources of data on post-1970 population change (Forstall, 1975). One must not lose sight of the fact that these are estimates, however, and not the result of a census or survey. Although there is reason to have confidence in the general trends, any individual county figure could be in error to a significant degree.

We begin this analysis by comparing annual rates of growth and net migration for groups of counties, differentiating metropolitan counties by size of SMSA, and nonmetropolitan counties by adjacency and by size of largest city in the county. Next, we examine the proportion of counties that are growing and the proportion gaining net migrants over each time period. Nonmetropolitan counties of the nation have been delineated into 26 subregions, and in the following section we compare their growth and migration patterns. Finally, we consider several county characteristics associated with increased or decreased growth in nonmetropolitan areas and discuss the implications of these trends. This research extends earlier work reported by the senior author (Beale, 1975).

Growth and Type of Residence

The remarkable recent reversal of long-term population trends is demonstrated by the growth of nonmetropolitan population of more than 5.6% between April, 1970 and July, 1974, compared with approximately 3.4% in metropolitan counties. Table 8.1 presents these results and also gives

TABLE 8.1.

Population and Net Migration Numbers and Percentages for Metropolitan and Nonmetropolitan Counties, United States 1950–1960, 1960–1970, and 1970–1974[a]

	Total	Metropolitan[b]	Nonmetropolitan
		(Numbers in thousands)	
Population			
1950	151326	100720	50605
1960	179311	127185	52126
1970	203301	148882	54419
1974	211392	153935	57457
Net migration			
1950–1960	2647	8950	−6302
1960–1970	3165	6015	−2850
1970–1974	2069	460	1609
Percentage change in population			
1950–1960	18.5	26.3	3.0
1960–1970	13.4	17.1	4.4
1970–1974	4.0	3.4	5.6
Percentage net migration[c]			
1950–1960	1.7	8.9	−12.5
1960–1970	1.8	4.7	− 5.5
1970–1974	1.0	.3	3.0

[a] The 3100 county units employed here include 24 election districts in Alaska. The independent cities in Virginia were combined with adjacent counties.
[b] Metropolitan counties as of September, 1974.
[c] Based on initial population.

net migration numbers and rates for the three time periods, 1950–1960, 1960–1970, and 1970–1974. In the 1950s more than 6 million people left the counties that were nonmetropolitan as of 1974. Increased retention is evident in the 1960s when the amount of outmigration was more than halved, and in the 1970–1974 period there was a net immigration of more than 1.6 million persons to nonmetropolitan counties. Over the 24-year period the numbers of migrants into metropolitan areas dropped steadily. There was a small net inmovement of people to metropolitan areas in 1970–1974, less than one-third of that to nonmetropolitan areas. Net inmovement could occur in both categories because the total population grew partly by net inmigration from abroad.

A common first reaction to these data and the basic change they indicate is to ask whether the higher nonmetropolitan growth and increase through net migration is not just spreading suburbanization into adjacent metropolitan counties. Answering this question requires a detailed consideration of county location both inside and outside metropolitan areas. The results are presented in Table 8.2. Here and in subsequent tables annual rates of population change and net migration are presented to facilitate comparisons between the two 10-year and the one 4¼-year time periods.[3]

Among metropolitan categories there has been a shift down the size scale in the pattern of growth and gain due to net migration. In the 1950s fringe counties of SMSAs of 1 million or more were growing twice as rapidly as the other groups of metropolitan counties, whereas in the 1970–1974 period they were equalled by SMSAs having less than 250,000 population. The core counties of SMSAs of 1 million grew somewhat less rapidly than the smallest SMSAs between 1950 and 1960, but in the most recent period they ceased to grow at all, and were the only group, metropolitan or nonmetropolitan, that had a negative net migration. Small SMSAs (with fewer than 250,000 people) on the other hand had an increase in the rate of net inmigration, comparing 1970–1974 with 1960–1970.

Nonmetropolitan counties grew less than one-half of 1% a year in the 1960s, but more than 1¼% per year in the early 1970s. The classification of nonmetropolitan counties by adjacency clearly shows that recent growth includes, but is not limited to, metropolitan spillover. The growth of adjacent counties due to net migration, 1 million, is five-eighths of the total of 1.6 million acquired by nonmetropolitan counties. But spillover is not the complete phenomenon. Nonmetropolitan counties that are not adjacent to SMSAs grew more rapidly (and gained more through net migration) than did metropolitan areas. Because a 1974 SMSA designation is used, one might expect in comparing the three time periods that the metropolitan and suburban development of the past 25 years would have caused an increase in the growth advantage of adjacent location. In com-

---

[3] The formulas used to yield annual rates are as follows:

$$\text{Rate of population growth: } \frac{P_2 - P_1}{k(\frac{1}{2})(P_2 + P_1)}\ (100)$$

$$\text{Rate of net migration: } \frac{N}{k(\frac{1}{2})(P_2 + P_1)}\ (100)$$

P_1 and P_2 are the populations at the beginning and end of the time interval, respectively; k is the time interval (10 or 4¼); and N is the number of net migrants (see Shryock et al., 1971, pp. 377–380).

Table 8.2.

Annual Rates of Population Change and Net Migration, by Metropolitan and Nonmetropolitan Location Categories, United States 1950–1960, 1960–1970, and 1970–1974

County characteristic and location	Annual rate of population change			Annual rate of net migration			Number of counties
	1950–1960	1960–1970	1970–1974	1950–1960	1960–1970	1970–1974	
United States	1.69	1.25	.92	.16	.17	.23	3100
Metropolitan	2.32	1.57	.79	.78	.44	.07	629
SMSAs 1 million up							
Core counties	1.70	1.07	−.09	.35	.05	−.69	48
Fringe counties	4.41	2.88	1.54	2.75	1.66	.79	129
SMSAs 250,000 to 1 million	2.37	1.61	1.21	.70	.42	.42	261
SMSAs less than 250,000	2.08	1.43	1.45	.35	.18	.60	191
Nonmetropolitan	.30	.43	1.27	−1.23	−.54	.67	2471
Adjacent	.54	.71	1.42	−.92	−.23	.82	969
SLP 10,000 up[a]	1.11	1.03	1.40	−.40	.01	.72	259
2500 to 10,000	.02	.36	1.39	−1.39	−.50	.87	460
Less than 2500	−.39	.22	1.67	−1.81	−.62	1.18	250
Not adjacent	.05	.14	1.13	−1.53	−.85	.52	1502
SLP 10,000 up[a]	1.04	.63	1.20	−.65	−.53	.44	271
2500 to 10,000	−.45	−.18	.92	−1.98	−1.05	.41	597
Less than 2500	−.99	−.37	1.39	−2.45	−1.17	.97	634

[a] SLP stands for population size of largest place in the county as of 1970.

paring adjacent and nonadjacent counties, however, the differential in population growth and net migration is less in 1970–1974 than in 1960–1970.

To what extent are nonmetropolitan growth and inmigration associated with local urbanizatiòn or the potential development of new metropolitan areas? To examine this question, we classified nonmetropolitan counties, both adjacent and not adjacent to SMSAs, according to the size of the largest incorporated center in the county in 1970. During both 1950–1960 and 1960–1970, counties with larger communities grew more or declined less than other counties and showed a similar relationship with their annual rates of net migration. This was true both for adjacent and nonadjacent counties, with adjacent counties having higher rates within size of place categories. In other words, the pattern of results reveals both a size of place effect and an adjacency effect, consistent with the view that both local urbanization and metropolitan expansion fostered county population increase.

For 1970–1974, however, this pattern is quite different. Within size of place groups, adjacent counties still show higher rates than those not adjacent to SMSAs. But completely rural counties (those with no town of 2500) had the highest rate of population change and net migration in both adjacent and nonadjacent locations. The 629 rural counties *not* adjacent to a SMSA together had a higher rate of inmigration than *any* metropolitan category, and higher than any nonmetropolitan group except for the 274 adjacent rural counties. Among nonadjacent counties, the next highest population change and net migration rates were for those having cities of over 10,000 population. Among adjacent counties, however, the size of place differential is just reversed from that of the previous 2 decades, with counties having places over 10,000 showing the lowest rates, those with places 2500 to 10,000 next, and rural counties with largest place under 2500 showing the highest annual rates of population change and net migration in the entire table.

There is considerable variation among counties that may be obscured by these rates for various aggregates. About 600 nonmetropolitan counties were declining in population in 1970–1974, but this was less than one-half the nearly 1300 counties declining in the 1960s, or the 1457 declining in the 1950s. The percentage of counties growing in population and the percentage gaining by net migration are given in Table 8.3. Four out of 10 nonmetropolitan counties were growing in the 1950s, about one-half in the 1960s, and three-fourths in the early 1970s. Even more striking is the increase in the proportion of nonmetropolitan counties gaining by net migration, from 12 to 22 to 63%. The differentials in proportions by location are consistent with the annual rates in Table 8.2. Note that in 1970–1974

TABLE 8.3.

Percentage of Counties Growing and Percentage Gaining through Net Migration, by Metropolitan and Nonmetropolitan Location, United States 1950–1960, 1960–1970, and 1970–1974

	1950–1960	1960–1970	1970–1974	(N)
Percentage of counties growing				
Metropolitan	89	91	83	629
Nonmetropolitan	41	47	75	2471
Adjacent	51	60	82	969
Not adjacent	34	40	71	1502
All counties	50	56	77	(3100)
Percentage of counties gaining by net migration				
Metropolitan	59	61	64	629
Nonmetropolitan	12	23	63	2471
Adjacent	16	30	67	969
Not adjacent	9	18	60	1502
All counties	21	31	63	(3100)

well over one-half of the counties in all locations were growing, and also well over one-half were gaining net migrants. Differentials, particularly between metropolitan and nonmetropolitan counties, are considerably less than before, although an individual county still is slightly more likely to grow or gain net migrants if it is metropolitan.

A Subregional Comparison

Our concern thus far has been with general patterns within the nation as a whole. Yet we know there are important economic and social differences between geographic subareas of nonmetropolitan America and that these differences influence population trends. For another study, we delineated 26 subregions by grouping together State Economic Areas reasonably similar in economy, history, physical setting, settlement patterns and culture (Beale and Fuguitt, 1975). These subregions are shown in Figure 8.1, and in Figures 8.2 and 8.3 we present for them the annual rates of nonmetropolitan population change and net migration over 1950–1960, 1960–1970, and 1970–1974.

Considering first the old trend, prior to 1970, several patterns are evident. Extensive rural outmigration continuing through both decades char-

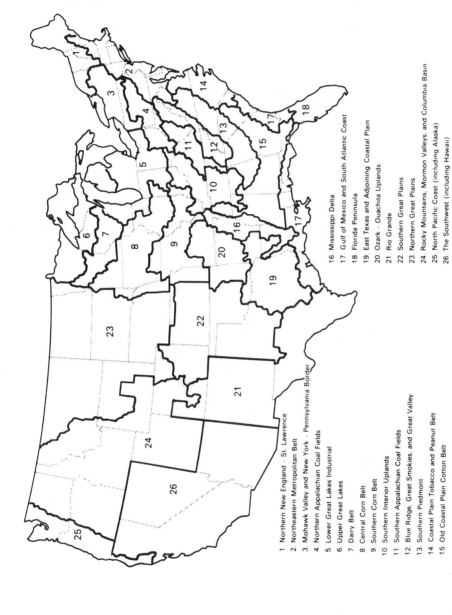

1. Northern New England - St. Lawrence
2. Northeastern Metropolitan Belt
3. Mohawk Valley and New York - Pennsylvania Border
4. Northern Appalachian Coal Fields
5. Lower Great Lakes Industrial
6. Upper Great Lakes
7. Dairy Belt
8. Central Corn Belt
9. Southern Corn Belt
10. Southern Interior Uplands
11. Southern Appalachian Coal Fields
12. Blue Ridge, Great Smokies, and Great Valley
13. Southern Piedmont
14. Coastal Plain Tobacco and Peanut Belt
15. Old Coastal Plain Cotton Belt
16. Mississippi Delta
17. Gulf of Mexico and South Atlantic Coast
18. Florida Peninsula
19. East Texas and Adjoining Coastal Plain
20. Ozark - Ouachita Uplands
21. Rio Grande
22. Southern Great Plains
23. Northern Great Plains
24. Rocky Mountains, Mormon Valleys, and Columbia Basin
25. North Pacific Coast (including Alaska)
26. The Southwest (including Hawaii)

Figure 8.1. Subregions for the analysis of United States nonmetropolitan population change.

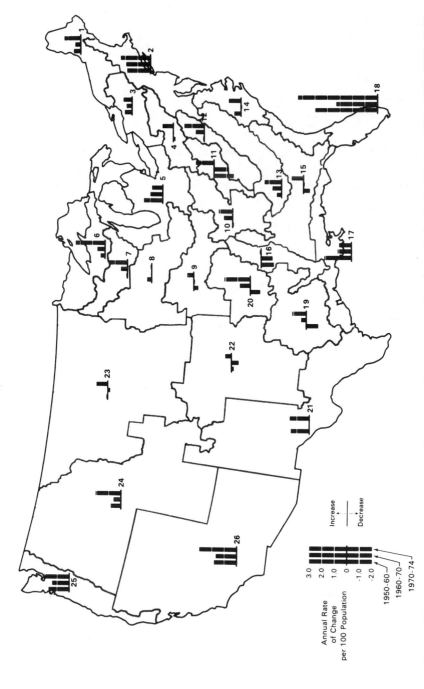

Figure 8.2. Annual rates of nonmetropolitan population change, subregions of the United States, 1950–1960, 1960–1970, 1970–1974.

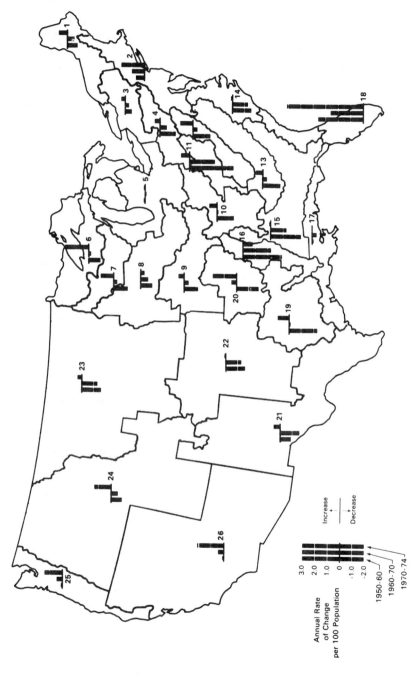

Figure 8.3. Nonmetropolitan annual net migration rates, subregions of the United States, 1950–1960, 1960–1970, 1970–1974.

acterized several subregions. In the northern and southern Great Plains (Subs. 22, 23) population declined in both decades, but rates of outmigration were lower in the latter decade. This area of commercial grain and cattle agriculture has the nation's greatest number of declining counties. The old Cotton Belt subregions with a large black population (Subs. 15 and 16) have a pattern similar to that in the Great Plains. These subregions had nonmetropolitan population decline in both decades, although both this decline and net migration loss were less in the second decade. The Southern Appalachians (Sub. 11), widely recognized as a rural problem area, had the largest rates of population decline and net outmigration for 1950–1960 and 1960–1970 among all 26 subregions, although again losses were less in the 1960s than the 1950s.

Another pattern is exemplified by three turnaround subregions in the South (Subs. 10, 19, and 20). These predominantly white areas were well along in their shift from agriculture by 1960. During the succeeding decade they had rapid nonagricultural economic growth, being major beneficiaries of the decentralization trend of manufacturing that took place in the 1960s. The Ozark–Ouachita area also had extensive development of reservoir centered recreation and retirement districts. These areas all went from population decline in the 1950s to growth in the 1960s. The Ozark–Ouachita subregion went from negative to positive net migration as well, with the other two moving from large to small negative net migration figures.

The Upper Great Lakes and the Dairy belt (Subs. 6 and 7) showed a marked increase in nonmetropolitan population growth, and corresponding decline in net outmigration, for 1960–1970 as compared with 1950–1960. Such increased growth was a turnaround for these northern areas, many of which had suffered widespread earlier decline from the exhaustion of timber and mining resources or from farming adjustments. Exurban sprawl around the Twin Cities area was no doubt one factor in the Dairy subregion, but increased retirement and recreation settlement, along with some gain in manufacturing employment, are considered major factors in the postwar growth of these upper middle west areas.

The Blue Ridge and Southern Piedmont areas (Subs. 12 and 13) also increased in population growth in the 1960s compared with the 1950s. Most other areas, however, went in the other direction, with lower growth rates in the 1960s than the 1950s. The Coastal Tobacco and Peanut Belt (Sub. 14) went from growth to decline, as did the Northern Great Plains already mentioned. The largest decline, however, was found in the Rio Grande subregion (Sub. 21), which went from 1.5% growth per year in the 1950s to essentially zero in the 1960s. Parts of this region went through exceptional growth from military or mining developments in the 1950s, followed by comparative stability or outright decline in the 1960s.

The Northeastern Metropolitan Belt (Sub. 2), Florida (Sub. 8), the Northern Pacific Coast (Sub. 25), and the Southwest (Sub. 26) all had rapid nonmetropolitan population increase between 1950 and 1970, and were the only subregions with net migration gain over both decades.

Turning now to the most recent period, 1970–1974, Figures 8.2 and 8.3 clearly show that the recent upsurge in nonmetropolitan growth is not restricted to a few selected areas of the nation. All 26 subregions experienced population growth between 1970 and 1974, and in 24 of the 26, the rate of growth was higher than in the 1960s. The only exceptions were the Lower Great Lakes Industrial Belt (Sub. 5) and the Gulf of Mexico and South Atlantic Coast (Sub. 17). In the 1960s, 7 subregions were declining in population, and they all reversed from decline to growth in 1970–1974. These include the Northern and Southern Great Plains (Subs. 22 and 23), the Southern Corn Belt (Sub. 9), the Mississippi Delta (Sub. 16), the Cotton Belt (Sub. 15), the Coastal Plain Tobacco and Peanut Belt (Sub. 14), and the Southern Appalachians (Sub. 11). The turnaround areas of the 1960s, moreover (Subs. 10, 19, and 20) accelerated their growth, with annual rates approximately twice as great or more in 1970–1974 as in 1960–1970. After no growth in the 1960s, the Rio Grande (Sub. 21) bounced back with a higher rate of growth in the early 1970s than in the 1950s.

Perhaps the most noticeable feature of the net migration map is the orderly progression over the three periods, found in 22 of the 26 subregions, toward less outmigration or more inmigration. Although most subregions were losing net migrants in the 1960s, this period had increased retention of the population compared with the 1950s, in the sense that either net outmigration was less or net inmigration was more. The trend from the 1950s to the 1960s anticipated the major switch from outmigration to inmigration in the latest period, when the number of subregions gaining net migrants was 23 compared with 5 in 1960–1970. The only 2 areas with net migration losses in the most recent period, the Mississippi Delta and the Cotton Belt (Subs. 16 and 15), both still have a large black population.

Some County Characteristics Associated with Growth

One major social trend in the United States since World War II has been expansion and development of institutions of higher learning. Many of these institutions are located in nonmetropolitan areas and represent an important economic resource and stimulus for population growth. Possible indirect effects also should not be overlooked. These institutions have greatly increased the availability and quality of higher education in nonmetropolitan areas and have made the affected communities more attractive for other development.

TABLE 8.4.

Annual Rates of Population Change and Net Migration by Presence of a Senior State College in the County, Net Inmigration at Retirement Ages, and Concentration of Military Personnel, Nonmetropolitan United States 1950–1960, 1960–1970, and 1970–1974

County characteristic and location	Annual rate of population change			Annual rate of net migration			Number of counties
	1950–1960	1960–1970	1970–1974	1950–1960	1960–1970	1970–1974	
Presence of senior state college in county							
County is adjacent to SMSA							
State college	.88	1.46	1.74	–.61	.40	1.02	75
No	.50	.59	1.37	–.96	–.33	.79	894
County not adjacent to SMSA							
State college	.84	1.00	1.47	–.76	–.13	.72	111
No	–.09	–.03	1.05	–1.67	–.99	.48	1391
Net inmigration rate, 1960–1970, for white persons 60 years old and over in 1970							
County is adjacent to SMSA							
15% or more	2.11	2.89	4.43	.89	2.17	4.09	89
10–14%	.43	1.13	2.16	–1.06	.15	1.50	72
Other	.43	.47	1.03	–1.05	–.49	.40	808
County not adjacent to SMSA							
15% or more	.54	1.60	3.19	–.78	.80	2.73	118
10–14%	.02	.63	1.76	–1.45	–.23	1.27	90
Other	.02	–.01	.88	–1.59	–1.02	.26	1294
Percentage of total population who are military personnel							
10% or more	4.53	2.08	–.30	2.08	.13	–1.86	28
Less than 10%	.23	.39	1.31	–1.21	–.55	.65	2443

The first panel of Table 8.4 classifies counties according to adjacency and presence of a 4-year state college. Counties with state colleges had higher growth rates in all three time periods than those that do not. The effect of having a state college against lacking one appears to be greatest on county growth and net migration in the 1960s and least in the 1970–1974 period.

Eventually, counties with senior state colleges may experience a drop in students if the decline in the birth rate since 1960 leads to reduced college enrollments. But communities and counties containing state colleges are unlikely to return to their earlier size and status.

An increasingly important factor in nonmetropolitan development has been the growth of recreation and retirement activities, often occurring together in the same localities. Recreational employment is not easily determined from available data, but by means of net migration estimates by age it is possible to identify counties receiving significant numbers of retired people. Using unpublished estimates prepared by Gladys Bowles of the Economic Research Service, counties were identitied in which there was a net inmigration, 1960 to 1970, of 10 to 14%, or 15% or more, of white residents who were age 60 and over in 1970. There is a strong consistent association between the migration of older people and total population growth and net migration, for both adjacent and nonadjacent counties. Overall growth rates since 1970 are very rapid in the primary retirement counties, with an annual growth of more than 4% in the adjacent class and 3% in the nonadjacent class. Such rates lead to substantial changes in the scale and character of communities if sustained for very long.

In contrast to the lessening import of having a college, the growth differential associated with net migration of older people is greater in 1970–1974 than in 1960–1970. Nonadjacent counties with less than 10% migration of older people had a low rate of population growth and net migration in the early 1970s, but these figures were still above the rates for all metropolitan counties. (There is negligible overlap between the state college and retirement counties.)

Military activity was a major rural growth industry in the period following World War II. Military bases were disproportionately located in nonmetropolitan areas, and they employed many civilians as well as military personnel. Since 1970 the number of armed forces personnel stationed in the United States has declined about 20%. We have identified nonmetropolitan counties—there are only 28 in all—where 10% or more of the total 1970 population consisted of military personnel. Table 8.4 shows that these counties grew very rapidly in the 1950s, less so in the 1960s, and actually declined in the 1970s. Decade percentage change figures for

1950–1960 and 1960–1970 were 59 and 23%, respectively. These counties also shifted from gain to loss due to net migration, with a net outmovement of 92,000 people over 1970–1974.

We also have considered two other variables known to be associated with nonmetropolitan population loss, black population and agricultural employment. Among the most uniformly heavy losers of population in prior decades were the nonmetropolitan counties of the South having a predominantly black population. Table 8.5 gives annual rates of population change and net migration for nonmetropolitan counties in the Census South classed by the percentage of the population black at the beginning of each decade. In counties with more than 40% of their population black, there is outmigration over each time period and generally a decline in population as well. But the rate of outmigration is greatly reduced in 1970–1974, compared with earlier years. In the 1950s and 1960s counties with very low proportions of blacks (less than 5%) also were declining and losing due to net migration. Most rapid growth or slowest decline was among the counties from 5 to 40% black. A new pattern emerged in the early 1970s, however. Among counties adjacent to SMSAs, those with less than 5% of their population black were growing rapidly and gaining from net migration. In nonadjacent counties also, the group with lowest proportions black were growing and gaining net migrants, more rapidly than counties with higher percentages of blacks. Many counties in the southern subregions of population turnaround have a very low proportion black.

TABLE 8.5

Annual Rates of Population Change and Net Migration for Counties Classified by Percentage of the Population at the Beginning of Each Decade Who Are Black, Nonmetropolitan South, 1950–1960, 1960–1970, and 1970–1974

Percentage population black in county	Annual rate of population change			Annual rate of net migration		
	1950–1960	1960–1970	1970–1974	1950–1960	1960–1970	1970–1974
Adjacent to SMSA						
0–4	−.18	.34	1.60	−1.75	− .59	1.01
5–19	.20	.99	2.04	−1.36	− .04	1.37
20–39	.47	.53	1.46	−1.25	− .55	.78
40 up	−.27	−.33	.59	−2.30	−1.63	− .23
Not adjacent to SMSA						
0–4	−.81	.06	1.46	−2.30	− .91	.95
5–19	−.12	.72	1.09	−1.67	− .28	.40
20–39	.04	.31	1.13	−1.75	− .81	.38
40 up	−.35	−.69	− .06	−2.45	−2.00	− .89

TABLE 8.6

Annual Rates of Population Change and Net Migration for Counties Classified by Percentage of the Employed Population Who Are in Agriculture at the Beginning of Each Decade, Nonmetropolitan United States 1950–1960, 1960–1970, and 1970–1974

Percentage of employed in agriculture in the county	Annual rate of population change			Annual rate of net migration		
	1950–1960	1960–1970	1970–1974	1950–1960	1960–1970	1970–1974
Adjacent to SMSA						
0–4	− .20	1.02	1.42	−1.58	.08	.75
5–9	1.38	1.01	1.42	.00	.02	.81
10–19	1.12	.90	1.60	− .30	− .03	1.08
20–29	.99	.35	1.04	− .47	− .54	.51
30–39	.38	.01	.45	−1.09	− .93	.14
40 up	− .54	− .74	− .08	−2.10	−1.79	− .90
Not adjacent to SMSA						
0–4	− .49	.05	1.23	−2.23	−1.16	.46
5–9	.85	.66	1.47	− .82	− .47	.84
10–19	.88	.59	1.10	− .65	− .37	.57
20–29	.55	.06	.47	−1.02	− .79	.12
30–39	.20	− .54	− .01	−1.34	−1.37	− .20
40 up	− .90	−1.12	− .02	−2.47	−2.00	− .31

As the demand for farm labor has decreased, nonmetropolitan counties in the United States with a high proportion of their workforce employed in agriculture have tended to have substantial population loss. Counties were classed by the percentage of the employed persons engaged in agriculture at the beginning of each decade (Table 8.6). Counties with more than 40% of their workforce in agriculture had a net migration loss over all three time periods, and generally experienced population decline as well, although there is improved population retention and a lower rate of outmigration in the 1970–1974 period. In the 1950s for both locations and also in the 1960s for those not adjacent to an SMSA, counties with less than 5% of the workforce in agriculture also declined in population or lost migrants, but by 1970–1974 these counties had relatively high rates of growth and gain due to net migration. This pattern is rather like that just described for the proportion black in the South. Over the nation it is often the areas with little farming activity (and a small black population) that have scenic qualities, including wilderness and lakes or reservoirs, and thus are attractive for recreation activities and retirement residents. Many such areas also have gained new manufacturing employment in recent years.

Attracting new industry has been a cornerstone in rural development programs aimed at reversing population decline. Indeed, the decentralization trend in U. S. manufacturing has been a major factor in transforming the rural and small town economy, especially in the upland parts of the South. To test the assumption often made that manufacturing is associated with nonmetropolitan growth, we have classified nonmetropolitan counties in Table 8.7 by the percentage of employed population in manufacturing at the beginning of each decade. For the first 2 decades there is a consistent stepwise relationship in the expected direction. Whether adjacent or not adjacent to an SMSA, counties have higher rates of growth (or lower decline) in population and net migration the higher the proportion employed in manufacturing.

With the new trend in 1970–1974, however, this is not the case, for counties intermediate in manufacturing concentration show the greatest gains in population and net migration. Thus although growth in manufacturing has been important in the revival of nonmetropolitan population growth, the recent shift in population trends has not been focused on areas already heavily dependent on manufacturing. Nor did we find 1970–1974 growth to be greatest in counties with the largest percentage increase in the number employed in manufacturing over 1960–1970 (tabulation not

TABLE 8.7

Annual Rates of Population Change and Net Migration for Counties Classified by Percentage of Employed Population Who Are in Manufacturing at the Beginning of Each Decade, Nonmetropolitan United States, 1950–1960, 1960–1970, and 1970–1974

Percentage of employed in manufacturing in the county	Annual rate of population change			Annual rate of net migration		
	1950–1960	1960–1970	1970–1974	1950–1960	1960–1970	1970–1974
Adjacent to SMSA						
0–4	.21	.07	1.69	−1.46	−1.30	.82
5–9	.36	.79	1.87	−1.15	− .22	1.13
10–19	.15	.73	2.09	−1.23	− .15	1.62
20–29	.79	.57	1.31	− .54	− .27	.80
30 up	.98	.80	1.07	− .52	− .17	.41
Not adjacent to SMSA						
0–4	− .34	− .52	.41	−2.08	−1.57	− .32
5–9	− .18	− .36	1.52	−1.80	−1.47	.83
10–19	.10	.32	1.10	−1.41	− .64	.52
20–29	.47	.41	1.22	− .96	− .41	.72
30 up	.65	.44	1.05	− .86	− .58	.48

included here). There is evidence that growth in employment in trade and other nongoodsproducing sectors has recently become more important in nonmetropolitan areas. Data on covered social security employment show that manufacturing jobs comprised just 18% of all nonmetropolitan employment growth between 1969 and 1973, compared with 50% from 1962 to 1969.

We have shown that southern nonmetropolitan counties with a high percentage black, and all nonmetropolitan counties with a high percentage of their workforce in agriculture and/or a low percentage in manufacturing have had net outmigration and slow growth or decline over the three time periods. A significant trend during this time has been a decline in the proportion of nonmetropolitan people who live in these types of counties. In the South in 1950, 23% of the nonmetropolitan population lived in counties in which more than 4 out of 10 persons were black, whereas 15% did so in 1970. The proportion of the U.S. nonmetropolitan population living in counties with more than 4 out of 10 employed persons in agriculture dropped from 31 to less than 1% over this 20-year interval. In 1950, 39% of the nonmetropolitan population lived in counties with fewer than 1 out of 10 employed persons in manufacturing, but this figure dropped to 18% by 1970. We entered the 1970s, then, with a considerably lower proportion of nonmetropolitan people living in traditional settings of population decline. This shift in population composition facilitated the recent growth in many parts of nonmetropolitan America.

Conclusion

The United States has entered a period of greatly reduced growth for its major metropolitan areas and of largely unpredicted demographic revival for most of its rural and small town areas. How long this will last is unknown, but the effect is already significant and none of us has ever seen its like before. The net movement into the nonmetropolitan areas is now as rapid as the movement out of them was in the 1960s, although not yet as strong as the high tide of metropolitanization of the 1950s.

Our presentation of the geographic dimensions of recent change reveals the pervasive nature of the emergent trend. The new pattern is not merely a heightened metropolitan sprawl; neither is it a feature of a few areas or a limited number of circumstances.

We have not attempted here to go deeply into the causes of the phenomenon, or to evaluate its effects. However, we have no hesitation in asserting that noneconomic factors are playing a critical role in the new trend. Will the shift in the direction of net migration result merely in an

urbanization of more sections of the country or a greater contextual rural-
ization of a larger segment of the population? Perhaps both will occur,
although we found that in contrast with earlier times the most rapid nonmetropolitan growth in the 1970s was in entirely rural counties. Under
conditions of general affluence, low total population increase, easy access
to all areas, modernization of rural life, and large metropolitan concentrations in which the advantages of urban life are seen to be diminished, a
downward shift to smaller communities may be both feasible and desirable.

As Hawley points out, the historical basis of much of our knowledge of
population trends has meant that one component after another of that
knowledge has tended to become obsolete before it has been perfected.
We believe that today the rules of reference for our thinking about the
residential distribution of the population are changed just as surely as the
events of the late 1940s shocked a reluctant demographic fraternity into a
reapprasial of the possibilities in fertility trends. We also strongly suspect
that, as with the postwar baby boom, trends of the type described here are
unlikely to be limited to only one nation in the Western world. At least for
the United States in the early 1970s, migration and population growth are
not simply part of an irreversible trend of metropolitan concentration reflecting the inexorable force of advantages of scale.

ACKNOWLEDGMENTS

The maps were prepared by the Cartographic Laboratory of the University of Wisconsin–Madison. The assistance of Vera Banks and David Brown, of the Economic Development Division, USDA, and Philip Groth, Louisiana State University, and Mary Jacobs,
the University of Wisconsin–Madison, is gratefully acknowledged.

References

Beale, C. L.
   1975   The Revival of Population Growth in Nonmetropolitan America. Economic Re-
           search Service, U. S. Department of Agriculture, ERS-605.
Beale, C. L., and G. V. Fuguitt
   1975   "Population trends of nonmetropolitan cities and villages in subregions of the
           United States." Center for Demography and Ecology Working Paper 75-30.
Forstall, R. L.
   1975   "Trends in metropolitan and nonmetropolitan population growth since 1970."
           Paper presented at the NICHD Conference on Population Distribution, Belmont
           (Baltimore, Maryland).
Hines, F. K., D. L. Brown, and J. M. Zimmer
   1975   Social and Economic Characteristics of the Population in Metro and Nonmetro
           Counties, 1970. Economic Research Service, U. S. Department of Agriculture,
           Agricultural Economic Report No. 272, March.

Shryock, H. S., J. S. Siegel, and associates
1971   *The Methods and Materials of Demography.* Washington, D. C.: U. S. Government Printing Office.

U. S. Bureau of the Census
1962   "Components of population change, 1950 to 1960, for counties, standard metropolitan statistical areas . . . . ," *Current Population Reports,* Series P-23, No. 7, November.

1975a   "Estimates of the population of . . . ." *Current Population Reports,* Population Estimates and Projections, Series P-25, Nos. 596 (Maryland), 597 (Washington), 599 (New York), 602 (Oregon), 604 (Alaska), and 609 (Texas).

1975b   "Estimates of the population of . . . ." *Current Population Reports,* Federal–State Cooperative Program for Population Estimates, Series P-26, Nos. 94–138 for individual states except those reported in P-25 Series listed above.

III
SOCIAL MOBILITY

9

Mobility and Stratification:
An Overview

DAVID D. McFARLAND

As the author of an overview chapter, I take my task to include: discussion of how mobility and stratification, the topic of this section, relates to social demography, the topic of the entire volume; discussion of the place of this section's chapters within the larger body of earlier, current, and needed research on mobility and stratification; and, more generally, discussion of the current state, trends, and prospects of research on mobility and stratification. Clearly a single chapter-length work cannot give exhaustive treatment of all these matters, but I will at least touch on each.

Social Demography and Social Stratification:
Definitions and Relationship

Demography, like any other field of study, consists of a body of knowledge and speculation and a set of research tools. Demographic knowledge and speculation pertain to the size of a population; its composition by age, sex, and region; and changes therein through the processes of fertility, mortality, and migration. Specifically demographic research tools—as

Social Demography

contrasted with those demography shares with other fields—include life table analysis, cohort analysis, standardization and decomposition of differences, and stable population techniques.

Social demography, then, might be defined as consisting of that body of work relating demography, thus defined, to other fields in the social sciences. This would include work on nondemographic determinants of demographic phenomena, such as Beckman's work in this volume on the effects of decision-making processes on fertility (see Chapter 4). It would also include work on demographic determinants of nondemographic phenomena, such as Keyfitz's (1973) study, which subsequently I shall discuss further, of the effects of different mortality levels on opportunity for advancement within an organizational hierarchy. And it would include the application of demographic tools to nondemographic problems, such as Featherman and Hauser's use of decomposition techniques to study not differences in fertility or mortality, but rather differences in educational or occupational attainment (Chapter 10 of this volume).

Social stratification concerns the unequal distribution of things that are widely desired, such as money or deference. *Social mobility* concerns change over time in an individual's attainment, or change from generation to generation in a family's attainment, of things that are widely desired.

Education and occupation—both of which are widely desired either for their own sakes or as means to more remote ends—are central to the Chapter 10 by Featherman and Hauser, and Chapter 11 by Winsborough. Age, one of the central variables of demography as narrowly defined here, plays a central role in these chapters, as does the notion of changing composition of a population, although they focus primarily on composition according to race, education, and occupation rather than on composition according to the more narrowly demographic characteristics of age, sex, and region. Furthermore, demographic techniques are employed; in particular, standardization and decomposition of differences and cohort analysis.

Thus the chapters by Featherman and Hauser and by Winsborough fall within social demography, as I have defined it, on two different grounds. First, they relate narrowly demographic variables (in particular, age or birth cohort) to variables of concern in the social stratification field (in particular, education and occupation). Second, they utilize specifically demographic research tools (in particular, cohort analysis and standardization and decomposition of differences) on problems that are not narrowly demographic—that do not lie within demography as I have defined it.

Chapter 12 by Singer and Spilerman, although a purely technical exposition devoid of substantive content, pertains to a technique that has been

used—and misused—in studying both the narrowly demographic phenomenon of migration and the phenomenon of social mobility. Thus its
inclusion may be justified on the grounds that it contributes to the development of demographic methods which elsewhere in the literature, although not in this paper itself, have been put to use on problems in the
social stratification area.

Other scholars might define demography, and likewise social stratification, differently than I have just done. But at least my definitions provide
one reasonable account of how it is that a demography conference happens to include a couple of papers on educational and occupational attainment and a paper on a particular branch of probability theory, namely
Markov processes.

To avoid possible misunderstanding, I should explicitly note that social
stratification, the topic of this session, does *not* fall completely within social demography. Many specialists in stratification have no demographic
training; Hope (1972), for example, was trained as a psychometrician. Indeed, many universities are organized in a manner that discourages contact between demographers and stratification specialists. At Harvard, for
example, demography is within the School of Public Health, which is or-
ganizationally distinct and physically isolated from the Sociology Department. Even in the University of Wisconsin where demography is within
the Sociology Department and where (subject to that one limitation) the
term *demographer* is used in the broadest possible sense (roughly, any
sociologist who can count), there exist nondemographers studying social
stratification.

Furthermore, a goodly number of stratification specialists would reject
not only the notion that their field is a subfield of social *demography,* but
also the notion that it is a subfield of social *science.* They do not study
such phenomena as occupational attainment, but rather such phenomena
as "oppression" by the "monopoly capitalist class." Their norms are primarily those of political advocacy rather than those of scientific investigation. (They commonly argue, however, with some justification in my
opinion, that self-proclaimed followers of the norms of scientific investigation do not follow those norms either, that the real difference is not
whether one's political values do or do not affect one's research, but
rather whether one's political values appear in one's work explicitly, or
only implicitly and covertly.) Thus their writing includes relatively more
political rhetoric and relatively less empirical evidence than stratification
work of social demographers—and their value-laden statements are explicit and intentional, rather than unwitting departures from the norms of
scientific impartiality.

However, this dichotomy, like most dichotomies, does not work very well in actual practice. Scientists, as well as political advocates, have values, and their work too contains value statements—only usually in less explicit form. Hauser and Featherman (1975, p. 3), for example, at one point shift from the value-neutral term *inequalities* to the value-laden term *inequities,* and also characterize social inequalities as constituting "social problems." Their paper implicity contains the value premise that reduction of inequality is desirable. Now I have no particular quarrel with that premise—I merely want to point out that it falls in the realm of political values, not in the realm of scientific facts or hypotheses. But Hauser and Featherman were mentioned only because they provide an example readily at hand; the practice of implicitly including political values in one's research is really quite widespread among social scientists. This is one reason for my assertion that there is not as great a gap as often supposed between political advocates and social scientists who both proclaim interest in social stratification.

A second reason is that one sometimes observes great similarities in the treatment of factual matters among scholars who differ greatly in the amount and nature of political rhetoric in their work. When it comes to questions of fact, we now have very similar questions being studied by sociologists of such disparate political views as Laumann and Zeitlin. Both are at work determining just which individuals and groups wield most power and influence, what interactions and bonds unite them, what mechanisms they collectively use to maintain their power and influence, and so on. (See Laumann, 1973; Laumann and Pappi, 1973; Zeitlin, 1974; Zeitlin *et al.,* 1974.) Such similarities in the treatment of factual questions should not be overlooked; one should definitely look beyond differences in rhetoric.

A third and final reason for my assertion that the political advocates and the social scientists are not as far apart as commonly supposed relates to a trend I think I see. (Here I remind you that the overview chapter is supposed to detect trends and otherwise comment on the future of the research area.) This trend is the increasing incidence in sociological writings of explicitly stated social goals and attention to possible means of attaining those goals.

There are at least three distinguishable manifestations of this trend. First, it appears in the increasing attention given to "policy implications" of research. A cynic may discount this as motivated by desires to find new funding sources in the face of cutbacks by sources that have been funding "pure research," and by desires to find new types of employment for people with doctorates in the face of a declining academic job market; but whatever the motivation may be, the effects of increasing attention to policy implications will be an important aspect of social research in the foreseeable future. Second, this trend appears in the "social indicators" movement. A *social indicator*, according to one widely quoted definitional statement (U. S. Department of Health, Education, and Welfare, 1969, p. 97) "is in all cases a direct measure of welfare and is subject to the interpretation that, if it changes in the 'right' direction, while other things remain equal, things have gotten better, or people are 'better off'." Thus a listing of social indicators constitutes a setting forth of social goals. Third, this trend appears in a shift in emphasis among mathematical sociologists and others who utilize formal models, a shift away from "descriptive" models, which merely tell how things are, and away from "predictive" models, which typically tell how things would be in the future were present trends to persist, and toward "normative" or "purposive" models, which tell how one might best go about trying to influence the future in the pursuit of explicitly stated goals.

Comparative Social Stratification

Featherman (1974) published a cautiously optimistic paper on the second generation of national mobility studies then underway or in the planning stage. The various investigators were meeting and exchanging ideas, all of which was taken as a basis for optimism about eventual, if not immediate, comparability across nations.

Comparability may indeed eventually be achieved, but it is by no means the automatic consequence of a few meetings of people who share the same research interest. Two powerful enemies of comparability are firmly entrenched in the system of science.

First, the notion of progress in technique and the accompanying urge always to use the best techniques currently available create tremendous pressure *not* to strictly replicate previous studies, for that would require using crude tools when better tools are now available. And in sociology newer tools measure phenomena *differently,* not just to a few more significant digits of accuracy.

Second, the reward structure of science does not adequately reflect the scientific importance of what is all too frequently discounted as "mere" replication, and regarded as a task only slightly more elevated than that of writing introductory textbooks. The emphasis placed on "original" research at "the frontiers of knowledge" implies a corresponding deemphasis on replication studies. In addition, replication is sometimes much more difficult than it might seem in that the documentation of earlier studies is often severely deficient.

An example of the results of such forces may be seen in the evolution of the goals of the Oxford study of social mobility conducted by Gold-thorpe, Hope, and others. In the first volume of papers, Hope (1972, p. 1) stated the main goals of the project as a comparison of present British mobility patterns with, on the one hand, earlier British mobility patterns as observed by Glass (1954), and with, on the other hand, U. S. mobility patterns as observed by Blau and Duncan (1967). Yet only 2 years later those goals had slipped from sight; Goldthorpe and Hope (1974) instead constructed from scratch a new scale for occupations, a scale that is poorly suited for making either of the two comparisons previously considered of central importance. Their scale is, insofar as I can tell, a good one—much better than either the Hall–Jones scale or the Duncan Scale (see my review, McFarland, 1975). In particular, Hope and Goldthorpe went to some lengths in their attempt to minimize what had been an important problem with previous occupational scales, namely the internal heterogeneity of the occupational categories to which scale values are assigned. Nevertheless, the new scale creates serious problems for anyone wishing to interpret observed differences between two mobility studies: To what extent are they real differences in mobility patterns, and to what extent are they artifacts of differences in the two occupation scales along which mobility was measured in the two studies?

Comparability requires that one carefully duplicate the procedures used by previous investigators, resisting the strong temptation to invent new procedures, no matter how much better the new procedures might be. Some investigators may decide that the value of a careful replication of previous studies exceeds the value of a noncomparable study using improved procedures; other investigators may decide the opposite; but only in very special cases may one investigator have it both ways.

It is perhaps worthy of mention, in the midst of demographers who tend to be quantitatively oriented, that *qualitative* conclusions are much more readily compared than quantitative results. For example, estimation of the Blau–Duncan model on Yugoslavian data to obtain results that would be meaningfully comparable to those from U. S. data would probably be out of the question at present, even though Caserman (1973) and Saksida *et al.* (1974) have begun publishing quantitative results of their study. Yet certain qualitative comparisons may readily be made. For example, it is quite clear that despite years of a socialist political system, women in Yugoslavia are still discriminated against in the occupational sphere, just as women in the U. S. have been (Mezhnarich and Josifovski, 1974).

Comparative studies, whether the comparisons be between nations or over time within a single nation, are fraught with difficulties, and quantitative studies that are truly comparable remain mainly in the realm of hopes rather than in the realm of actual accomplishments.

Mortality as a Determinant of Social Mobility

There is an anomaly about a review of social demography, which has chapters on a marginal topic such as social stratification while having none on a core demographic topic such as mortality. I am not prepared to rectify fully the situation, but I will make a token gesture in that direction by mentioning the relationship between mortality and opportunity for social mobility.

Mortality facilitates upward mobility, not only for those departed who move from earth to heaven, but also for those left behind who are promoted to fill the positions previously held by the departed, for those promoted to fill the positions previously held by those promoted to fill the positions previously held by the departed, and so on, as far as one wishes to trace the chain of promotions generated by a death. Mortality does not facilitate upward mobility, however, in cases where the dead are persons who would otherwise have been one's benefactors rather than one's competitors. These matters have been the subject of several investigations, some primarily theoretical and others primarily empirical.

White (1970) has been the main advocate among sociologists for what he calls the vacancy chain approach to social mobility. He has emphasized the importance of considering the chain of upward moves by different persons, all of which are generated by a single death (or retirement), rather than considering the sequence of upward moves by a single person during the course of his career. (Perhaps it should be mentioned that not all of the moves White observed were clearly "upward," there being no really clearly defined hierarchical ordering of pastorates within the church denominations he studied.)

Keyfitz (1973), in his paper on individual mobility in a stationary population, provided a theoretical analysis of the rather remarkable extent to which plausible variations in mortality affect the speed with which an individual advances relative to other members of the population—always subject to the proviso that mortality claims only his competitors and not the focal individual himself. Keyfitz showed that plausible variations in mortality could determine whether it required several years or several decades to reach a specified fractile on the seniority distribution.

Mortality of those who would otherwise have been one's benefactors does not facilitate upward mobility. In particular, the absence of a father during one's formative years has substantial negative effects on one's educational attainment (note the effects of the "broken family" variable in the analyses by Featherman and Hauser in Chapter 10).

The Organization as a Context for Mobility

One point on which there appears to be some growing agreement is that students of social mobility should not confine themselves entirely to national samples. For at least some purposes one is better off focusing on smaller, more tightly interdependent social systems, ones whose personnel are less diverse than the populace at large, and perhaps ones that have some centralized personnel planning and policymaking.

An interesting puzzle I sometimes assign to my students is to resolve the apparent discrepancy between a paper by Hodge (1966) and one by Vroom and MacCrimmon (1968), both of which use Markov models in relation to the concept of "careers." Hodge uses a Markov chain as a "baseline" model for careers; that is, observed deviation from, rather than observed fit to, a Markov chain is the empirical finding Hodge takes as providing evidence that men experience careers as opposed to haphazard moves from job to job. Vroom and MacCrimmon take a Markov chain as both a "descriptive" model of careers and a "predictive" model of careers; that is, a model that both corresponds to previous moves of career men and is anticipated to correspond to their future moves. Vroom and MacCrimmon take the predictions of a Markov chain to describe careers, while Hodge takes observed *deviations from* the predictions of a Markov chain to describe careers.

Now this question is an ideal essay question, in that it involves a large number of subtleties, more than any one student is likely to include in his answer. But one set of differences is crucial. The population considered by Vroom and MacCrimmon is that of the managerial personnel of a single firm, while the personnel considered by Hodge constitute roughly a representative sample of urban U. S. males. Correspondingly, the classifications used by Vroom and MacCrimmon are much finer than those used by Hodge. This makes a great difference on the question of how well the Markovian postulate holds in the two studies: the "current state" of a Vroom and MacCrimmon subject (for example, Engineering, level 2) tells a great deal more about that person than does the "current state" of a Hodge subject (for example, upper white-collar). Furthermore, the "current state" of a Vroom and MacCrimmon subject tells something about his past: Someone currently in Engineering, level 2, is highly likely to have previously been in Engineering, level 1; this is in contrast to the

Hodge study where, for example, the fact that someone is currently in upper white-collar does not make it particularly likely that he has previously been in lower white-collar. The point is that by focusing on a smaller, more tightly interdependent social system, one may observe both subtle status distinctions and interdependencies that would be lost in a study of the populace at large.

The individual firm, of course, is not necessarily always the most appropriate unit of study. Sometimes a more comprehensive unit, such as an industry, would be appropriate. Lane (1975) reports significant industry-to-industry differences in the patterns of occupational attainment. And the personnel employed in a single industry are at least somewhat more homogeneous than the populace at large. Earlier, Lane (1968) has found some nontrivial differences in the mobility patterns in different cities, suggesting regions or cities as desirable units of study.

White, in the vacancy chain work cited earlier, considers a single organization at a time—and not the entire organization, but only a specific type of worker within that organization. Thus every person under consideration might reasonably aspire eventually, if not immediately, to hold any position under consideration. He considered only priests, presumedly aspiring to move to more desirable parishes; choir directors, whether or not they aspired to become priests, were excluded.

Even this restriction, however, did not produce a mobility process with a clean structure, presumably because there did not exist a clearcut hierarchical ordering of parishes according to desirability. (For further comment on White's work, see McFarland 1974a,b.) Brown (1972), in his study of the mobility of educational administrators within public school systems, had similar results: Some elementary principals became secondary principals, and vice versa, there being no fully clear ordering according to preferability between the two. Stewman (1975) in a study of the Michigan state police system did observe a mobility process with a clean structure: One either retained his previous rank or was promoted to the next higher rank; the remaining entries of the mobility matrix were zero or negligible. (Stewman's matrix reminds the mathematical demographer of the population projection matrix, which has zero entries except in the top row and one of the diagonals.) Stewman has found that mobility within a single organization, in his case a rigidly hierarchical one, behaves much more systematically than does mobility within the populace at large. One research strategy may be to resolve a single complex structure into an aggregate of several much simpler structures. Stewman has found one simply structured component of social mobility, but it remains to be seen whether the residual may similarly be decomposed into simply structured components.

Purposive Action in Social Mobility Models

The single most important recent development among mathematical sociologists concerned with social mobility is in my opinion the explicit introduction of purposive action into the models. It is one thing to use mathematical models merely to *describe* the existing degree of inequality while remarking in the text that a reduction of inequality would be desirable. But it is something quite different to use mathematical models *normatively,* that is, to derive from the mathematical models guidance as to what steps one should take in order to pursue his stated goals most effectively. Featherman and Hauser state (although not fully explicitly) the goal of reducing social inequality, but they provide no explicit statements as to what actions, among those that could be taken, would be most effective in pursuing that goal (Chapter 10).

In a paper that has been circulated since 1968 Coleman (1973) called for the incorporation of what he called "extremal principles," according to which some quantity is maximized or minimized or held constant. The principle of utility maximization, which is central to economic theory, was one he cited as exemplary.

Some sociologists would consider this development an important one primarily because of its potentially terrible implications for the discipline. Here is Coleman, a very prominent sociologist, giving up the claim of any distinctly sociological methods or perspective, and instead urging that we mimic the economists. Now it is one thing to include a few dead economists in accounts of the intellectual ancestry of present-day sociology (Max Weber's professorship was, after all, in economics rather than in sociology), but it is something quite different, and dangerous, to propose that sociologists should base their models on principles from economics rather than on principles from sociology.

To our good fortune, however, David Bartholomew is neither a sociologist nor an economist, so he has been free to pursue interesting problems without regard to their status vis à vis the disciplinary boundary separating sociology from economics. Some of the results of his work and that of others are contained in a new chapter in the second edition of his book, *Stochastic Models for Social Processes* (Bartholomew, 1973, Ch. 4).

Instead of using models solely or mainly to describe how the mobility process has been working, we now can use models to guide efforts at modifying the mobility process so as to make it work differently in the future. To be more specific, Bartholomew considers a graded social system and the allocation of people to the several grades, along with personnel flows involving recruitment of newcomers, movement among grades, and loss of personnel, in a context where some unspecified actor is presumed to desire to control the "structure" of the system ("structure" here referring to the proportional distribution of persons among grades) and also is presumed to be able to manipulate either recruitment parameters or internal movement parameters of the system. (Many business firms would have a vice president for personnel, or someone with a similar title, who meets this description, but it is by no means clear that there exists any actor, individual or collective, who meets this description when the system in question is the labor force for an entire nation. Thus we underline the observation made earlier, that a single organization is sometimes a better object of study than is a national sample.)

The problems Bartholomew considers are whether and how an existing structure may be maintained or a different, desired structure may be attained, by appropriate changes in the values of the manipulable quantities. Bartholomew's chapter gives some results which, to me at least, are not at all obvious. Consider a social system whose internal mobility is fixed at rates given in a matrix P, and whose size is also fixed. Calculate the matrix $(I - P)^{-1}$, and divide through by its row totals to make each row sum to unity. Treat each row as the coordinates of a point in the space of all possible structures for the system under consideration. Then the initial structure can be maintained only if it lies in the convex hull of the set of points thus obtained (Bartholomew, 1973, p. 103). The theorem just paraphrased makes use of some mathematics that are nontrivial (or at least not nearly as trivial as squaring a matrix to predict what will happen during a time interval twice as long) to yield some nonobvious results.

The full potential of purposive models in sociology has barely begun to be realized. In large part this is because few sociologists are very familiar with the mathematics involved. But in even greater part it is because the mere setting up of a substantive problem for analysis along these lines is itself a quite formidable task. First one must specify the person or collectivity to be treated as a purposive actor. Second, one must identify the goals to be pursued and the tradeoffs among them. Third, one must identify variables that are subject to manipulation by the actor under consideration. Fourth, one must develop a model with which to anticipate the effects which would be produced on the goal-related variables by the various possible actions that might be taken regarding the manipulable variables.

Who, precisely, is in a position to do something about the extent of social inequality in the contemporary United States? What variables are subject to his (or, more likely, their collective) control? These are not easy questions; yet they must be answered before one may bring purposive models to bear on the matter of social inequality. Even more difficult is the question: What additional, and potentially conflicting, goals are also being sought by the actor in question, and what sorts of tradeoffs among competing goals would the actor consider appropriate? For example, how much persistence of inequality would one be willing to put up with in return for a specified increase in the minimum standard of living in the society? This latter question is the subject of a book-length essay recently published by a leading U. S. economist (Okun, 1974), an essay whose length is indicative of the degree of difficulty inherent in such questions.

Much remains to be done before we can realize the potential of purposive models in this area. At this point we may, nevertheless, take heart in the fact that such work has begun.

Continuous-Time Markov Models

Let me return now to Chapter 12 by Singer and Spilerman. Earlier in my remarks it was characterized as a purely technical chapter devoid of substantive content, whose inclusion in a conference on social demography can be justified only by reference to the fact that elsewhere in the literature, although not in this chapter itself, the Markov models that are the topic of this chapter have been put to use in the study of both migration and social mobility, as well as a variety of other processes.

Chapter 12 deserves to be read, or rather to be studied in detail, by mathematically oriented social scientists in several different disciplines, wherever continuous-time Markov models are being used or being considered for possible use. Its relevance is by no means limited to social mobility, or even to social demography.

People who use mathematical models to study stratification and mobility generally use one or other of two types of models, either path analysis and its regression-based relatives, or Markov models with their base in matrix algebra. The former models treat social status as a continuous variable, while the latter treat it as a discrete variable composed of a number of mutually exclusive and exhaustive categories or "states." The former is used in most of the work by Duncan and his students, including Featherman and Hauser. The latter is used by a number of authors including Bartholomew (1973), Blumen et al. (1955), Boudon (1973), Brown (1972, 1975), Coleman (1964), Ginsberg (1971, 1972a, b), Henry (1971), Hodge (1966), Land (1969), Lieberson and Fuguitt (1967), Matras (1960, 1961, 1967), McGinnis (1968), Morrison (1967), Prais (1955a, b), Singer and Spilerman (1974), Stewman (1975), and White (1970), as well as the present author (McFarland 1970, 1973, 1974b, c).

Markov models themselves may be distinguished by their treatment of the "time variable ("time" appears in quotation marks because in many cases the so-called "time" variable does *not* correspond to time in the ordinary sense, as measured on clocks and calendars; see McFarland, 1974b). Some treat only discrete points on the "time" variable, while others incorporate "time" as a continuous variable. Discrete-time formulations have been used in most applications of Markov models, at least in sociological studies, but Singer and Spilerman urge upon us the virtues of continuous-time Markov models.

Singer and Spilerman display exemplary care in their handling of some subtle and often neglected issues in the mathematical analysis of social data such as the question of whether the solution of a set of equations is unique. But the models they urge upon us are enormously more complex and mathematically difficult than sociologists, even demographers, are accustomed to dealing with, and the kinds of longitudinal data for which they are best suited are available only from a few expensive data collection projects.

I should like to caution the reader against behaving like the little child in the story, who received a hammer for Christmas and promptly discovered that literally *everything* around the house needed hammering. Singer and Spilerman in this chapter and other work have presented us with a splendid new tool, but we need not discard all the tools with which we are familiar nor apply a single tool to every task. Additions to the contents of the social scientist's toolbox are welcome even if the customary tools remain suitable for much of our work.

References

Bartholomew, D. J.
  1973   *Stochastic Models for Social Processes*. 2nd ed. New York: Wiley.
Blau, P. M., and O. D. Duncan
  1967   *The American Occupational Structure*. New York: Wiley.
Blumen, I., M. Kogan, and P. J. McCarthy
  1955   *The Industrial Mobility of Labor as a Probability Process*. Ithaca: New York State School of Industrial and Labor Relations.
Boudon, R.
  1973   *Mathematical Structures of Social Mobility*. Amsterdam: Elsevier.
Brown, D. J.
  1972   "The Organizational Mobility of Educational Administrators." Doctoral dissertation, University of Chicago.
  1975   "A simple Markovian model for general mobility: Some preliminary considerations." *Quality and Quantity* 9: 145–169.
Caserman, A.
  1973   "Patterns of career mobility in post-revolutionary society." Pp. 321–328 in W. Müller and K. U. Mayer (eds.), *Social Stratification and Career Mobility*. Paris: Mouton.

Coleman, J. S.
  1964   *Introduction to Mathematical Sociology.* New York: Free Press.
  1973   "Theoretical bases for parameters of stochastic processes." Pp. 17–28 in R. E. A. Mapes (ed.), *Stochastic Processes in Sociology.* (The Sociological Review Monograph 19.) Keele, England: University of Keele.
Featherman, D. L.
  1974   "Toward comparable data on inequality and stratification: Perspectives on the second generation of national mobility studies." *The American Sociologist* 9: 18–25.
Ginsberg, R. B.
  1971   "Semi-Markov processes and mobility." *Journal of Mathematical Sociology* 1: 233–262.
  1972a "Critique of probabilistic models: Application of the semi-Markov model to migration." *Journal of Mathematical Sociology* 2: 63–82.
  1972b "Incorporating causal structure and exogenous information with probabilistic models: With special reference to choice, gravity, migration, and Markov chains." *Journal of Mathematical Sociology* 2: 83–103.
Glass, D. V., ed.
  1954   *Social Mobility in Britain.* London: Routledge & Kegan Paul.
Goldthorpe, J. H., and K. Hope
  1974   *The Social Grading of Occupations: A New Approach and Scale.* Oxford: Clarendon Press.
Hauser, R. M., and D. L. Featherman.
  1975   "Equality of access to schooling: Trends and prospects." Working Paper 75-17. Center for Demography and Ecology, University of Wisconsin, Madison.
Henry, N. W.
  1971   "The retention model: A Markov chain with variable transition probabilities." *Journal of the American Statistical Association* 66: 264–267.
Hodge, R. W.
  1966   "Occupational mobility as a probability process." *Demography* 3: 19–34.
Hope, K.
  1972   *The Analysis of Social Mobility.* Oxford: The University Press.
Keyfitz, N.
  1973   "Individual mobility in a stationary population." *Population Studies* 27: 335–352.
Land, K. C.
  1969   "Duration of residence and prospective migration: Further evidence." *Demography* 6: 133–140.
Lane, A.
  1968   "Occupational mobility in six cities." *American Sociological Review* 33: 740–749.
  1975   "Industry as a context for occupational achievement." Unpublished manuscript.
Laumann, E. O.
  1973   *Bonds of Pluralism: The Form and Substance of Urban Social Networks.* New York: Wiley.
Laumann, E. O., and F. U. Pappi
  1973   "New directions in the study of community elites." *American Sociological Review* 38: 212–230.
Lieberson, S. and G. V. Fuguitt
  1967   "Negro-white occupational differences in the absence of discrimination." *American Journal of Sociology* 73: 188–200.

Matras, J.
1960	"Comparison of intergenerational occupational mobility patterns." *Population Studies* 14: 163–169.
1961	"Differential fertility, intergerational mobility, and change in the occupational structure." *Population Studies* 15: 187–197.
1967	"Social mobility and social structure: Some insights from the linear model." *American Sociological Review* 32: 608–614.

McFarland, D. D.
1970	"Intragenerational social mobility as a Markov process: Including a time-stationary Markovian model that explains observed declines in mobility rates over time." *American Sociological Review* 35: 463–476.
1973	"Circulation of elites and constraints on intergenerational status transmission." *International Review of Modern Sociology* 3: 152–167. [Reprints with corrections of numerous printing errors are available from the author.]
1974a	"Review of *Chains of Opportunity: System Models of Mobility in Organizations,* by H. C. White." *American Journal of Sociology* 79: 1343–1345.
1974b	"Substantive contributions of Markov models to the study of social mobility." Pp. 5–28 in R. Ziegler (ed.), *Anwendung Mathematischer Verfahren zur Analyse Sozialer Ungleichheit und Sozialer Mobilität.* Kiel, W. Germany: Soziologisches Seminar der Christian-Albrechts-Universität.
1974c.	"On the relationship between mathematical models and empirical data, and the relationship between duration of stay and subsequent mobility." *American Sociological Review* 39: 883–885.
1975	"Review of *The Social Grading of Occupations,* by J. H. Goldthorpe and K. Hope." *Quantitative Sociology Newsletter* 15: 78–81.

McGinnis, R.
1968	"A stochastic model of social mobility." *American Sociological Review* 33: 712–722.

Mezhnarich, S., and I. Josifovski
1974	"Social change and intergenerational mobility of women: The case of a postrevolutionary (equility oriented) society." Pp. 275–325 in *Some Yugoslav Papers Presented to the VIII World Congress of the International Sociological Association.* Ljubljana, Yugoslavia: University of Ljubljana.

Morrison, P. A.
1967	"Duration of residence and prospective migration: The evaluation of a stochastic model." *Demography* 4: 553–561.

Okun, A. M.
1974	*Equality and Efficiency: The Big Tradeoff.* Washington: The Brookings Institution.

Prais, S. J.
1955a	"Measuring social mobility." *Journal of the Royal Statistical Society* 118(Series A): 55–66.
1955b	"The formal theory of social mobility." *Population Studies* 9: 72–81.

Saksida, S., A. Caserman, K. Petrovic, and I. Josifovski
1974	"Social stratification and mobility in Yugoslav society." Pp. 211–274 in *Some Yugoslav Papers Presented to the VIII World Congress of the International Sociological Association.* Ljubljana, Yugoslavia: University of Ljubljana.

Singer, B., and S. Spilerman
1974	"Social mobility models for heterogeneous populations. Pp. 356–401 in H. Costner (ed.), *Sociological Methodology—1973–1974.* San Francisco: Jossey-Bass.

Stewman, S.
  1975   "Two Markov models of open system occupational mobility: Underlying concep-
         tualizations and empirical tests." *American Sociological Review* 40: 298–321.
U. S. Department of Health, Education and Welfare
  1969   *Toward a Social Report*. Washington: U. S. Government Printing Office.
Vroom, V. H., and K. R. MacCrimmon
  1968   "Toward a stochastic model of managerial careers." *Administrative Science
         Quarterly* 13: 26–46.
White, H. C.
  1970   *Chains of Opportunity: System Models of Mobility in Organizations*. Cambridge:
         Harvard University Press.
Zeitlin, M.
  1974   "Corporate ownership and control: The large corporation and the capitalist
         class." *American Journal of Sociology* 79: 1073–1119.
Zeitlin, M., R. E. Ratcliff, and L. A. Ewen
  1974   "The 'inner group': Interlocking directorates and the internal differentiation of
         the capitalist class in Chile." Presented to the annual meeting of the American
         Sociological Association, Montreal.

10

Changes in the Socioeconomic Stratification of the Races[1]

DAVID L. FEATHERMAN and ROBERT M. HAUSER

Classical sociological theories about advanced industrial societies commonly propose that particularistic standards, such as those based on kinship, race, and ethnicity, eventually give way to universalistic, meritocratic practices and institutions (for example, Levy, 1966). Such transitions follow ineluctably from the functional "requirements" of industrial societies—those of factory production, the formal prerequisites of schooling for employment and jobs, and the character of technical knowledge. Consequently, proponents of theories of industrialization argue that

[1] Reprinted with permission from the *American Journal of Sociology,* Volume 82, Number 3 (November 1976), pp. 621–651. © 1976 by The University of Chicago Press.

Earlier versions of this paper were presented at the Conference on Social Demography, University of Wisconsin–Madison, July 1975, and at the San Francisco meetings of the American Sociological Association, August 1975. This work was supported by the National Science Foundation (GI-44336), by the National Institute of Child Health and Human Development (HD-05876), by the College of Agricultural and Life Sciences of the University of Wisconsin–Madison, and by the Institute for Research on Poverty with funds granted by the Department of Health, Education, and Welfare pursuant to the Economic Opportunity Act of 1964.

modern societies tend toward common institutional forms and styles (for example, Feldman and Moore, 1962). Critics of these ideas about convergence note the importance of indigenous culture and political history for understanding the alterations of social structure under industrialization (for example, Goldthorpe, 1964; Bell, 1973, Ch. 1). Others question the verifiability of the theses of industrialization and convergence, arguing that they are definitions rather than testable theories (Garnsey, 1975).

The predictions of the industrialism thesis notwithstanding, racial inequalities persist throughout modern American society, and they invite explanation. During the 1960s the civil rights movement, the war on poverty, and ghetto riots were among the more visible signs of the salience of race as a social attribute, but these events in themselves tell us little about changes in the socioeconomic life chances of blacks and whites. Neo-Marxist analysts (for example, Hechter, 1971, 1974) point to the resurgence of ethnic and racial consciousness in the United States and other advanced nations. They argue that racial inequalities and cleavages play an important part in maintaining the social relations of capitalist industrial economies (Bonacich, 1976). Indeed, some view racial conflicts in this country as arising from the same "colonization" of the black minority as putatively took place among "peripheral" ethnics by "core" elites in Latin America (Blauner, 1969).

Thus, theoretical as well as political or ameliorative interests point to the importance of monitoring racial inequalities and their sources. In this chapter we present new data on trends in occupational inequality and stratification among black and white men in the United States, and we explore briefly the implications of our findings for theories of societal development and ethnic relations.

Recent studies of school and residential segregation in major cities find little amelioration since the mid-1950s (Farley and Taeuber, 1974), despite the enactment of civil rights legislation in the 1960s, the general rise in the socioeconomic circumstances of blacks in the past 20 years (Farley and Hermalin, 1972), and the substantial potential for residential integration that follows from these economic trends (Hermalin and Farley, 1973). These concrete realities take on greater significance when seen against apparent shifts in white attitudes toward racial integration (Greeley and Sheatsley, 1971; Hermalin and Farley, 1973). Of course, disjunctures between public opinion and behavior are nothing new, but they underscore the concern expressed by social commentators (U. S. National Advisory Commission on Civil Disorders, 1968) and social scientists alike about the potential volatility of racial relations in this country and about the tendency of the races to remain apart, residentially, if not also in terms of public attitudes and sentiments (Campbell, 1971; Schuman and Hatchett, 1974).

Whether we speak of the quality of housing, of employment status, of educational attainment, of occupational level, or of earnings, the importance of socioeconomic standing for the assessment of race relations must not be minimized. Life styles, public attitudes, and political activities reflect socioeconomic circumstances, and civil disorder (at least its severity) seems to covary with racial inequalities in strategic socioeconomic conditions (Morgan and Clark, 1973).

More generally, the ethnic dimension is fundamental to social structure as well as to the political climate of the society. Among major axes of social differentiation (for example, age, sex, class), ethnicity (of which race is an instance) is unique in its potential for political mobilization, with movements to create and maintain separate nation-states serving as clear illustrations (Lieberson, 1970). In addition, ethnic inequality and stratification affect other elements of social structure. For example, they can alter relations among economic classes (Barth, 1969; Bonacich, 1976; Hechter, 1971, 1974) or they can provide for differential patterns and rates of industrial or occupational growth (Hodge and Hodge, 1965). Consideration of the racial dimension in studies of inequality and stratification in the United States is essential for understanding and interpreting changes in allocative social processes.

In this chapter, we examine changes in the occupational standing of black and white men between 1962 and 1973. For each race separately, and then for both in comparison, we describe shifts in the occupational socioeconomic status of men in the experienced civilian labor force. We attempt to account for occupational changes and differentials in terms of changes and differentials in family background and educational attainment. We also examine the allocative life-cycle processes which relate family background and schooling to current occupational positions. These allocative processes are an important source of social differentiation and inequality, and we refer to them as processes of socioeconomic stratification (Duncan, 1968c). In the early 1960s processes of stratification were different for black and white men, defining a situation of unequal opportunity for socioeconomic achievement for blacks and whites (Duncan, 1967, 1968a). Whether these allocative processes have converged toward a uniform pattern is as important as whether the racial gap in occupational status has narrowed over the decade. Each datum refers to a different feature of status inequality in American society; changes in status levels need not imply change in stratification processes, and vice versa.

Recent assessments of socioeconomic trends for the races have noted selective improvements for blacks, both in absolute and relative terms (U. S. Bureau of the Census, 1975; Farley and Hermalin, 1972). A few studies have analyzed change in terms of compositional shifts in socioeconomic background or schooling (Hauser and Featherman 1974a, 1974b).

In the past decade blacks gained ground on whites in schooling, occupational status, and income, but the improvements were relatively greater for the young and in some instances occurred only among women. With respect to occupations, both black and white men experienced net upward status shifts in both the manual and nonmanual categories of the experienced civilian labor force, a decline in farming and self-employment, and an increase in salaried professional and managerial roles. These shifts were less a response to changes in the socioeconomic background or schooling of recent cohorts than to changes in labor markets and patterns of career mobility. For example, white men, but not blacks, need more formal education to hold the same jobs that same-aged cohorts held a decade ago. However, black men are still consigned to occupations of lower status than white men of similar social background and educational attainment.

These generalizations about the sources of changing socioeconomic distributions for the races could only be tentative, for they rested upon inferences or projections from baseline studies. For example, Hauser and Featherman (1974b) used the 1962 Occupational Changes in a Generation (OCG) survey (Blau and Duncan, 1967) to estimate the occupational destinations of black and white cohorts in 1972 as if they had experienced the same allocative processes as men of the same age in 1962. From discrepancies between projected destination distributions and observed distributions in the March 1972 Current Population Survey (CPS), Hauser and Featherman inferred that change in racial stratification had occurred. Such indirect techniques of measuring change and of attempting to explain it are no longer necessary for the 1960s. New data about the socioeconomic origins and destinations of black and white men are available from the 1973 replicate of the 1962 OCG survey. These data provide direct evidence about change in stratification processes and outcomes among black and white men. They also permit some intriguing speculations about the course of racial inequality and about the evolving roles of families and schools in a maturing, post-industrial economy.

Data

The 1962 OCG survey and its 1973 replicate were carried out in conjunction with the March demographic supplement to the Current Population Survey (CPS) (Blau and Duncan, 1967; Featherman and Hauser, 1975). The 1962 survey had a response rate of 83% to a four-page questionnaire which was left behind by the CPS interviewer. More than 20,000 men aged 20–64 in the civilian noninstitutional population responded. In 1973, the eight-page OCG questionnaire was mailed out 6 months after the

March CPS and was followed by mail, telephone, and personal callbacks. The respondents, 88% of the target sample, included more than 33,500 men aged 20–65 in the civilian noninstitutional population. Also, in the 1973 sample, blacks and persons of Spanish origin were sampled at about twice the rate of whites, and almost half the black men were interviewed personally. In this chapter we shall make age-constant, intercohort comparisons among men in the postschooling, economically active years. We limit our analysis to men aged 25–64 in the experienced civilian labor force in March 1962 or March 1973, that is, men who were employed and those who were unemployed but had previously held a job. In both OCG samples, women are represented only through husbands. That is, socioeconomic background characteristics of women were elicited only if they were married and living with husbands in the OCG samples. Elsewhere, we have compared the educational and occupational attainments and earnings of male and female married, spouse-present populations (Featherman and Hauser, 1976).

We have made extensive efforts to establish the comparability of measurements in the 1962 and 1973 OCG surveys (Featherman and Hauser, 1975). Both surveys were carried out by the U. S. Bureau of the Census using its standard field methods and editing, coding, and weighting procedures. For the items on which this report is based, the CPS and OCG questions and questionnaire layouts were almost identical in 1962 and in 1973. Although 1970 census occupation coding materials were in use at the time of the 1973 survey, we arranged for occupation and industry reports to be coded using 1960 census coding materials.

Yet some failures of replication were inevitable, and we have attempted to explore their effects and draw attention to them where they may affect our conclusions. For example, we thought that the quality of the survey data for blacks might be better in the supplementary sample of men interviewed personally than in the basic sample. This might have affected comparisons of blacks and whites in 1973 and comparisons of blacks between 1962 and 1973. However, our examination of black men in the basic sample in 1973 and of those in the supplementary sample revealed no substantial differences between the two. Another unavoidable methodological change was a modification of the wording of the class-of-worker item, intended to improve the measurement of self-employment.

Intercohort Shifts in Occupational Socioeconomic Status

Reports of current (March or last) occupation, industry, and class of worker and corresponding reports for the OCG respondent's father (or

other family head) when the respondent was about 16 years old were
coded into seven-digit 1960 census codes, and these were mechanically
transformed into values of Duncan's (1961) socioeconomic index (SEI)
for occupations. Thus, our measure of occupational standing does not
refer to the prestige of the jobholder or of incumbents in his occupation,
but to the average educational and income level of occupational incumbents. We believe that occupational socioeconomic status is the major dimension along which occupational positions persist from generation to
generation (Featherman *et al.*, 1975); for further discussion of the measurement and scaling of occupations, see Featherman and Hauser (1973).
As noted above, if the respondent's father was absent, "father's" occupation refers to that of the mother or other household head; about one-
third of black men and one-sixth of nonblack men said they did not live
with both parents most of the time up to age 16.

Following a well-established pattern, the net intercohort shifts in current occupational socioeconomic status have been upward for both whites
(Table 10.1) and blacks (Table 10.2) at all ages. For whites aged 25–64 in

TABLE 10.1

**Means and Standard Deviations of Occupational Status Variables: Nonblack Men
Aged 25–64 in the Experienced Civilian Labor Force, March 1962 and March 1973**

Age	1962		1973		Arithmetic change	
	Mean	Standard deviation	Mean	Standard deviation	Mean	Standard deviation
Total, 25–64						
Father's occupation	28.09	21.27	30.15	22.57	2.06	1.30
Current occupation	39.25	24.44	42.58	25.22	3.33	0.78
25–34						
Father's occupation	30.36	21.75	33.96	23.93	3.60	2.18
Current occupation	40.37	24.96	42.74	24.95	2.37	−0.01
35–44						
Father's occupation	28.74	21.78	30.13	22.42	1.39	0.64
Current occupation	40.66	24.71	44.59	25.45	3.93	0.74
45–54						
Father's occupation	26.56	20.45	28.01	21.41	1.45	0.96
Current occupation	38.11	23.57	43.13	25.27	4.02	1.70
55–64						
Father's occupation	25.86	20.44	26.52	20.92	0.66	0.48
Current occupation	36.89	24.23	38.63	24.88	1.74	0.65

TABLE 10.2

Means and Standard Deviations of Occupational Status Variables: Black Men Aged 25–64 in the Experienced Civilian Labor Force, March 1962 and March 1973

Age	1962		1973		Arithmetic change	
	Mean	Standard deviation	Mean	Standard deviation	Mean	Standard deviation
Total, 25–64						
Father's occupation	16.15	12.88	15.95	13.72	−0.20	0.84
Current occupation	17.77	15.16	25.76	20.44	7.99	5.28
25–34						
Father's occupation	17.36	15.34	17.66	15.61	0.30	0.27
Current occupation	18.30	16.34	29.10	21.74	10.80	5.40
35–44						
Father's occupation	14.79	11.26	16.32	14.20	1.53	2.90
Current occupation	19.24	16.05	27.66	21.34	8.42	5.29
45–54						
Father's occupation	16.24	11.58	14.39	11.90	−1.85	0.32
Current occupation	17.19	13.85	23.43	18.66	6.24	4.81
55–64						
Father's occupation	16.36	12.55	14.06	10.35	−2.30	−2.20
Current occupation	14.94	12.70	18.72	16.06	3.78	3.36

the experienced civilian labor force (ECLF), the increase of 3.33 points on the Duncan scale between 1962 and 1973 represented a shift of about 14% of the 1962 standard deviation. Larger than average intercohort improvements in current status were experienced by white men in the middle years, ages 35–54, while the youngest and oldest age groups had smaller gains. Among white men there were small upward intercohort shifts in the average status of father's occupation. These may be observed in comparisons across cohorts within either survey (read down the columns of the table) or across cohorts between surveys. Over the decade, inequality of occupational socioeconomic status remained virtually constant among whites, as shown by standard deviations in Table 10.1.

At every age, black men enjoyed larger absolute and relative upward shifts in current occupational status than did whites (Table 10.2). For example, the 8-point rise in average status among black men aged 25–64 was almost two and one-half times the gain for whites, and it represented an improvement equal to 53% of the black standard deviation in 1962. Absolute and relative gains varied inversely with age among blacks; the greatest gains occurred among young workers.[2] These changes seem unlikely to have followed from shifts in the socioeconomic circumstances of the families in which black men were reared, as net shifts in paternal (head's) status were very small and irregular (both between and within surveys). The variation in current occupational status increased for blacks at every age over the decade, and the size of this shift, too, varied inversely with age. Thus, greater status inequality within the black male labor force came along with higher levels of occupational standing.

Of course, gains for blacks must be viewed in the context of their historically subordinate status relative to whites. At every age, and both with respect to paternal and current occupational statuses, blacks in 1973 occupied a lower socioeconomic level than whites at any age 11 years earlier. Still, racial gaps in current occupational status have narrowed (Table 10.3). In 1962 the black average of current occupational status was more than 20 points below the white average at every age. By 1973, while the racial gap was still close to 20 points among men over 45 years old, it had narrowed to less than 14 points in the youngest cohort. The racial gap had closed by nearly 8.5 points on the Duncan scale at ages 25–34 and by 4½ points for all men aged 25–64. These declines are 38% and 22% of the respective racial gaps in 1962. At the same time, blacks appear to have lost ground relative to whites in socioeconomic background, as all but the cohort aged 35–44 in 1973 were reared in relatively less beneficial socioeconomic circumstances than blacks in 1962. Thus, racial differences in occupational status origins may remain an important source of current occupational status differentials between the races.

Historically, variation in current socioeconomic status has been greater for whites than blacks, reflecting greater differentiation in the white occupational distribution. Shifts in differential status inequality have occurred since 1962; the ratio of the black to white standard deviations (Tables 10.1 and 10.2) has risen from 0.62 to 0.81 for men aged 25–64

---

[2] In assessing shifts between the OCG surveys, it is important to remember that the civilian noninstitutional population of 1973 included a larger percentage of (especially younger) cohorts between the ages of 25 and 64 than in 1962. Better coverage in 1973 stems, in the main, from the fact that the armed forces had decreased in size. For example, coverage of men aged 25–34 in the 1962 OCG was 91.5%; in 1973, 94.5% of the men aged 25–34 were covered in the OCG sample under analysis. The bearing of more extensive coverage via a less extensive armed forces on our comparisons is difficult to assess, as the effects are apt to differ for the races. Moreover, our focus on the ECLF compounds the issue, inasmuch as young black men aged 25–34 were less likely to be in the labor force in 1973 than same-aged blacks in 1962. This is not merely of methodological interest: Our study excludes the substantial minority of young black men who are not in the labor force as conventionally measured.

TABLE 10.3

Racial Differences in Average Occupational Status and in Socioeconomic Variation: Men Aged 25–64 in the Experienced Civilian Labor Force, March 1962 and March 1973

Age	1962[a]		1973		Arithmetic change	
	Mean	Standard deviation	Mean	Standard deviation	Mean	Standard deviation
Total, 25–64						
Father's occupation	11.94	8.39	14.20	8.85	2.26	0.46
Current occupation	21.48	9.28	16.82	4.78	−4.66	−4.50
25–34						
Father's occupation	13.00	6.41	16.30	8.32	3.30	1.91
Current occupation	22.07	8.62	13.64	3.21	−8.43	−5.41
35–44						
Father's occupation	13.94	10.52	13.81	8.22	−0.13	−2.30
Current occupation	21.42	8.66	16.93	4.11	−4.49	−4.55
45–54						
Father's occupation	10.32	8.87	13.62	9.51	3.30	0.64
Current occupation	20.92	9.72	19.70	6.61	−1.22	−3.11
55–64						
Father's occupation	9.50	7.89	12.46	10.57	2.96	2.68
Current occupation	21.95	11.53	19.91	8.82	−2.04	−2.71

[a] Positive difference indicates higher value for whites; negative difference indicates higher value for blacks.

in the ECLF. Again, the convergence between the races is most apparent at younger ages.

Another way of describing the changes in occupational status differentials between the races is to note that black men in the ECLF of 1973 are more likely than those in the 1962 ECLF to have experienced intergenerational status mobility like that among whites. Table 10.4 reorganizes Tables 10.1 and 10.2 by comparing the status of a man's current occupation with that of his father's occupation as an index of status mobility in the life cycle (between age 16 and the survey date). In 1962, white men in every cohort held occupations which averaged 10 or more points higher in status than their fathers' occupations. Black men of all ages except 35–44 had not been able to advance in the status hierarchy much beyond the positions of their family heads. This is not to say that black men tended to "inherit" the occupations of their fathers by going into the same general line of work; if anything, the facts are to the contrary (see Duncan, 1968b;

TABLE 10.4

Average Intergenerational Occupational Status Mobility: Men Aged 25–64 in the Experienced Civilian Labor Force, by Color, March 1962 and March 1973

	1962		1973	
Age	Nonblack	Black	Nonblack	Black
Total, 25–64	11.16	1.62	12.43	9.81
25–34	10.01	0.94	8.78	11.44
35–44	11.92	4.45	14.46	11.34
45–54	11.55	0.95	15.12	9.04
55–64	11.03	−1.42	12.11	4.66

Hauser *et al.,* 1977). In 1973, the upward intergenerational mobility of whites continued in roughly the same amounts, but black men were far more likely to be upwardly mobile than their counterparts a decade earlier. In fact, at ages 25–34, the absolute amount of intergenerational mobility in the black population is greater than in the white population (11.44 versus 8.78 points on the Duncan scale). Thus, black men have begun recently to experience status mobility in their life cycles which resembles more closely that among whites. The importance of cohort replacement in social change is suggested by the inverse variation of intergenerational status gains with age among blacks in 1973. At the same time, some of the observed status gains relative to fathers may have occurred since 1962. We can make a crude comparison of earlier and later measurements on the same cohort by reading Table 10.4 diagonally (from upper left to lower right). For example, the status gain was 4.45 points among blacks aged 35–44 in 1962, but 9.04 points among black men aged 45–54 in 1973. If we assume that these figures refer to successive measurements of the same cohort, we must conclude that there was an intragenerational upward status shift of about 4.5 points between 1962 and 1973.

Intercohort Changes in Socioeconomic Background and Education

We have already commented on the rising occupational status origins of successive cohorts of white men and the absence of parallel shifts among black cohorts. In most other respects the social background of successive cohorts of both races has become more conducive to high levels of occupational achievement.[3] Between the cohorts aged 55–64 and those aged 25–34 in the 1973 survey, the average educational attainment of fathers rose from 7.31 years to 9.89 years among white men and from 4.94 years to 7.64 years among black men. Between these same cohorts the average number of siblings declined from 4.30 to 3.18 among white men and from 5.32 to 5.07 among blacks. The proportion of nonblack men whose fathers were farmers fell from 34% to 14% among nonblacks and from 59% to 26% among blacks. However, between these two cohorts there was virtually no change in the proportions of blacks or whites raised in broken families; among whites the shares were 15% in the oldest cohort and 13% in the youngest. Thirty-two percent of both black cohorts were raised in broken families. Obviously, these trends have not eliminated racial differences in socioeconomic origins. These and other trends and differentials in social background are treated in detail by Hauser and Featherman (1976).

Trends in socioeconomic background are dwarfed by the large and regular increases in educational attainment among men of both races (not tabulated here). In 1962 the oldest cohort of black workers averaged 5.4 years of schooling, but by 1973 the youngest cohort of black workers had completed an average of 11.6 years of school. Among whites also the educational change was impressive: from an average of 9.6 years among the oldest men in 1962 to an average of 12.7 years in the youngest 1973 cohort. Overall, the schooling of the average black worker rose from 8 to 10 years between 1962 and 1973, while that of the average white rose from 11 to 12 years. Growth in educational attainment was accompanied by a narrowing of the educational distribution. Among white male workers the standard deviation of educational attainment fell from 3.6 years in the oldest 1962 cohort to 2.8 years in the youngest 1973 cohort. Among black men there was a parallel decline in educational inequality; the standard deviation of schooling was 3.8 years among the oldest black men in 1962 and 2.6 years among the youngest black men in 1973. Elsewhere, we have

---

[3] Paternal education is scaled in years completed according to the following recode of class intervals: no school, 0.0 years; elementary (1–4), 3.3 years; elementary (5–7), 6.3 years; elementary (8), 8.0 years; high school (1–3), 9.9 years; high school (4), 12.0 years; college (1–3), 13.8 years; college (4), 16.0 years; college (5 or more), 18.0 years. Number of siblings is the number of respondent's brothers and sisters. Farm origins is a dummy variable, with a score of one indicating that respondent's father was a farmer, farm manager, farm laborer, or farm foreman. Broken family is a dummy variable, with a score of one indicating that the respondent was not living with both parents (however, respondent defined the situation) most of the time up to age 16. Respondent's education is in single years, as reported to the CPS.

shown that greater educational equality was produced by a combination of reduced effects of social background and increased equality among men with the same social background (Hauser and Featherman, 1976).

Racial differentials in educational attainment seem to be disappearing. Whereas the black–white difference in mean education was 3.0 years in 1962 for men aged 25–64 in the ECLF, the gap was 2.0 years in 1973. At ages 55–64 the racial gap in average educational attainment narrowed from 4.2 years in 1962 to 3.2 years in 1973, and among young men (aged 25–34) it closed by half, from 2.3 years in 1962 to 1.2 years in 1973. Indeed, in 1973 there was no difference in the average length of schooling between young black and white men with the same socioeconomic background (Hauser and Featherman, 1976). Thus, declining racial differentials in schooling, especially at the youngest ages, parallel observed declines in occupational socioeconomic differentials and may help to explain them. We defer a discussion of the contributions of intercohort shifts in family socioeconomic factors and education to racial differentials in occupational status until we have looked at change over the decade in the process of occupational stratification.

Processes of Socioeconomic Allocation in 1962 and 1973

In Tables 10.5 and 10.6 we have elaborated a "basic" model of occupational stratification (Blau and Duncan, 1967, Ch. 5) to include a somewhat broader array of family background factors. Table 10.5 gives estimates of the reduced-form equation relating five exogenous, predetermined family factors to occupational socioeconomic status. Table 10.6 reports estimates of our final equation, which includes education as a regressor. We do not include first job in our model, as this item was not comparable between the 1962 and 1973 surveys (see Featherman and Hauser, 1975; the education equation in our model is analyzed in Hauser and Featherman, 1976).

In the reduced-form equation for current occupational status (Table 10.5) we find the now rather familiar pattern of relationships between family background and occupational status among white men in the 1962 ECLF. Both father's occupation and education made positive contributions to occupational standing, even if these were small in metric terms. Large numbers of siblings, farm origins, and rearing in a broken family all had negative effects. About 21% of the variance in occupational status was explained by these five family factors. Among blacks in 1962, only farm origins and paternal education had statistically significant effects on occupational status. Overall, the five family factors accounted for a mere

8% of the variance, but among blacks aged 25–44 the larger handicap of farm origins increases R^2 to about .11.[4] While occupational status was more closely linked to family background among white than among black men in 1962, there was also greater variability in occupational standing among white than among black men with the same social background. (These two findings are not inconsistent because the total variability in occupational standing was much greater among white than black men.) The standard errors of estimate (standard deviations about the regression line) of occupational status were about 22 points on the Duncan SEI scale for white men at every age, but for black men they varied inversely with age from 12.8 points for the cohort aged 55–64 to 15.6 points for the cohort aged 25–34. Thus, net of social background, white men had more diverse status opportunities than blacks, but the variation by age among blacks suggested a movement toward the white pattern.

By 1973, the articulation of family background and occupational status had decreased slightly at all ages among whites, while it had increased among blacks except at ages 35–44 (compare R^2 values in 1962 and 1973 by age within race in Table 10.5). Conditional inequality of occupational socioeconomic status (see the standard errors of estimate) increased within both races, but more for blacks than for whites. Still, the diversity of status opportunities remained greater among whites than blacks at every age in 1973. Because the conditional inequality of occupational status increased substantially among black men, the changes in R^2 between 1962 and 1973 understate the increasing effects of socioeconomic background on occupational status among black men. That is, "class" factors are becoming more important in explaining the distribution of occupational status in the black population.

Among whites there were small, and in some cases irregular, changes in the effects of specific background variables on occupational status; among all men 25–64 years old the effect of every variable except number of siblings declined absolutely between 1962 and 1973. With the exception of farm origin, the bearing of each family factor on black occupational status increased (absolutely) over the decade. Thus, the several regression coefficients, as well as variance components, suggest a convergence between the races in patterns of occupational stratification. This is most apparent among men aged 25–34 in 1973. In that cohort the effects of

[4] Analysis of remeasurement data from the 1973 OCG survey shows that the depressing effects of random measurement error on these regression coefficients are larger among black than among white respondents (Bielby *et al.*, 1977). Consequently, our comparisons of black and white regression equations for 1962 and for 1973 probably overstate racial differences in the occupational achievement process. Obversely, the convergence in achievement processes between black and white men may be closer than that reported below.

TABLE 10.5

Regression Analysis of Current Occupational Status on Family Background Factors: Men Aged 25–64 in the ECLF, by Color, March 1962 and March 1973[a]

Population	Predetermined variables					R^2	Constant	SEE
	Father's occupational status	Father's education	Siblings	Farm origin	Broken family			
1962								
Total, 25–64								
Nonblack	0.286 (0.016)	0.873 (0.080)	-1.097 (0.105)	-5.949 (0.662)	-3.245 (0.743)	.209	31.00	21.75
Black	0.067 (0.052)	0.563 (0.175)	-0.221 (0.261)	-4.978 (1.318)	-0.506 (1.354)	.080	17.06	14.61
25–34								
Nonblack	0.265 (0.029)	1.173 (0.162)	-1.306 (0.207)	-5.502 (1.388)	-4.011 (1.466)	.216	28.54	22.13
Black	0.051 (0.086)	0.837 (0.369)	0.046 (0.417)	-6.822 (2.720)	-0.556 (2.781)	.110	13.89	15.64
35–44								
Nonblack	0.277 (0.028)	0.985 (0.146)	-1.167 (0.195)	-6.456 (1.225)	-3.372 (1.370)	.224	31.79	21.79
Black	0.124 (0.115)	0.569 (0.362)	-0.506 (0.415)	-7.464 (2.522)	-1.367 (2.667)	.117	20.43	15.33
45–54								
Nonblack	0.331 (0.031)	0.586 (0.149)	-0.921 (0.203)	-5.113 (1.247)	-1.225 (1.408)	.195	30.77	21.18
Black	0.039 (0.114)	0.264 (0.346)	-0.313 (0.462)	-2.765 (2.718)	0.112 (2.631)	.033	18.31	13.90
55–64								
Nonblack	0.254 (0.041)	0.786 (0.195)	-1.006 (0.255)	-7.316 (1.559)	-4.438 (1.850)	.191	32.79	21.85
Black	0.134 (0.119)	0.348 (0.376)	0.138 (0.466)	-1.024 (2.915)	-1.717 (2.911)	.047	11.78	12.75

1973

Total, 25–64								
Nonblack	0.249	0.866	−1.266	−4.789	−2.472	.181	33.76	22.83
	(0.010)	(0.056)	(0.077)	(0.494)	(0.533)			
Black	0.200	1.062	−0.513	−5.009	−1.946	.138	20.87	19.01
	(0.043)	(0.160)	(0.188)	(1.198)	(1.148)			
25–34								
Nonblack	0.232	1.020	−1.454	−1.616	−2.711	.175	29.98	22.68
	(0.018)	(0.108)	(0.148)	(1.043)	(1.001)			
Black	0.246	1.180	−0.930	−3.861	−1.303	.167	21.87	19.97
	(0.070)	(0.340)	(0.344)	(2.395)	(2.095)			
35–44								
Nonblack	0.232	1.030	−1.379	−5.882	−3.078	.196	35.51	22.83
	(0.020)	(0.112)	(0.149)	(0.988)	(1.048)			
Black	0.177	0.918	−0.526	−4.764	−2.621	.099	23.84	20.40
	(0.088)	(0.361)	(0.389)	(2.522)	(2.388)			
45–54								
Nonblack	0.260	0.965	−1.162	−4.924	−3.172	.182	34.58	22.87
	(0.021)	(0.111)	(0.147)	(0.918)	(1.017)			
Black	0.162	0.732	−0.197	−4.034	−3.113	.081	20.98	18.03
	(0.092)	(0.288)	(0.367)	(2.227)	(2.210)			
55–64								
Nonblack	0.270	0.883	−1.053	−7.691	−0.631	.199	32.26	22.29
	(0.026)	(0.130)	(0.172)	(1.054)	(1.236)			
Black	0.092	0.979	−0.144	−6.349	0.396	.132	16.95	15.16
	(0.111)	(0.332)	(0.386)	(2.429)	(2.409)			

[a] Approximate standard error in parentheses; SEE = standard error or estimate.

TABLE 10.6

Regression Analysis of Current Occupational Status on Family Background Factors and Education: Men Aged 25–64 in the ECLF, by Color, March 1962 and March 1973[a]

Population	Predetermined variables						R^2	Constant	SEE
	Father's occupational status	Father's education	Siblings	Farm origin	Broken family	Education			
1962									
Total, 25–64									
Nonblack	0.167 (0.014)	0.072 (0.072)	-0.242 (0.095)	-3.000 (0.587)	0.576 (0.657)	3.597 (0.587)	.387	-3.47	19.14
Black	0.046 (0.050)	0.196 (0.175)	-0.112 (0.207)	-1.424 (1.351)	0.418 (1.301)	1.272 (0.175)	.160	6.91	13.97
25–34									
Nonblack	0.122 (0.025)	0.271 (0.141)	-0.332 (0.180)	-3.606 (1.179)	-1.762 (1.229)	4.435 (0.165)	.437	-16.28	18.76
Black	0.025 (0.082)	0.347 (0.366)	-0.066 (0.396)	-3.212 (2.697)	0.287 (2.640)	1.830 (0.405)	.207	-0.72	14.81
35–44									
Nonblack	0.151 (0.025)	0.135 (0.131)	-0.253 (0.173)	-3.344 (1.066)	-0.379 (1.191)	3.978 (0.154)	.420	-7.81	18.85
Black	0.063 (0.113)	0.329 (0.356)	-0.318 (0.405)	-4.111 (2.619)	-0.284 (2.595)	1.153 (0.330)	.181	10.41	14.80
45–54									
Nonblack	0.189 (0.028)	-0.103 (0.135)	-0.181 (0.182)	-2.247 (1.109)	1.039 (1.247)	3.494 (0.160)	.373	-1.49	18.70
Black	0.078 (0.110)	-0.070 (0.344)	-0.108 (0.446)	1.421 (2.853)	0.917 (2.525)	1.271 (0.358)	.123	6.51	13.29
55–64									
Nonblack	0.157 (0.038)	0.058 (0.182)	-0.381 (0.234)	-5.283 (1.413)	-1.405 (1.632)	2.998 (0.191)	.341	7.67	19.73
Black	0.022 (0.115)	0.140 (0.357)	0.158 (0.436)	2.054 (2.856)	-0.677 (2.739)	1.418 (0.390)	.175	4.42	11.93

1973

									SEE
Total, 25–64									
Nonblack	(0.153) (0.009)	−0.112 (0.051)	−0.284 (0.068)	−1.399 (0.433)	0.848 (0.467)	4.258 (0.062)	.377	−10.98	19.91
Black	0.164 (0.039)	0.293 (0.151)	−0.322 (0.170)	−0.286 (1.118)	−0.382 (1.042)	2.666 (0.156)	.297	−3.62	17.18
25–34									
Nonblack	0.135 (0.015)	−0.052 (0.097)	−0.318 (0.131)	−1.566 (0.901)	0.184 (0.868)	4.897 (0.124)	.384	−22.53	19.60
Black	0.151 (0.063)	0.623 (0.278)	−0.620 (0.310)	0.213 (2.182)	−0.756 (1.878)	3.827 (0.372)	.332	−19.34	17.90
35–44									
Nonblack	0.122 (0.018)	0.055 (0.100)	−0.277 (0.131)	−2.877 (0.849)	0.204 (0.118)	4.300 (0.900)	.412	−12.18	19.52
Black	0.144 (0.076)	0.100 (0.323)	−0.149 (0.339)	−0.089 (2.234)	0.328 (2.092)	3.487 (0.322)	.323	−10.97	17.71
45–54									
Nonblack	0.161 (0.019)	0.028 (0.100)	−0.359 (0.130)	−0.903 (0.808)	0.664 (0.893)	4.183 (0.119)	.378	− 9.04	19.94
Black	0.116 (0.084)	0.001 (0.274)	0.090 (0.333)	−0.294 (2.060)	−1.527 (2.005)	2.406 (0.282)	.252	0.38	16.29
55–64									
Nonblack	0.170 (0.024)	0.067 (0.120)	−0.261 (0.156)	−3.832 (0.951)	2.109 (1.105)	3.601 (0.140)	.365	− 3.34	19.84
Black	0.076 (0.105)	0.535 (0.325)	−0.060 (0.364)	−3.774 (2.342)	1.367 (2.275)	1.506 (0.299)	.235	5.62	14.26

[a] Approximate standard error in parentheses; SEE = standard error of estimate.

father's occupational status and educational attainment were virtually
identical for white and black men, and only the racial differences in the
effects of number of siblings and farm origin were as large as one standard
error of the black regression coefficient. Again, these similarities in regression slopes do not imply equality of occupational status levels between blacks and whites, but they do indicate growing similarity in the
process of occupational achievement. Even outside the group aged 25–34
the regression coefficients for black men are more comparable to the
white values than in 1962. One other noteworthy change is the declining
influence of farm background for both whites and blacks in the two youngest cohorts.

In Table 10.6 educational attainment of the respondent is added to the
occupational status equation. Readers familiar with the 1962 OCG findings will remember that education was a major factor in the basic model of
socioeconomic achievement (Blau and Duncan, 1967, Ch. 5). For virtually all cohorts in both races, the addition of education to the set of family background regressors nearly doubled the explained variance in occupational status. About 39% of that variance for whites and 16% for blacks
was explained by family factors and schooling.

Of course, the introduction of education into the model of stratification
altered the reduced-form coefficients for family effects on achievement in
1962. In brief, the effect of each family factor was reduced, signaling the
importance of schooling as an intervening mechanism (as well as a direct
causal agent) of status transmission (Alwin and Hauser, 1975). That is,
family socioeconomic resources and related factors were converted into
occupational status by means of differential educational attainment of offspring. An illustration of this role of education is the reduction by about
50% of the handicap of farm origin for whites when education is entered
into the equation (compare 1962 panels by age and race in Tables 10.5 and
10.6). Larger reductions occurred for older white men. Among blacks
most (70%) of the negative effect of farm origin was associated with the
lower educational attainments of black farmers' sons in 1962. Excepting
the persistent influence of father's occupational status and farm origin,
virtually all of the effects of socioeconomic origins on occupational status
were explained by differential schooling in 1962. These same explanatory
relationships reappear in the 1973 data. Schooling mediates much of the
influence of socioeconomic background on occupational status among
men of both races throughout the economically active years (compare
1973 panels by age and race in Tables 10.5 and 10.6).

Perhaps the most important intercohort change in the occupational
achievement process is the increasing effect of educational attainment.
For white men aged 25–64 in the 1962 ECLF, each additional year of

schooling was worth 3.6 points of occupational status on the Duncan scale; for black men, each additional year was worth only one-third as much, 1.3 points. Similar racial differentials in occupational effects of schooling occurred at every age in 1962. By 1973, the effect of an additional year of schooling on the occupational statuses of whites aged 25–64 in the ECLF had increased 18% (to 4.3 points); among blacks it had more than doubled (to 2.7 points). In relative terms, the return to schooling increased for blacks to 63% of its value for whites. The effect of schooling on occupational standing increased between successive cohorts among black and white men at every age. Among white men, but not among blacks, the greater returns to schooling appear primarily to reflect cohort replacement. That is, returns to schooling do not appear to have changed within cohorts over the decade; the effect of years of schooling is about the same for the cohorts aged 35–64 in 1973 as for the respective cohorts aged 25–54 in 1962. On the other hand, among black men the effect of years of schooling was roughly twice as large at ages 35–44 and 45–54 in 1973 as it was at ages 25–34 and 35–44, respectively, in 1962. Thus, among black men career mobility as well as cohort replacement appear to be factors in the increasing effect of schooling on occupational status.

As a consequence of these changes, younger blacks and whites experienced much more similar occupational returns to each year of schooling in 1973 than in 1962. In fact, for young workers, especially those aged 25–34, the stratification process was far less differentiated by race than a decade earlier. Apart from the remaining difference in the education coefficient (about 1 point on the SEI scale per year of schooling), the net effects of family factors are rather similar, if not in absolute size, at least in that they are uniformly small and not significantly different from one another (compare the racial differences with the standard errors of the coefficients among blacks). At least at these younger ages, there is evidence of convergence in the allocative mechanisms, though not of complete equality of occupational opportunity.

As returns to schooling have increased, so has the proportion of explained variance in occupational status attributable to education net of family background. About 38% of the variance in white occupational status and 30% of that in black attainment was explained in 1973. Note that R^2 *decreased* trivially over the decade for whites ($R^2 = .387$ versus $.377$) and *increased* substantially for blacks ($R^2 = .160$ versus $.297$). Of the explained variance, 52% and 54% are assignable to the effect of schooling net of social background for whites and blacks, respectively. (The figure for both races in 1962 was 48%.)

Despite the increased effects of schooling, the conditional inequality in occupational status increased between 1962 and 1973. That is, the variation in occupational status net of family background and schooling increased among black as well as white men and at every age (compare standard errors of estimate between years in Table 10.6). While critics of educational credentialism argue that reliance on schooling as a criterion for employment creates a needless and rigid link between schooling and jobs, the data show that variations in occupational standing have increased along with the effects of schooling.

The possible convergence of blacks and whites in processes of stratification appears to result from two opposite trends. First, among whites there has been a modest weakening of stratification—the linking of status in one generation to that in the next. This has occurred without reducing occupational inequality and in conjunction with a greater role of education (relative to family background) in the generation of socioeconomic differences. Mechanisms which allocate whites in the occupational hierarchy became more egalitarian and meritocratic and less deterministic by the early 1970s than they had been in the early 1960s.

For blacks, there has been a second, more noticeable, and perhaps more socially significant change. The capacity of both families and schools to provide resources which black men can convert into occupational achievements has grown. The tighter articulation between family background and achievement has fashioned a pattern of intergenerational stratification for younger blacks which resembles that among younger white men. It is ironic that parity between black and white men in the achievement process may occur as a consequence of greater socioeconomic ascription within the black population. At the same time, the effect of education on occupational status has increased absolutely and relative to that of the family since 1962, and there is growing inequality in the statuses of black men of similar social origins and schooling. Thus, as intergenerational stratification has increased for blacks, the process has also become more meritocratic, for educational credentials meant more to a black man in 1973 than in 1962.

Sources of Change in Socioeconomic Status

For both black and white men the average socioeconomic status of occupations rose between 1962 and 1973. To what can we attribute this pattern of change? In particular, can intercohort shifts in status be explained by changes in family factors and educational attainment? In seeking answers to these questions we have standardized our data on the 1973 regression equations for each race separately. (For an alternative standardization see Hauser and Featherman, 1974b.) For example, among blacks aged 25–34, the intercohort shift in mean socioeconomic status was 10.8 SEI points (Table 10.2). To decompose this difference, we insert the means of the family background variables for 25- to 34-year-old black men in 1962 into the reduced-form regression for blacks aged 25–34 in 1973 (from Table 10.5). The estimated socioeconomic score is 0.78 points lower than the observed mean in 1973, indicating that about 7% of the intercohort change is associated with shifts in family factors for this age between 1962 and 1973 (see Table 10.7). We then insert the 1962 means of the family factors and educational attainment into the full 1973 regression

TABLE 10.7

Components of Intercohort Change in Occupational Socioeconomic Status: Men Aged 25–64 in the Experienced Civilian Labor Force, by Color, March 1962 and March 1973[a]

Age and component	Black		Nonblack	
Total, 25–64				
Family factors[b]	1.06	(13)	1.86	(56)
Education	4.68	(59)	3.07	(92)
Residual	2.25	(28)	−1.60	(−48)
Intercohort change	7.99	(100)	3.33	(100)
25–34				
Family factors	0.78	(7)	2.78	(117)
Education	7.12	(66)	2.01	(85)
Residual	2.90	(27)	−2.42	(−102)
Intercohort change	10.80	(100)	2.37	(100)
35–44				
Family factors	1.32	(16)	1.75	(45)
Education	6.48	(77)	4.23	(108)
Residual	0.62	(7)	−2.05	(−52)
Intercohort change	8.42	(100)	3.93	(100)
45–54				
Family factors	0.15	(2)	1.58	(31)
Education	3.74	(60)	3.93	(78)
Residual	2.35	(38)	−0.49	(−10)
Intercohort change	6.24	(100)	5.02	(100)
55–64				
Family factors	0.88	(23)	0.92	(53)
Education	2.85	(75)	3.96	(228)
Residual	0.05	(1)	−3.14	(−180)
Intercohort change	3.78	(100)	1.74	(100)

[a] Numbers in parentheses are percentages.

[b] Includes paternal (head's) occupational status and education, number of siblings, farm origins, and broken family.

equation (from Table 10.6) for blacks aged 25–34. The estimated socio-economic score is an additional 7.12 points below the observed 1973 mean; thus, shifts in educational attainment over the decade, net of family factors, account for some 66% of the intercohort change in occupational achievement among black men aged 25–34. The remaining 27%, or 2.90 points on the Duncan scale, represents change in occupational opportunities between 1962 and 1973. Of course, these components of change may vary if other variables are added to the regression model or if a different regression equation, for example the 1962 one, is taken as the standard. For this reason our calculation might better be regarded as a mental experiment than as a statistical estimate in the usual sense. We have carried out this indirect regression standardization for each age group in the white and black samples.

For blacks, shifts in family background account for only a small portion of total intercohort changes in occupational status—about 13% for men aged 25–64 (see Table 10.7). A larger percentage of change comes from rising levels of schooling—between 60 and 75%—and there is less age variation in this percentage than for the family background components taken as a block. Except at ages 45–54, roughly three-quarters of the rise in occupational status of black men results from increased levels of schooling and small net improvements in family background circumstances. The remaining quarter represents change in the occupational opportunities of black men with given socioeconomic origins and levels of schooling.[5] Compositional shifts in family factors and education come closest to explaining intercohort change in occupational status at ages 35–44 and 55–64.

For whites, the compositional changes in family factors and education are more than enough to account for the small intercohort rises in average occupational status. This fact is apparent from the negative signs of the residual components in Table 10.7. For example, among men aged 25–64, intercohort increases in average schooling account for nearly all (92%) of the total intercohort gain in occupational status. Coupled with rising socioeconomic levels of parents, this change could account for an upward status shift 148% as large as the observed intercohort shift. Thus, like blacks, whites have experienced changes in occupational opportunities which reflect more than compositional shifts in background and education. However, the net change for whites is a decline in mean occupa-

---

[5] Since effects of family background and schooling on occupational status increased among black men between 1962 and 1973, choice of 1973 regressions as the standard yields smaller residual components of change in status opportunities than would standardizations based on the 1962 regressions. Compare Hauser and Featherman (1974b, Table 2).

tional socioeconomic status. That is, white men of all ages in 1973 could expect to hold lower average socioeconomic statuses at each level of schooling and social background than their counterparts in 1962 (compare Hauser and Featherman, 1974b). Unlike whites, blacks in 1973 did not have to acquire more education just to stay at the same occupational levels as same-aged men in 1962. Obversely, the schooling of white, but not of black, occupational incumbents was upgraded at each age between 1962 and 1973. We shall comment later on the significance of these differentials, especially since these shifts in occupational opportunities are coupled with intercohort increases in the occupational returns to each year of additional schooling for both whites and blacks.

Compositional differences in family background and schooling account for most of the racial differentials in mean occupational status in both 1962 and 1973, as shown in Table 10.8. Here we standardize on the age-specific regression equations for whites from Tables 10.5 and 10.6 for each year, inserting the black age-specific means into the white equations. The logic of these interracial comparisons is the same as in the decompositions of intercohort changes within races. As in previous use of this procedure (Duncan, 1968a, 1968c; Hauser and Featherman, 1974b), we interpret residual racial differences as conservative estimates of racial discrimination in the labor market.[6] Obviously, "discrimination" measured in this way may be confounded with effects of omitted variables, such as differences between the races in culture or ability (to the extent that they are not represented by family background and educational attainment).

Racial differences in family background accounted for about an 8-point occupational status differential between black men in 1973 as in 1962 (see Table 10.8). At no age in either year was this component of the racial gap larger than 9.5 SEI points or smaller than 7.0 SEI points. Differences in years of schooling accounted for smaller status differentials between the races in 1973 than in 1962. This is not a trivial finding, for the narrowed racial gap in schooling is partly compensated for in these calculations by the increased status returns to schooling in 1973 relative to 1962. The size of the racial gap in occupational status attributable to schooling varied directly with age in 1962. This age pattern was even stronger in 1973 because the effect of schooling on the occupational status gap declined most

---

[6] Use of regression equations for white men as the standard is conservative because the generally steeper slopes in white than in black equations lead to smaller estimates of racial "discrimination" than would standardization on the equations for blacks. Also, use of the white equations as the standard is more nearly correct, for response error leads to larger downward biases in regression coefficients estimated for black than for white men (Bielby *et al.*, 1977).

TABLE 10.8

Components of Racial Socioeconomic Differences: Men Aged 25–64 in the Experienced Civilian Labor Force, by Age, March 1962 and March 1973[a]

Age and component	1962		1973	
Total, 25–64				
Family factors[b]	8.04	(37)	8.37	(50)
Education	7.90	(37)	2.55	(15)
Residual	5.54	(26)	5.90	(35)
Racial difference	21.48	(100)	16.82	(100)
25–34				
Family factors	8.44	(38)	9.53	(70)
Education	5.06	(23)	−1.04	(−8)
Residual	8.57	(39)	5.15	(38)
Racial difference	22.07	(100)	13.64	(100)
35–44				
Family factors	8.70	(41)	8.39	(50)
Education	6.85	(32)	4.39	(26)
Residual	5.87	(27)	4.15	(24)
Racial difference	21.42	(100)	16.93	(100)
45–54				
Family factors	7.03	(34)	8.72	(44)
Education	6.58	(31)	5.88	(30)
Residual	7.31	(35)	5.10	(26)
Racial difference	20.92	(100)	19.70	(100)
55–64				
Family factors	8.14	(37)	8.55	(43)
Education	7.74	(35)	6.90	(35)
Residual	6.07	(28)	4.46	(22)
Racial difference	21.95	(100)	19.91	(100)

[a] Numbers in parentheses are percentages.
[b] Includes paternal (head's) occupational status and education, number of siblings, farm origins, and broken family.

at the younger ages. Residual or discriminatory differentials in status between the races also declined inversely with age. Taken together, these two changes produced a direct variation of the total racial gap with age which was absent in 1962. These changes are obscured when the components are obtained for men throughout the working ages, for in the aggregate the effect of schooling differences on the racial gap has declined, but not the effects of discrimination and family background. These changes in the size of specific components of racial differences in occupational status have increased the relative importance of family background as a factor in the racial gap. In the aggregate, family background explained 37% of the racial gap in 1962 and 50% in 1973. Similar shifts occurred at ages 35–64, and the change was even more marked at ages 25–34.

Last, what portion of the declining racial gap in occupational status (seen most clearly among men in their early work careers) is associated with changing differentials in family socioeconomic statuses and schooling? What portion represents "true" change in the occupational positions accessible to black and white men? Table 10.9 shows our analyses of these questions. We have used the age-specific regressions for whites in 1973 as the standard. Into these equations we have inserted the changes in the mean racial differences over the decade, following our earlier pattern. To interpret Table 10.9, we observe that the racial gap in occupational sta-

TABLE 10.9

Components of Change in Racial Differences in Occupational Status: Men Aged 25–64 in the Experienced Civilian Labor Force, March 1962 and March 1973

Age and component	SEI points
Total, 25–64	
Family factors[a]	0.95
Education	−3.32
Residual	−2.29
Net change	−4.66
25–34	
Family factors	2.31
Education	−5.15
Residual	−5.59
Net change	−8.43
35–44	
Family factors	0.15
Education	−5.39
Residual	0.75
Net change	−4.49
45–54	
Family factors	1.08
Education	−1.46
Residual	−0.84
Net change	−1.22
55–64	
Family factors	0.46
Education	−2.79
Residual	0.29
Net change	−2.04

[a] Includes paternal (head's) occupational status and education, number of siblings, farm origins, and broken family.

tus for ages 25–64 narrowed by 4.66 points between 1962 and 1973. We estimate that the gap would have increased by about 1 unit on the SEI scale (0.95) if one took into account only the changes in racial differentials in family factors; but net of those changes, we note a decline of 3.32 points in the gap owing to shifts in schooling differentials. The difference between these net amounts and the observed total change of −4.66 SEI points is −2.29, or the decline in the gap attributable to changes in the differential occupational opportunities of black and white men. This aggregate decomposition is a bit misleading, for with the exception of men aged 25–34, change in the educational differences between the races is sufficient to account for the narrowing socioeconomic gap between black and white occupations. Among men aged 35–44, for example, a decline of 5.39 points is expected as a result of changing differentials in schooling, and this is larger than the observed decline of 4.49 SEI points. If changes in the educational differentials between the races serve to reduce occupational status differentials, the changing racial differences in family background serve to limit such improvements in the social standing of blacks. At every age the relative gains of whites in family contexts favorable to socioeconomic advancement partly offset the declines in racial occupational differences which stem from education.

For the youngest workers (aged 25–34), the shift toward greater educational equality also accounts for a large part of the declining occupational difference (5.15 SEI points), but it is smaller than the very large net decline in the occupational gap (8.43 points) at these ages. Only among the youngest workers did a decline in labor market discrimination appear to account for a substantial component (5.59 SEI points) of the reduction in black–white occupational status differentials. Interestingly, this is also the age at which the process of occupational stratification has shown the clearest signs of convergence between the races. Thus, changes both in levels of occupational standing and in processes of socioeconomic stratification have been most evident among young workers.

Summary, Interpretations, and Speculations

In the decade between 1962 and 1973 both white and black males in the experienced civilian labor force enjoyed a general rise in the socioeconomic status of their occupations. Among whites, the gains were concentrated in the middle years of the work career; blacks in the early career experienced the largest improvements in average status. Relative to whites, black workers in 1973 had gained ground, closing the socioeconomic status gap by about 22%, with greater equality of attainments among men aged 25–34. Still, occupational statuses of blacks in 1973 fell below the average attainments of whites at every age in 1962.

Through the succession of cohorts, the socioeconomic circumstances of black and white families of origin improved, as did levels of schooling, and this created more favorable environments for the social promotion of cohorts in the later period. These more favorable conditions for achievement do not account fully for intercohort shifts in occupational status for either race, indicating that occupational opportunities were changing.

Change in the process of stratification has followed different patterns for blacks than for whites. Having been reared in farm families represents less of an occupational handicap for both races in 1973 than in 1962, and the socioeconomic status returns to educational achievement for men of equivalent social backgrounds are greater in the 1970s than in the last decade. The increased occupational value of each additional year of schooling is more noticeable among blacks than whites and more evident among younger than older workers. Taken as a block, family factors play a somewhat less substantial role in the occupational attainments of whites than in 1962, and the relative importance of education (vis-à-vis the family) has increased. However, the occupational statuses of whites in 1973 vary more within levels of socioeconomic background and schooling than in 1962. Thus, the process of occupational stratification has become more meritocratic and perhaps more random (with respect to the family and schooling) for whites. Schooling remains the single most important element of status allocation, and indeed the value of each additional year of education has increased for whites. At the same time, whites are unable to convert their educational attainments into occupational statuses at the same level as did men of equivalent schooling in 1962. Therefore, downward shifts in education-specific occupational attainments have occurred since 1962, even as the socioeconomic differentials between educational levels have risen.

If the process of stratification has become somewhat more random for whites over the decade, it has grown more deterministic for black men in the ECLF, as both socioeconomic background and, especially, schooling are more tightly linked to occupational statuses.[7] Families and schools apparently have begun to function in the socioeconomic life cycles of blacks as they did for whites in earlier years. The greatest racial similarities in status allocation appear among workers in the early careers, the same group for whom the racial gap in occupational socioeconomic status has

---

[7] Within these categories of family and schooling, however, occupational achievement was less determinate in 1973 than in 1962, even as in both years achievement was more determinate for blacks than whites.

shrunk the most since 1962. Over the decade, increases in the value of each additional year of education have been large for blacks—nearly 50%. These substantial gains have not eliminated the racial difference in returns to schooling, but neither have blacks experienced the downward shift in education-specific occupational status which has occurred among whites.

The racial gap in mean socioeconomic status has declined, and similarities in the process of status allocation for young men of both races are greater, but blacks still experience occupational discrimination. There has been little change since 1962 in the percentage of the racial gap which we have designated as discrimination. Changes in educational differentials account for a significant portion of the declining gap at all ages. But it is among workers in their early careers that such compositional sources are least able to account for the narrowing (notable at ages 25–34) of the mean socioeconomic levels of the races. Among these young workers, changes in differential occupational opportunities, together with the near disappearance of racial differences in education, combine to reduce the occupational status differentials between whites and blacks.

What do these various trends and changes signify for racial or ethnic relations in the United States? Unfortunately, there is no simple answer. Even with respect to the limited issue of the "structural integration" (Hechter, 1971) of blacks into the economy, the data are equivocal. On the one hand, the process of stratification appears to be moving toward a racially homogeneous pattern, as younger workers seem to be experiencing quite similar allocation from socioeconomic origins to schooling and then into the occupational hierarchy. Differentials in process and level of occupational attainment persist, even among the young, but gaps have declined and inequality of opportunity has diminished. Black families seem increasingly able to transfer their socioeconomic status to sons. Put another way, economic classes are more visible among the black population now than they were a decade ago. In addition, young black men have achieved near equality of schooling with whites, and relative to conditions for blacks over a decade ago, increments to regular or formal education provide better jobs at each level of schooling and for each additional year completed.

On the other hand, differentials in returns to education and family resources remain, as do gaps in average occupational status, especially among older men. Discrimination in the labor market, although perhaps smaller in absolute size, is not significantly less as a proportion of the total gap in occupational status than it was a decade ago. In addition, a more favorable socioeconomic position relative to whites has not led automatically to less discrimination against blacks in other components of the quality and style of life, as exemplified by the persistence of segregated housing. And, even though young blacks in the civilian labor force have gained ground on their white contemporaries, the likelihood of a young black being in the labor force was less in 1973 than in 1962. In sum, the evidence for a consistent trend in structural integration of the races is mixed. It confounds the always problematic associations among cultural, structural, and political integration (Hechter, 1971) and makes predictions about change in racial relations impossible.

Surely racial stratification and inequality persist, even in these "post-industrial" United States. Even so, trends in stratification of the races reveal evidence for increased economic rationality which places constraints on the effective ability of the white majority to control the socioeconomic well-being of the black minority or to institutionalize the existing stratification system. Proponents of the thesis of industrialism (see Treiman, 1970 for an overview)—the view that social change in the United States occurs primarily through industrial transformation and evolution—might be heartened by the diminished role of family factors as education becomes more effective in allocating men to occupational positions in the socioeconomic hierarchy. In that sense, stratification has grown more universalistic. The process is more rational in that, for example, it responds to larger cohorts of highly educated whites by raising the educational prerequisites for each occupation (see Smelser and Lipset, 1966; Thurow and Lucas, 1972). Educational upgrading of the occupational hierarchy in the last decade is consistent both with the view that credentialism is rampant (for example, Berg, 1970) and with the contention that economic change since 1962 has increased the premium for higher productivity.[8] This pre-

---

[8] Competing explanations of these trends in terms of productivity versus credentialism effects are difficult if not impossible to adjudge. We do note that for whites the predictive power (in R^2) of the family-plus-education equation is less for 1973 than for 1962. In addition, occupational inequality within categories of family and education has hardly changed for whites. Had credentialism grown as a tendency over the period, we might have expected (1) between-education variation to increase (it did) and (2) within-education variation to decrease (it did not). Were productivity relationships at work, we might have expected both within- and between-variation to rise, as both education and other skill-related characteristics (not indexed by formal schooling) have become more closely associated with occupational differences. The same line of argument leads to an expectation that on-the-job training and other skills have become more central in earnings differentials within jobs. We report on these analyses elsewhere (Featherman and Hauser, 1978, Chs. 5 and 6); here we merely note that male earnings were less determined by family, schooling, and occupational level in 1973 than in 1962 (controlling also for weeks worked), even as the (constant) dollar returns to each year of schooling have increased in the period. While somewhat equivocal in meaning, these data are not inconsistent with the view that productivity relationships, not credentialism, were the major force behind the rising returns to schooling between 1962 and 1973.

mium takes the form of greater occupational and earnings differences among persons at each educational level than a decade earlier as, for example, those with higher education are recruited into growth industries, especially in the tertiary sector (see Bell, 1973, Ch. 3).

Blacks have shared in these putative transformations of the economy and in the process of socioeconomic stratification. Because educational achievements of blacks became more important in status allocation over the decade, proportionately less of the variance we can explain in occupational attainment in 1973 reflects ascribed (family) factors. Increasing mean levels of schooling have not raised the educational prerequisites for occupations for blacks as they have for whites: black men at each educational level were able to obtain higher-status jobs in 1973 than they could in 1962. At the same time, each increment of schooling brought greater returns than a decade ago. Blacks have become more internally differentiated by occupation, creating more distinctive economic strata within the race, with education serving as an effective mechanism allocating persons to jobs. The converging educational achievements of the races have provided a major impetus to the decline in occupational inequality between black and white men, and at the younger ages declining labor market discrimination has also narrowed the racial gap in occupational status.

In all of these contemporary shifts and changes in socioeconomic stratification we find little support for applying to ethnic relations in modern America a theory which casts the differential achievements of majority and minority groups in terms of "core" and "peripheral" classes or one which emphasizes racist tendencies, whether de jure or de facto, to the neglect of other tendencies in the allocation of statuses (cf. Hechter, 1971, p. 42). Indeed, such theories are frequently designed to account for the stability of positions of super- and subordination rather than for change in the process of stratification. Our analysis of change in racial stratification shows that whites in 1973 faced less favorable circumstances than in 1962, especially as they attempted to convert their schooling into jobs and occupational statuses. In that respect, the relative improvement of the occupational standing of blacks has occurred at the expense of whites.

Whatever the source of ascendancy of whites over blacks, whatever the basis of current inequities in economic power, whites have not been able to monopolize the advantages of socioeconomic change since 1962. Stratification of the black population between generations is beginning to follow a pattern of relationships which tends to characterize majority populations in many industrialized nations (see Featherman et al., 1975 for a treatment of some of these commonalities). Meanwhile, white families have not effectively insulated their offspring from the occupational consequences of a burgeoning supply of highly educated workers. As parents of higher socioeconomic means become less able to guarantee the educational attainments of their offspring (Hauser and Featherman, 1976) and as family factors grow less powerful in the occupational allocation of whites, the efficacy of both race and class as sources of status inequality declines.

ACKNOWLEDGMENTS

We thank Peter J. Dickinson and Neil D. Fligstein for technical assistance and Christopher S. Jencks and Ross M. Stolzenberg for friendly critcism. Any opinions, findings, conclusions or recommendations are those of the authors and do not necessarily reflect the views of the National Science Foundation or other agencies supporting this work.

References

Alwin, D. F., and R. M. Hauser
  1975   "The decomposition of effects in path analysis." *American Sociological Review* 40 (February): 37–47.
Barth, F.
  1969   *Ethnic Groups and Boundaries*. Boston: Little, Brown.
Bell, D.
  1973   *The Coming of Post-industrial Society*. New York: Basic Books.
Berg, I.
  1970   *Education and Jobs: The Great Training Robbery*. New York: Praeger.
Bielby, W. T., R. M. Hauser, and D. L. Featherman
  1977   "Response errors of black and nonblack males in models of the intergenerational transmission of socioeconomic status." *American Journal of Sociology* 82 (May): 1242–1288.
Blau, P. M., and O. D. Duncan
  1967   *The American Occupational Structure*. New York: Wiley.
Blauner, R.
  1969   "Internal colonization and ghetto revolt." *Social Problems* 16 (Spring): 393–408.
Bonacich, E.
  1976   "Advanced capitalism and black/white relations in the United States: A split labor market interpretation." *American Sociological Review* 41 (February): 34–51.
Campbell, A.
  1971   *White Attitudes toward Black People*. Ann Arbor, Mich.: Institute for Social Research.
Duncan, O. D.
  1961   "A socioeconomic index for all occupations." Pp. 109–138 in A. J. Reiss (ed.), *Occupations and Social Status*. New York: Free Press.
  1967   "Discrimination against Negroes." *Annals of the American Academy of Political and Social Science* 371 (May): 85–103.
  1968a   "Inheritance of poverty or inheritance of race?" Pp. 85–110 in D. Moynihan (ed.), *On Understanding Poverty*. New York: Basic Books.
  1968b   "Patterns of occupational mobility among Negro men." *Demography* 5 (1): 11–22.

1968c "Social stratification and mobility: Problems on the measurement of trend." Pp. 675–719 in E. B. Sheldon and W. E. Moore (eds.), *Indicators of Social Change*. New York: Russell Sage.

Farley, R., and A. Hermalin
1972 "The 1960s: A decade of progress for blacks?" *Demography* 9 (August): 353–370.

Farley, R., and A. F. Taeuber
1974 "Racial segregation in the public schools." *American Journal of Sociology* 79 (January): 888–905.

Featherman, D. L., and R. M. Hauser
1973 "On the measurement of occupations in social surveys." *Sociological Methods and Research* 2 (November): 239–251.
1975 "Design for a replicate study of social mobility in the United States." Pp. 219–251 in K. C. Land and S. Spilerman (eds.), *Social Indicator Models*. New York: Russell Sage.
1976 "Sexual inequalities and socioeconomic achievement in the U. S., 1962–1973." *American Sociological Review* 41 (June): 462–483.
1978 *Opportunity and Change*. New York: Academic Press.

Featherman, D. L., F. L. Jones, and R. M. Hauser
1975 "Assumptions of social mobility research in the United States: The case of occupational status." *Social Science Research* 4 (December): 329–360.

Feldman, A., and W. E. Moore
1962 "Industrialization and industrialism: Convergence and differentiation." In *Transactions of the Fifth World Congress of Sociology*. Washington, D. C.: International Sociological Association.

Garnsey, E.
1975 "Occupational structure in industrialized societies: Some notes on the convergence thesis in the light of soviet experience." *Sociology* 9 (September): 437–458.

Goldthorpe, J. W.
1964 "Social stratification in industrial society." In P. Halmos (ed.), *The Development of Industrial Societies*. Vol. 8. Keele: University of Keele.

Greeley, A. M., and P. B. Sheatsley
1971 "Attitudes toward racial integration." *Scientific American* 225 (December): 13–19.

Hauser, R. M., and D. L. Featherman
1974a "White-nonwhite differentials in occupational mobility among men in the United States, 1967–1972." *Demography* 11 (May): 247–265.
1974b "Socioeconomic achievements of U. S. men, 1962 to 1972." *Science* 185 (July): 325–331.
1976 "Equality of schooling: Trends and prospects." *Sociology of Education* 49 (April): 99–120.

Hauser, R. M., D. L. Featherman, and D. P. Hogan
1977 "Sex in the structure of occupational mobility in the U. S., 1962." Pp. 99–122 in R. M. Hauser and D. L. Featherman, *The Process of Stratification: Trends and Analyses*. New York: Academic Press.

Hechter, M.
1971 "Towards a theory of ethnic change." *Politics and Society* (Fall): 21–44.
1974 "The political economy of ethnic change." *American Journal of Sociology* 79 (May): 1151–1178.

Hermalin, A. I., and R. Farley
1973 "The potential for residential integration in cities and suburbs: Implications for the busing controversy." *American Sociological Review* 38 (October): 595–610.

Hodge, R. W., and P. Hodge
  1965   "Occupational assimilation as a competition process." *American Journal of Sociology* 71 (November): 249–264.
Levy, M., Jr.
  1966   *Modernization and the Structure of Societies*. Princeton, N. J.: Princeton University Press.
Lieberson, S.
  1970   "Stratification and ethnic groups." Pp. 172–181 in E. O. Laumann (ed.), *Social Stratification: Research and Theory for the 1970s*. Indianapolis: Bobbs-Merrill.
Morgan, W. R., and T. N. Clark
  1973   "The causes of racial disorders: A grievance-level explanation." *American Sociological Review* 38 (October): 611–624.
Schuman, H., and S. Hatchett
  1974   *Black Racist Attitudes: Trends and Complexities*. Ann Arbor, Mich.: Institute for Social Research.
Smelser, N. J., and S. M. Lipset
  1966   *Social Structure and Mobility in Economic Development*. Chicago: Aldine.
Thurow, L. C., and R. E. B. Lucas
  1972   *The American Distribution of Income: A Structural Problem*. Washington, D. C.: U. S. Government Printing Office.
Treiman, D. J.
  1970   "Industrialization and social stratification." Pp. 207–234 in E. O. Laumann (ed.), *Social Stratification: Research and Theory for the 1970s*. Indianapolis: Bobbs-Merrill.
U. S. Bureau of the Census
  1975   "The Social and Economic Status of the Black Population in the United States, 1974." *Current Population Reports*. Special Studies, Series P-23, no. 54. Washington, D. C.: U. S. Government Printing Office.
U. S. National Advisory Commission on Civil Disorders
  1968   *Report of the National Advisory Commission on Civil Disorders*. New York: Bantam.

11

Statistical Histories of the Life Cycle of Birth Cohorts: The Transition from Schoolboy to Adult Male[1]

HALLIMAN H. WINSBOROUGH

Two closely related ideas are important in understanding the dynamics of social and demographic change in modern societies. They are the idea of a life cycle and the idea of a cohort or "generation." This chapter is an initial report on a research project whose aim is to construct statistical histories of the life cycle of annual birth cohorts in the United States from around 1900 to the present. The aim of the project is to produce as coherent a description of how members of each cohort have lived out their lives as can be generated at present from publicly available data sources.

This chapter will present the conceptual background of the project and some examples of the findings to date. The project as a whole will draw data from the decennial censuses, Vital Statistics Reports, the National

[1] Aspects of this research were supported by the National Science Foundation (SOC75-20409), the Population Research Center grant (5PO1-HD05876) awarded to the Center for Demography and Ecology at the University of Wisconsin by the Center for Population Research of the National Institute for Child Health and Human Development and by a grant from the Research Committee of the Graduate School, The University of Wisconsin–Madison. Some of the data used in this paper derive from the Occupational Changes in a Generation II Survey which was supported under a grant from the Division of Social Systems and Human Resources, RANN-NSF (GI-31604X).

231

Longitudinal Survey of Labor Market Experience (NLS), the various national fertility surveys, and the Current Population Surveys (CPS) and their supplements. Of particular importance are the two Occupational Changes in a Generation supplements to the CPS. Data from the latter supplement will predominate in the examples of results to date.

In the project as a whole, six aspects of the life cycle of cohorts will be investigated. They are:

1. The background of the cohort
2. The family, childhood, and education of the cohort
3. The process of getting started in adult life
4. Career and family building
5. The end of childraising and the later career
6. The terminal years—retirement, widowhood, morbidity, and mortality

The preliminary findings presented in this chapter will focus on the transition from the second to the third of these stages as it operates for males. It is this transition that moves male cohort members from the status of schoolboy to that of fully adult member of our society. The findings presented will show how the joint action of several secular trends has operated to markedly change the length of time it takes a cohort to move through the series of steps that constitute this transition.

The chapter will proceed as follows: First, it will discuss the idea of a life cycle, the idea of a cohort, and the relationship between them. Then, it will present an argument about why a descriptive study of the life cycles of cohorts seems appropriate at this time. Finally, it will present data on the transition from schoolboy to adult male in the hope that findings from this investigation are concrete evidence of the utility of the approach.

Conceptual Background

THE IDEA OF A LIFE CYCLE

The notion that individuals in a given society live out their lives according to a partly biologically and partly socially determined pattern is an old one in Western thought.[2] It is also an old idea that societies differ in the way an individual's progress through his appointed years is organized. In a stable society this organizational pattern is thought to be an important

---

[2] The Sphinx's riddle answered by Oedipus is, perhaps, the oldest available expression of the idea.

aspect of culture that may interact with other aspects.[3] As societies change there may develop a lack of fit between the organization of the life cycle and other aspects of culture. In the course of his discussion of the idea of a "typical biography," Redfield discusses the impact of this kind of disjuncture on individuals as follows:

> The more important characteristics of the human career in societies that have changed rapidly and are continuing to change is that the career of any one kind of person, man or woman, factory worker or business man, becomes within itself inconsistent and inconclusive. The purposes that are created in early life as to material success are not always the purposes that the individual finds he can realize; or the ideals and purposes of mutual help and sacrifice for the community are not the ideals and purposes which he may be called upon to realize in his working life. The ends of life become obscure. Educated women find themselves doing many things which are immediately necessary but that do not seem to be directed toward significant ends. People develop wants whose satisfaction brings no satisfaction. Such characteristics of the human career in the more modern societies demand a view of the community that is more than its conception as social structure; the biographic dimension is a form of description and investigation which exposes these characteristics to our notice and that calls upon us to devise ways more precisely to define and to explain them [Redfield, 1955, p. 63].

In modern society, of course, many aspects of social structure, as well as individual expectations, wants, and needs, depend on the orderliness of the life cycle. Special institutions exist to "process" people through various life cycle stages. As life cycle patterns are disturbed by time-specific events such as wars or depressions, and as patterns undergo modification over time, clear institutional and even societal difficulties may be experienced. The current uncertainty about future college enrollment is perhaps an example that will strike home to readers of this chapter.

Knowledge of relatively stable components of the life cycle in modern society has been a necessary basis for important models of social processes as well as for the orderly operation of the social system. The Blau–Duncan model of social mobility depends on the fact that, by and large, people in modern society complete their education prior to their major involvement in the labor force (Blau and Duncan, 1967). Models of fertility behavior frequently depend on the fact that most people marry prior to having children (Coale and Trussell, 1974). Clearly, there exist societies or parts of societies in which these assumptions about the life cycle do not obtain. Analysis of Latin American fertility is complicated by a "disorderly" pattern of consanguineous unions (Stycos, 1968, especially Chapters 12 and 13), while the "disorderly" arrangement of child-having and

---

[3] Consider, for example, Durkheim's discussion of initiation rites or the lack of them in *The Elementary Forms of the Religious Life*, 1954, p. 383 and following.

labor force participation for women in American society defies neat modeling (Sweet, 1973).

In summary, then, there exists in social science the idea that:

1. Life cycles exist as patterns of what happens in a lifetime.
2. Life cycles may vary from society to society.
3. Life cycles may be disrupted by time-specific events.
4. Life cycles may change within a given society in response to other social changes.
5. Disruption or change in the life cycle has ramifications for other aspects of social structures.

THE IDEA OF COHORTS

The second idea that is important for understanding social and demographic change is the notion of a cohort or "generation." The basic idea is that individuals born at about the same time in a society—a birth cohort or "generation"—form an important social aggregate. Mannheim (1952, pp. 289–290), for example, asserted that the logical status and social importance of the cohort is roughly co-equal with that of a social class, an idea which he took quite seriously.

Two corollaries to the cohort idea are important. First is the notion that the thing that makes a cohort or "generation" unique is that it experiences similar conditions at similar life cycle stages as it moves through its lifetime and that this sharing of experiences sets it off both objectively and subjectively from other cohorts. Objectively it may be important that circumstances encourage a given cohort to marry early or late and that subsequent nuptial, fertility, or even labor force behavior of the cohort is likely to be modified thereby (Ryder, 1964, 1965). Subjectively it may be that a cohort's set of shared experiences creates in its opinion, subjective experiences, and artistic products an internal logic difficult to appreciate or understand by members of other cohorts.

The second corollary idea about cohorts is that the population of a society at a given point in time can be seen as a set of cohorts, each cohort being represented as persons of a particular age. Thus the current state of the population with respect to any aggregate rate or mean may be most intelligible in terms of the cohort-specific processes then underway. Ryder (1962) has coined the phrase "demographic translation" to describe the analytic process of moving between a series of cohorts and a series of cross-sectional rates. Thus high aggregate fertility in the cross section may perhaps be understood in terms of the "catching up" of older cohorts who have previously delayed child-having and the concurrent early fertility of younger cohorts. It is important in this corollary that not only the cross-sectional state of the population is to be understood in cohort terms, but also that aggregate change can be usefully described in terms of:

1. Changing within-cohort behavior
2. The replacement, over time, of older cohorts with more recently born ones

In the foregoing paragraphs, I have used the concepts of *cohort* and *generation* synonymously, a usage in keeping with the older sociological literature as well as with the popular understanding of the terms. More precise current usage reserves the term *generation* to indicate biological progeny. I shall henceforth use that term in the more modern way.

The point of making this distinction is that the progeny of a single birth cohort are spread over many subsequent birth cohorts; a single birth cohort represents end points of individual generations of varying length. This fact is of considerable social importance. Demographers are familiar with the observation that a perturbance in the birth rates of a stable population causes an irregularity in the age distribution that, although reflected in the size of birth cohorts including the progeny of the original one, "smooths out" over time in a fashion controlled by the distribution of generation lengths in the population (Keyfitz, 1968, especially pp. 59–73). If women all had their children at exactly the same age, call it a, an irregularity in the age distribution would reappear in *every* ath birth cohort. Thus the fact that generation is *not* a function that maps from one birth cohort into one and only one subsequent cohort is the fact that permits the age distribution of a stable population to "forget" the perturbation of the past.

A similiar process must operate for many intergenerationally transmitted social characteristics. To take a fanciful example, suppose the fact of beginning life in a depression causes certain birth cohorts to transmit to their children a "cautious" approach to life that would lead to a dearth of entrepreneurship in the generation of the children. The fact that the individual generations are not all of the same length saves the society from continually repeated "busts" in entrepreneurship. This intercohort spreading of intergenerationally transmitted characteristics, then, is an important aspect of human society that may permit reequilibration after an important historical event.[4]

___

[4] For further discussion of the impact of this process, see Matras (1973). For a revealing analysis of the difference between cohort and generation effects, see Duncan (1975).

THE RELATIONSHIP BETWEEN LIFE CYCLES, GENERATIONS, AND COHORTS

The relationship between the idea of a life cycle and the idea of a cohort can be stated succinctly. If the idea of a life cycle is a concept applying to an aggregate, then it is a cohort which lives out an actual life cycle.

The tripartite relationship between life cycles, cohorts, and generations is somewhat more specific and complex. It is the distribution of fertility implied in the life cycle pattern of a cohort that determines the spread of lengths of individual generations and hence the rate at which a given cohort's intergenerationally transmitted characteristics are diffused among subsequent cohorts.

Overview and Justification of the Project

Given the foregoing as a cursory conceptual background, the purpose and motivation of this project can be stated briefly. The aim of the project is to draw together from publicly available sources, material to describe the life cycle of various cohorts in the United States and to document the changes in them.

The motivation for, and strategy in, undertaking such a descriptive project at this time can be summarized as follows. I take it as given that increasing our understanding about how social changes takes place is a good thing. Clearly many kinds of things can be thought of as representing social change. This descriptive work will focus on those kinds of change that are made manifest through the changed behavior of individuals as they live out their life cycle. Thus a large class of changes—for example, changes in laws, in patterns of governance, and in institutional arrangements—are represented only as they impinge on and modify the pattern of individual behavior in the course of living out a life. But surely it is just these modifications of the pattern of life that will be perceived in the population as the most salient kind of changes. Furthermore, insofar as such changes affect fertility or the arrangements for child care, their ramifications can spread through the cohort structure, creating changes in subsequent generations. Finally, they represent an important class of social changes in their own right that affect as well as respond to changes in other sectors of the social world. Thus the class of social changes represented by changes in the life cycle seems worth investigation.

But why undertake a *descriptive* study focusing on the cohort process? For some kinds of social change, noncohort analytic models may be more useful. Whatever may eventually prove to be the most useful analytic device for understanding a specific kind of change, however, it is clear that the mechanism through which that change will become apparent is the process of within or between cohort change. Thus the cohort approach seems a "natural" vehicle for organizing description because it is related to the mechanism for making the change manifest. Such a description, then, may aid understanding in its own right, prod intuition to construct more useful models, and provide a body of data that other scholars may use for analysis.

As a final point of justification, I argue that a project of this kind is timely and appropriate to the present state of interest in, and development of, knowledge about social change. The project is prima facie the creation of a set of social indicators using the cohort idea. It is different from much of the work on social indicators that use the cohort idea, however, in two important ways. First, much of the work on social indicators and most of the work on cohort analysis per se has focused on the analysis of one variable at a time. Thus we know a good deal about many important life cycle events each taken singly. But an important point in both the life cycle and the cohort idea is that events later in the life cycle may be contingent upon the nature of the earlier events. The focus of this study is to reveal these dependencies by investigating not single life cycle events, but rather the pattern of events that taken together constitutes the life cycle itself.

The second difference between this project and past ones is as follows. There exist a number of important studies that focus on all or a part of the life history of a single or a few adjacent cohorts. (See, for example, Blum *et al.,* 1969; Elder, 1975; Flanagan *et al.,* 1971; Sewell and Hauser, 1975.) Some of the studies provide a richer list of variables than can be derived from public data in some areas of the life cycle. Because they focus on a single or a few adjacent birth cohorts, however, they provide only modest information on changes in the life cycle. This study of change in the life cycle, then, although necessarily less detailed than the single cohort studies, may serve as a useful context from which to inspect detailed data on single cohorts.

FROM SCHOOLBOY TO ADULT: CHANGES IN A LIFE CYCLE TRANSITION

As an example of the kind of work that this project hopes to accomplish, let us focus our attention on that complex time of life in which young males move through a series of steps from the dependent status of schoolboy to the mature status of employed, married adult. It is a commonplace observation that decisions made during this time of life are of considerable consequence for an individual's future. He decides how much schooling he will complete. He enters the labor force in a job of particular status at a particular time. He does his military service. He chooses to marry a particular person at a particular time. All of these decisions influence his later career. (See, for example, Duncan *et al.*, 1972, pp. 170–183, 205–224.) The question we pose here is not how these individual decisions influence subsequent individual events, but how cohorts move through the process. The basic question we ask is, "Have there been changes in the way cohorts of males make their transition?"

Information is available on several of the steps in this process from the OCG II file. We can find out when individuals left school from their response to the question, "In what month and year did you COMPLETE your highest grade of school?"

The survey also asked the individual to "Describe the FIRST, FULL-TIME CIVILIAN JOB you had AFTER you completed your highest grade in school," along with instructions "DO INCLUDE full-time work in a family business or farm even if you were working without pay. DO NOT COUNT military service." Subsequent to collecting information to yield occupation, industry and class-or-worker codes for this job, the survey asks, "In what month and year did you BEGIN this job," and includes instructions, "Report the month and year in which you ACTUALLY began this job EVEN IF you started the job before you completed your highest grade in school." From the responses to this question we probably have about as good a measure of the respondent's time of entrance to his first "real" job during an interruption in schooling and for some respondents the job reported may not have been very "real" in the sense of being the beginning of a career line. Nonetheless, this question probably provides the best data currently available on the date of entry to first job.

With respect to military service, the survey begins by asking, "Have you ever been on active service in the U. S. Armed Forces or spent at least two months on active duty in the Reserves or National Guard?" Of those responding affirmatively, the survey asks, "When did you FIRST enter active military service?" with responses elicited as to month and year of entry. Following this question and also asked of all persons reporting service is the question, "What was the date of your LAST separation from active service?" with the instructions, "DO NOT COUNT Reserve, National Guard, etc. after active service." From responses to this series of questions we can garner information on entry to and exit from the military.

Information on age at first marriage is also available from OCG II but I have here perferred to rely on 1970 Census material because the age-at-first-marriage volume contains a satisfactory table.

Clearly these data provide a good deal of information about how individuals move through some of the important steps leading to adult status.

How can we use these data to yield information about the transition process for birth cohorts? Suppose we say that a cohort has "begun" one of the steps in this process when 25% of its members have made the necessary transition. For example, let us say that the cohort has begun the process of leaving school when 25% of the cohort have completed their education and that the cohort has "completed" the process when 75% have taken the step—in this case, when 75% have completed their education. Suppose further that we call the difference between the age at which 75% have completed school and the age at which 25% have finished the "duration" of the school leaving process.

THE EXIT FROM SCHOOL PROCESS

Let us begin by inspecting quartiles in the age at school completion distribution for the various cohorts. Table 11.1 presents first, second, and third quartiles for this distribution. Figure 11.1 graphs these numbers by birth year. From Figure 11.1 we observe the rise in median age at completion of school, which is to be expected from our knowledge of the increasing grade completion levels. Median age moves from the 16th year of life for earlier cohorts to the 18th for more recently born ones. Figure 11.1 shows also the increase in the 25th percentile of age that might be expected from the increase in the youngest age at which children are permitted to leave school. Age at which 75% of the cohort have completed school shows a good deal of intercohort variation but also shows a rather clear jump for cohorts born after 1920. Subsequent to this jump, the 75th percentile seems to remain at a rather high level until cohorts born in the 1940s.

Figure 11.2 plots the duration of the school leaving process. The process appears to have decreased in length—primarily due to the rise in the first quartile—from the cohort of 1909 to the cohort of 1920; then duration jumps and remains high until after the cohorts most affected by the Korean War. Subsequently, duration declines rather markedly, due both to the increase in the 25th percentile level and to the decline in the 75th percentile.

Some further insight into the fluctuations in the 75th percentile of the age at completion distribution can be provided by investigating school interruptions. Data on school interruptions is available in the OCG II survey from response to the question, "BEFORE you completed your highest grade in regular school, did you ever DISCONTINUE YOUR SCHOOLING FOR 6 MONTHS OR MORE?" Figure 11.3 displays the proportion of cohort members responding affirmatively to this question. In this figure we see disruption rates rise very rapidly for cohorts subject

TABLE 11.1

Age by Which 25%, 50%, and 75% of Male Members of Annual Birth Cohorts Completed Schooling and Duration[a] of the School Leaving Process[b]

Birth year	25% completed	50% completed	75% completed	Duration
1953	16.67	17.98		
1952	16.77	18.49		
1951	16.87	18.88	21.65	4.78
1950	16.92	18.57	21.57	4.65
1949	16.83	18.79	22.52	5.69
1948	16.66	18.63	22.85	6.19
1947	16.78	18.77	23.55	6.77
1946	16.57	18.65	23.76	7.19
1945	16.41	17.95	23.55	7.14
1944	16.34	17.75	22.88	6.54
1943	16.44	18.35	23.88	7.44
1942	16.29	17.98	24.74	8.45
1941	16.38	17.92	23.67	7.29
1940	16.43	18.10	24.38	7.95
1939	16.17	18.18	24.36	8.19
1938	16.20	17.98	24.52	8.32
1937	15.91	17.99	25.09	9.18
1936	16.08	17.91	23.95	7.87
1935	16.22	17.99	24.81	8.59
1934	16.14	17.74	24.00	7.86
1933	16.00	18.05	25.50	9.50
1932	15.41	17.61	25.19	9.78
1931	15.43	17.54	24.90	9.43
1930	15.62	17.57	24.41	8.79
1929	15.45	17.72	24.65	9.20
1928	14.91	17.22	24.35	9.44
1927	15.08	17.22	23.94	8.86
1926	15.39	17.50	26.11	10.72
1925	15.11	16.86	24.17	9.06
1924	15.34	17.28	24.69	9.35
1923	15.37	17.40	26.31	10.94
1922	15.32	17.34	23.17	7.85
1921	15.32	17.62	25.47	10.15
1920	15.10	17.25	21.24	6.14
1919	14.94	17.40	22.20	7.26
1918	14.87	16.94	21.13	6.26
1917	15.11	17.28	22.33	7.22
1916	14.93	17.36	22.77	7.84
1915	14.72	17.28	22.95	8.23
1914	14.52	16.92	21.45	6.93
1913	14.14	16.73	21.60	7.46
1912	13.90	17.14	24.06	10.16
1911	13.84	16.74	21.27	7.43
1910	14.16	16.63	22.78	8.62
1909	13.78	16.67	23.11	9.33

[a] Duration is computed as the difference between age at the 75th and 25th percentile level.

[b] Source: Occupational Change in a Generation II Survey, March 1973.

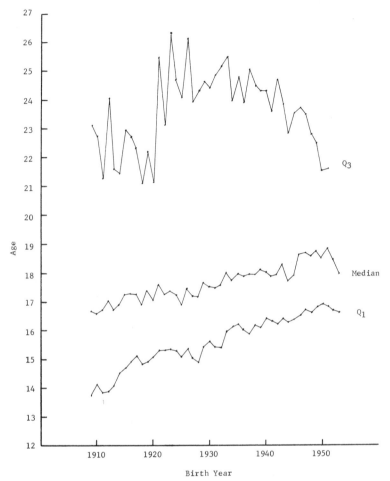

Figure 11.1. Quartiles of the age at school completion distribution by birth year.

to the draft at a young age in the Second World War. Although lower than World War II cohorts, Korean War and post-Korean War cohorts retain apparently elevated rates of school disruption. One suspects that this elevation is related to the "peacetime" draft. The dramatic decline in disruption for cohorts born around 1950 may signal a shift in the degree to which cohorts of men move through school in an uninterrupted manner without the uncertainties implied in the majority of peacetime draft regulations. One might, if he were willing to interpret the data in this way, forecast that duration of schooling is likely to decline even further in the future.

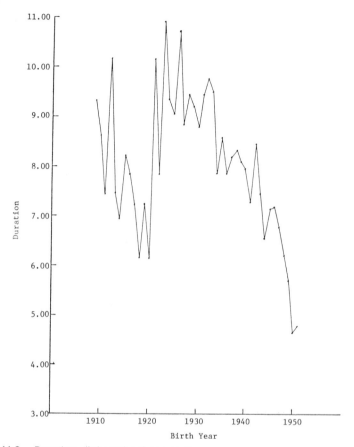

Figure 11.2. Duration of the school completion process.

Such a forecast is chancey for two reasons. First, its appropriateness depends on whether or not more recently born cohorts not in school in
March, 1973 may subsequently return. Further analysis of data on age at
first disruption—a variable available from the OCG II survey—may be
helpful in assaying the validity of this alternative explanation. Second, although cohorts from 1930 through 1948 retain fairly high and fairly constant disruption rates, the duration of the school leaving process dropped
rather markedly for the same cohorts. Thus it may be that those social
forces auguring for a more compact distribution of the cohort-specific
school completion process have been very nearly accommodated by
changing peacetime draft regulations.

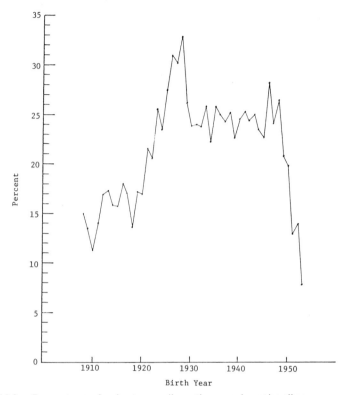

Figure 11.3. Percentage of cohort ever disrupting regular schooling.

ENTRANCE TO THE LABOR MARKET

Although the age at school completion distribution seems to show a good deal of complexity, the age at first job distribution seems, at first glance, more easily understood. Quartile levels of the process for this latter variable are presented in Table 11.2. Figure 11.4 presents a graph of the numbers. Median age at entry has risen somewhat from early cohorts: The first quartile, in general, shows a rising level of entrance to first job. Values rise rapidly for cohorts entering the labor market during the depression. Thereafter, values remain fairly constant until a modest decline for cohorts most affected by the World War II draft. There appears to be a jump after the last cohort to be of draftable age in World War II and a rather constant rise subsequently. Values for the 75th percentile level generally show a declining pattern. Values for this variable also exhibit

TABLE 11.2

Age by Which 25%, 50%, and 75% of Male Members of Annual Birth Cohorts Begin First Full-Time Job after Completing School, and Duration of the Labor Force Entry Process[a]

Birth year	25% completed	50% completed	75% completed	Duration[b]
1953	16.70	18.46		
1952	16.67	18.74		
1951	17.06	19.42		
1950	17.17	19.39	21.90	4.73
1949	17.01	19.46	22.58	5.57
1948	16.98	19.50	22.98	6.00
1947	17.06	19.98	23.71	6.65
1946	16.84	19.54	23.20	6.36
1945	16.63	18.94	23.10	6.47
1944	16.77	19.32	22.80	6.03
1943	16.75	19.45	23.03	6.28
1942	16.59	19.09	23.79	7.20
1941	16.66	19.25	23.53	6.87
1940	16.64	18.87	23.78	7.14
1939	16.66	19.42	24.35	7.69
1938	16.55	19.10	24.09	7.54
1937	16.16	19.56	25.31	9.15
1936	16.12	18.80	23.60	7.48
1935	16.50	18.80	24.39	7.89
1934	16.38	18.76	24.60	8.22
1933	16.18	19.30	24.37	8.19
1932	16.04	18.85	24.46	8.42
1931	16.03	18.77	25.64	9.61
1930	16.16	18.73	25.79	9.63
1929	16.21	18.68	24.71	8.50
1928	15.60	18.47	24.03	8.43
1927	15.58	18.89	23.96	8.38
1926	15.61	19.81	25.74	10.13
1925	15.87	19.29	24.97	9.10
1924	16.19	18.55	25.24	9.05
1923	16.18	18.94	26.37	10.19
1922	16.24	18.26	24.64	8.40
1921	16.26	18.59	26.14	9.88
1920	15.74	17.97	25.33	9.59
1919	15.75	18.31	26.52	10.71
1918	16.23	18.46	26.00	9.77
1917	15.91	18.77	25.64	9.73
1916	15.94	18.76	25.38	9.44
1915	16.09	18.86	26.50	10.41
1914	15.40	18.53	24.36	8.96
1913	14.90	18.20	25.60	10.70
1912	14.63	18.13	24.62	9.94
1911	14.30	17.44	22.96	8.66
1910	14.78	17.78	28.33	13.55
1909	14.52	17.51	24.50	9.98

[a] Source: Occupational Change in a Generation II Survey, March 1973.
[b] Duration is computed as the difference between age at 75th and 25th percentile level.

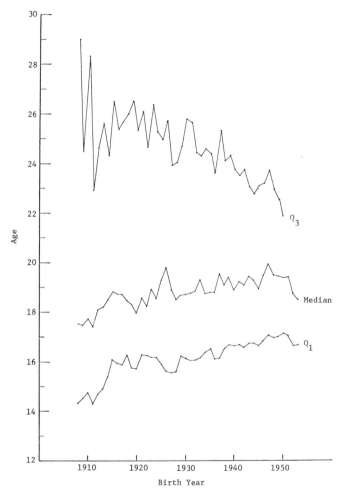

Figure 11.4. Quartiles of the age at first job distribution by birth year.

fluctuations similar to those for the median and lower quartile representing the impact of the depression and the second World War. In general, these patterns of the first quartile rise and third quartile decline yield
a decline in the duration of the entrance to the labor force process. Figure
11.5 graphs this rather dramatic shortening in the duration of the process.

About half of the men in the birth cohorts we have been investigating
spent some time in the armed forces. Cohort-specific proportions ever
serving in the armed forces are presented in column 1 of Table 11.3 and
graphed in Figure 11.6. More than 40% of cohort members served in the

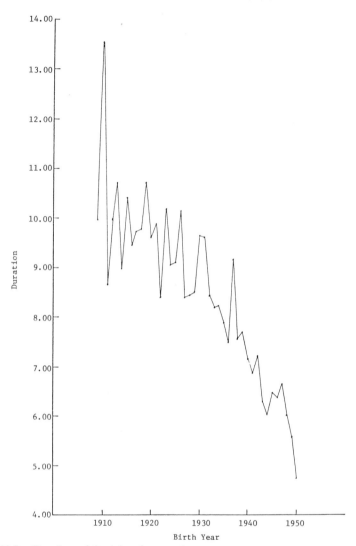

Figure 11.5. Duration of the labor force entrance process.

armed forces for each of the 34 cohorts from that of 1915 to that of 1949.
For the seven cohorts of 1941 through 1947, about 75% of cohort members served. For all but the earliest cohorts this period of service was contained within the time span of the transition from schoolboy to adult. Thus
entrance to and exit from the armed forces must be considered as a part of
the life cycle of the cohorts we are investigating. Table 11.3 presents,
along with the percentage of cohort members serving, the 25th and 50th

TABLE 11.3

Percentage Ever Serving in the Armed Forces; and for Those Who Served, 25th and 50th Percentiles for Age of First Entering and 50th and 75th Percentiles for Age of Last Separation by Birth Year[a]

Birth year	Percentage ever in	Ever entering		Ever leaving	
		25%	50%	50%	75%
1950	37.8	17.39	18.27	20.53	21.42
1949	41.6	17.56	18.48	20.92	23.00
1948	50.6	17.36	18.12	20.98	22.10
1947	55.1	17.48	18.41	21.19	22.65
1946	45.8	17.59	18.65	21.47	22.90
1945	42.9	17.11	19.14	21.65	23.71
1944	46.7	17.05	18.92	22.10	24.31
1943	40.6	16.65	18.03	21.70	23.77
1942	41.8	16.73	18.45	21.56	23.70
1941	42.0	17.18	18.82	21.93	23.96
1940	48.0	16.54	18.03	21.68	24.56
1939	49.1	16.66	18.21	21.72	24.02
1938	48.1	16.68	17.88	21.48	23.93
1937	48.6	16.55	17.96	21.89	24.11
1936	52.4	17.27	18.56	21.87	24.63
1935	55.9	17.26	18.80	21.85	23.73
1934	59.2	17.43	18.69	21.52	22.97
1933	63.7	17.07	18.52	21.48	22.93
1932	67.0	17.49	18.70	21.63	22.90
1931	66.2	17.10	19.18	22.08	23.53
1930	64.7	17.12	19.83	22.46	23.85
1929	62.3	16.40	18.60	22.40	23.90
1928	69.7	16.16	16.77	18.70	23.11
1927	77.7	16.16	16.72	18.78	20.19
1926	73.8	16.24	16.73	19.55	20.50
1925	73.9	17.02	17.45	20.33	20.85
1924	75.6	17.43	18.14	21.22	21.89
1923	75.2	18.19	18.79	22.12	22.75
1922	75.3	19.13	19.55	22.90	23.63
1921	74.2	19.87	20.48	23.86	24.57
1920	68.5	20.56	21.41	24.90	25.66
1919	66.7	21.30	22.20	25.79	26.54
1918	57.8	22.58	23.43	26.76	27.48
1917	53.3	23.67	24.57	27.84	28.51
1916	51.8	24.52	25.42	28.85	29.62
1915	41.2	25.40	26.42	29.78	30.49
1914	38.5	26.34	27.42	30.66	31.41
1913	36.7	27.98	28.72	31.82	32.55
1912	33.6	29.03	29.67	32.71	33.43
1911	27.8	29.81	30.70	33.74	34.55
1910	27.0	31.00	31.63	34.62	35.38

[a] Source: Occupational Change in a Generation II Survey, March 1973.

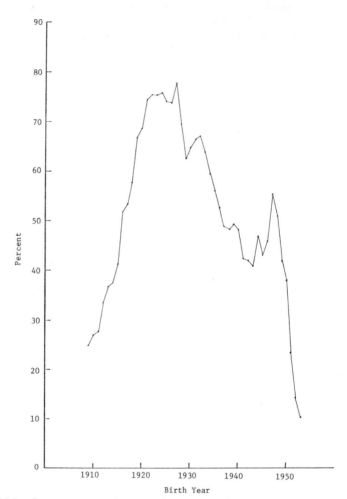

Figure 11.6.   Percentage ever in armed forces by birth year.

percentile levels of the age at entrance distribution and the 50th and 75th
percentile levels for the age at last separation for the cohort members who
served. Let us define the *duration* of the armed forces service stage of the
life cycle as the span of age between the 25th percentile for the age at entrance distribution and the 75th percentile for the age at separation distribution. This duration is graphed in Figure 11.7.

Three aspects of these data seem especially interesting. First is simply
the pervasiveness of military service as a component of the life cycle of
these men.

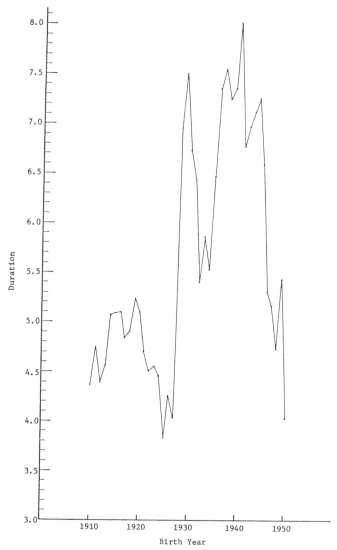

Figure 11.7. Duration of the armed forces process.

Second is the relatively smooth shape of the graph of the proportion ever serving by birth year. Contrast this rather smooth graph with that shown in Figure 11.8 which presents the number of military personnel on active duty from 1930 to 1972. Clearly a kind of demographic translation has been going on in which quite dramatic period shifts in the demand for military personnel are translated into a rather smoother set of cohort sat-

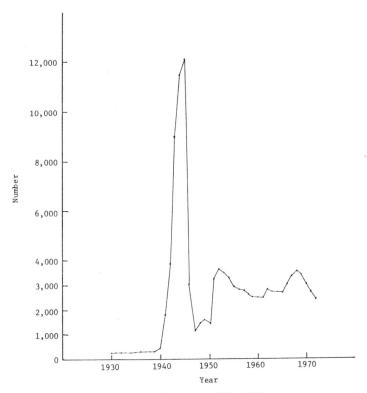

Figure 11.8. Military personnel on active duty, 1930–1972.

isfactions of time-specific demands. The capacity to produce a very large military force in the Second World War involved drawing on the potential for service in cohorts of men born earlier than those men of prime age for service at the onset of the war. During the Korean War one again finds a relatively more rapid rise in the size of the military than in the proportion of prime age cohorts called, suggesting the possibility of dependence on some potential for service in immediately earlier cohorts. It is interesting that the rise in military personnel during the Viet Nam War seems smoother than its impact on prime age cohorts. Certainly a careful understanding of the translation process would require aggregate period information on call-ups and discharges. It would also require a careful study of draft regulations. For example, it seems likely that the marked change in cohort rates for Viet Nam is a reflection of age preferences in draft regulations toward the end of this conflict.

The third interesting aspect of these numbers is the varying duration of the process of military service over cohorts. For cohorts serving in World

War II the duration of the service process is comparatively small. Those cohorts achieving prime age of service between World War II and the Korean War show a marked increase in duration. Duration drops for people of prime age during the Korean War and immediately after as the potential for service is rather quickly exhausted; it rises again for cohorts ripe for the post-Korean peacetime draft and falls again for cohorts of prime age in the Viet Nam conflict.

For some cohorts, then, the military service component of the life cycle drags out for as much as 8 years while for others it is relatively short. On the one hand, the lengthened duration of the process may have implied a greater choice in the time of the satisfaction of a man's military "obligation" and thus represents an advantage to cohorts attempting to make a relatively rapid transition to adulthood. On the other hand, this long duration means that some cohort members have spent a lot of time suffering uncertainty as to when, if at all, they will be required to satisfy that obligation.

AGE AT FIRST MARRIAGE

Finally, let us inspect the age at first marriage distribution by cohort. Recall that these data are derived from the 1970 Census rather than from the OCG II Survey. Table 11.4 presents 25th, 50th, and 75th percentiles of the distribution along with the calculation of the duration of the process. These percentiles are graphed in Figure 11.9 and the duration is displayed in Figure 11.10. The well-known cohort declines in age at first marriage appear in the graph for median age. Disruptions in a smooth decline appear for cohorts most subject to military service in World War II and in Korea. Perhaps less often observed is the diminution in the spread of this process. The duration of the first marriage process shifts from about 9 years for the cohort of 1911 to about 5 years for the cohorts of 1944 and 1945. The latter figure reflects a fairly rapid recent decline from a plateau of a duration of about 6 years, which existed from the cohort of 1922 to that of 1940.

In the foregoing discussion we have inspected some of the component processes involved in the transition from schoolboy to married adult. What can we say about the process as a whole? Let us begin by looking at Figure 11.11, which displays for selected cohorts the duration and median of each component process. In this figure age is arrayed on the x-axis. Birth years are arrayed on the y-axis. The top line for each birth year indicates the duration of the school exit process; the second indicates the entrance to first job duration; and the third indicates the duration of military service. The last line for each birth year indicates the duration of the first

TABLE 11.4

Age by Which 25%, 50%, and 75% of Male Members of Annual Birth Cohorts Married for the First Time, and Duration of First Marriage Process[a]

Birth year	25% completed	50% completed	75% completed	Duration[b]
1949	20.89			
1948	20.87			
1947	20.92	22.88		
1946	20.82	22.97		
1945	20.81	23.04		
1944	20.82	22.94	26.00	5.18
1943	20.94	22.98	26.12	5.18
1942	20.88	23.04	26.29	5.41
1941	20.80	23.01	26.46	5.66
1940	20.76	23.01	26.69	5.93
1939	20.80	22.94	26.55	5.75
1938	20.83	22.98	26.73	5.90
1937	20.79	23.03	26.73	5.94
1936	20.83	23.03	26.70	5.87
1935	20.93	23.16	26.89	5.96
1934	20.97	23.31	26.86	5.89
1933	21.01	23.48	26.96	5.95
1932	21.14	23.64	27.16	6.02
1931	21.19	23.75	27.45	6.26
1930	21.23	23.75	27.51	6.28
1929	21.30	23.70	27.56	6.26
1928	21.29	23.63	27.56	6.27
1927	21.34	23.69	27.59	6.25
1926	21.43	23.74	27.60	6.17
1925	21.69	23.90	27.63	5.94
1924	21.87	24.05	27.76	5.89
1923	21.85	24.43	28.00	6.15
1922	21.82	24.72	28.15	6.33
1921	21.88	25.06	28.46	6.58
1920	22.01	25.16	28.86	6.85
1919	22.26	24.98	29.10	6.84
1918	22.38	24.93	29.40	7.02
1917	22.45	25.17	29.75	7.30
1916	22.42	25.35	30.20	7.78
1915	22.54	25.65	30.70	8.16
1914	22.59	25.83	30.71	8.12
1913	22.64	25.90	30.98	8.34
1912	22.61	25.88	31.22	8.61
1911	22.73	26.08	31.89	9.16

[a] Source: Occupational Change in a Generation II Survey, March 1973.

[b] Duration is computed as the difference between age at the 75th and 25th percentile level.

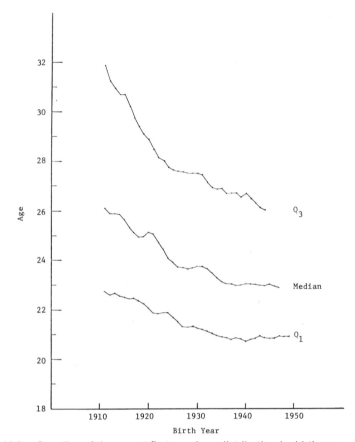

Figure 11.9. Quartiles of the age at first marriage distribution by birth year.

marriage process. The main impression one gains from this figure is one of the shortening of the process as a whole. That impression can be strengthened by reference to Figure 11.12, which shows the duration of the aggregate of the processes, that is, the distance in age between the 25th percentile of the school exit distribution and the 75th percentile of the first marriage process. For the earliest cohort this transition took about 18 years. For recent cohorts it took slightly less than 10 years. Thus the length of time a cohort is involved in this transition has almost halved. Furthermore, the decline in duration is remarkably smooth, especially given the variation among cohorts in the proportion ever in the armed forces.

In one sense this decline in duration is not especially surprising: We all know that median years of school completed has been rising and that age

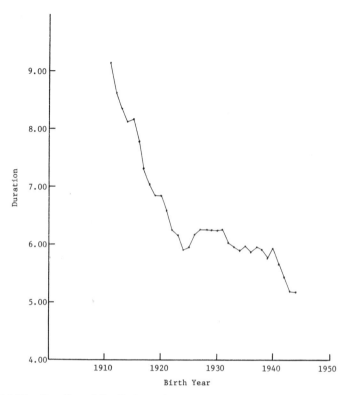

Figure 11.10. Duration of the first marriage process.

at first marriage has been declining. The decline in duration of the transition to adulthood is not entirely attributable to these shifts in the location of the distributions, however. Table 11.5 decomposes the total duration into components. One component is the difference between the medians of the age at first marriage and the age at leaving school distributions. This component represents about half of the duration of the process for most cohorts and the decline in this component yields about half of the decline in total duration. The remainder of total duration is due to the age difference between the 25th and 50th percentiles of the age at school exit distribution and between the 50th and 75th percentiles of the age at first marriage distribution. About two-thirds of this residual quantity is due to the upper tail of the age at first marriage distribution and two-thirds of the decline in duration attributable to "spread" is due to the age at marriage tail.

It seems reasonably clear, then, that the transition from schoolboy to married, employed adult has shortened markedly over the cohorts we

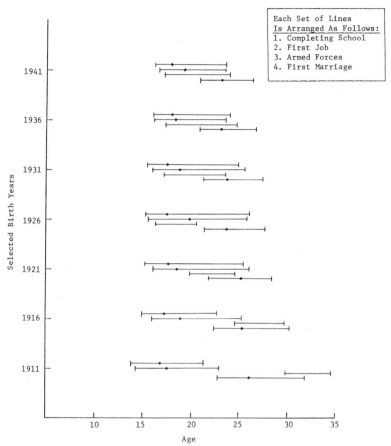

Figure 11.11. Quartiles of the age at school completion, first job, armed forces service, and first marriage distribution for selected birth years.

have been investigating. Not only has the total duration decreased, but also each of its component parts excluding armed forces service has decreased. This decrease has come about despite the addition of armed forces service as an important part of the "normal" experience during these ages.

What do these trends augur for the transition to be experienced by more recently born cohorts than those investigated in this study? On the one hand we know that age at first marriage is moving up, a fact that may suggest a lengthening of the process. On the other hand, we know that for many members of the cohorts studied, military service has delayed their transition somewhat. With the end of the draft and presuming no forth-

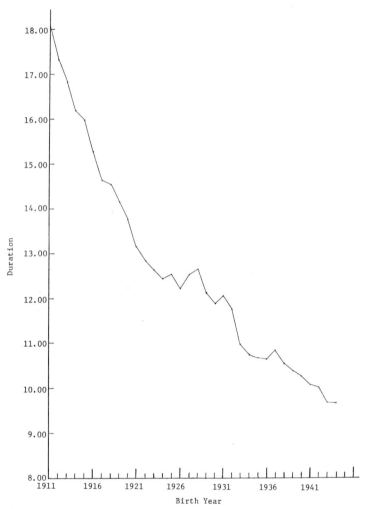

Figure 11.12.   Duration of the aggregate transition to maturity.

coming reinstatement of immediate call-ups, we might expect there to be more elbow room within durations of the kind observed for the recently born cohorts we have investigated. What will newer cohorts do with that elbow room?

Any forecast about the future duration of these life cycle transitions would require an explanation of why the overall process and its component parts have shortened in the past. I have no satisfactory explanation nor is it clear to me presently what form a testable explantaion would

TABLE 11.5

Total Duration of the Transition to Adulthood and Components of the Duration by Birth Year, 1911–1944

Birth year	Total dura- tion	Difference due to medians	Difference due to spread	Difference due to spread in lower tail	Difference due to spread in upper tail
1944	9.66	5.19	4.47	1.41	3.06
1943	9.68	4.63	5.05	1.91	3.14
1942	10.00	5.06	4.94	1.69	3.25
1941	10.08	5.09	4.99	1.54	3.45
1940	10.26	4.91	5.35	1.67	3.68
1939	10.38	4.76	5.62	2.01	3.61
1938	10.53	5.00	5.53	1.78	3.75
1937	10.82	5.04	5.78	2.08	3.70
1936	10.62	5.12	5.50	1.83	3.67
1935	10.67	5.17	5.50	1.77	3.73
1934	10.72	5.57	5.15	1.60	3.55
1933	10.96	5.43	5.53	2.05	3.48
1932	11.75	6.03	5.72	2.20	3.52
1931	12.02	6.21	5.81	2.11	3.70
1930	11.89	6.18	5.71	1.95	3.76
1929	12.11	5.98	6.13	2.27	3.86
1928	12.65	6.41	6.24	2.31	3.93
1927	12.51	6.47	6.04	2.14	3.90
1926	12.21	6.24	5.97	2.11	3.86
1925	12.52	7.04	5.48	1.75	3.73
1924	12.42	6.77	5.65	1.94	3.71
1923	12.63	7.03	5.60	2.03	3.57
1922	12.83	7.38	5.45	2.02	3.43
1921	13.14	7.44	5.70	2.30	3.40
1920	13.76	7.91	5.85	2.15	3.70
1919	14.16	7.58	6.58	2.46	4.12
1918	14.53	7.99	6.54	2.07	4.47
1917	14.64	7.89	6.75	2.17	4.58
1916	15.27	7.99	7.28	2.43	4.85
1915	15.98	8.37	7.61	2.56	5.05
1914	16.19	8.90	7.29	2.40	4.89
1913	16.84	9.17	7.67	2.59	5.08
1912	17.32	8.74	8.58	3.24	5.34
1911	18.05	9.34	8.71	2.90	5.81

take. The best I can offer is a crude speculation. Perhaps the cause of the dramatic shortening of the duration of the transition is precisely that factor which has seemed most likely to disrupt the smooth transition, that is, the relatively high and persistent probability of military service. Perhaps it is the case that the high probability that an individual's progress through the transition will be disrupted by military service has led to a closer calculation about how to make the component transitions, an overcompensation for the time that may be lost, and a pressure to get on with the business of getting started in life before the ax falls. If this explanation has any validity, then we may well see the duration of these transitions increase in the future. Not only might we expect some increase in the upper quartile of the age at marriage distribution, but we may also see an increasing spread in the age at completion of education distribution and the age at labor force entrance distribution. The timing of fertility with respect to the male life cycle may be similarly affected. Such changes, if they occur for the reasons stated, would *not* indicate a change in the value placed on maturity, the married state, or paternity. Rather they would represent a desire by cohort members to wend their way with more deliberateness through the difficult decisions involved in these transitions when not faced with the threat of military service.

What would be the implications of such a lengthening of the cohort transition into adult life? Working out the translation of these cohort changes into period changes in the enrollment rates for higher education, rates of entry into the labor force, and marriage rates is beyond the scope of this paper. It seems clear, however, that the outcome of such an exercise would yield a rather different projection of such rates than one made assuming no change in the timing of these events.

ACKNOWLEDGMENTS

The principal investigators of grant RANN-NSF (GI-31604X), D. L. Featherman and R. M. Hauser, very kindly provided access to these data shortly after they received them from the Census Bureau. Their good colleagueship in this matter and their cheerful willingness to discuss this paper and its data problems in an instance of the cooperative concern for the development of our discipline that makes working in demography a pleasure. Any misuses of these data are, of course, the sole responsibility of the author.

References

Blau, P. M., and O. D. Duncan
   1967   *The American Occupational Structure.* New York: John Wiley and Sons.
Blum, Z. D., N. L. Karweit, and A. B. Sørensen
   1969   "A method for the collection and analysis of retrospective life histories." Johns Hopkins University, Center for Social Organization of Schools, Report No. 48.
Coale, A. J., and T. J. Trussell
   1974   "Model fertility schedules: Variations in the age structure of childbearing in human populations." *Population Index* 40 (April): 85–258.

Duncan, O. D.
  1975 "Measuring social change via replication of surveys." Pp. 118–127 in K. C. Land and S. Spilerman (eds.), *Social Indicator Models*. New York: Russell Sage Foundation.
Duncan, O. D., D. L. Featherman, and B. Duncan
  1972 *Socioeconomic Background and Achievement*. New York: Seminar Press.
Durkheim, E.
  1954 *The Elementary Forms of the Religious Life*. London: George Allen and Unwin, Ltd.
Elder, G. H., Jr.
  1975 *Children of the Great Depression*. Chicago: University of Chicago Press.
Flanagan, J. C., M. F. Shaycroft, J. M. Richards, Jr., and J. G. Claudy
  1971 *Project Talent: Five Years After High School*. Pittsburgh: University of Pittsburgh Press.
Keyfitz, N.
  1968 *Introduction of the Mathematics of Population*. Reading, Mass.: Addison-Wesley.
Mannheim, K.
  1952 *Essays on the Sociology of Knowledge,* Ch. 7, "The problem of generations." London: Routledge and Kegan Paul, Ltd.
Matras, J.
  1973 *Populations and Societies*. Englewood Cliffs, N. J.: Prentice-Hall.
Redfield, R.
  1955 *The Little Community*. Chicago: University of Chicago Press.
Ryder, N. B.
  1962 "The translation model of demographic change." In Emerging Techniques in Population Research, Proceedings of the 1962 Annual Conference of the Milbank Memorial Fund, New York.
  1964 "Notes on the concept of a population." *The American Journal of Sociology* 69 (March): 447–463.
  1965 "The cohort as a concept in the study of social change." *American Sociological Review* 30 (December): 843–861.
Sewell, W. H., and R. M. Hauser
  1975 *Education, Occupation, and Earnings*. New York: Academic Press.
Stycos, J. M.
  1968 *Human Fertility in Latin America*. Ithaca, N. Y.: Cornell University Press.
Sweet, J. A.
  1973 *Women in the Labor Force*. New York: Academic Press.

12

Some Methodological Issues in the Analysis of Longitudinal Surveys[1]

BURTON SINGER and SEYMOUR SPILERMAN

In recent years there has been a considerable expansion in the availability of longitudinal data files. Sociological theory has always had the study of social change as its core, yet the majority of quantitative empirical researches have involved the analysis of cross-sectional data. Longitudinal studies, in particular multiwave panel studies, have not been very common. In part, this is because of the considerable cost involved in surveying a population sample at multiple points in time. It is also due to the fact that several years must usually elapse after the first interview for the longitudinal aspect of the data to become sufficiently detailed so that patterns of change can be detected and studied. However, stimulated by a recent concern with the development of social indicators and by a related

[1] Reprinted with permission from *The Annals of Economic and Social Measurement*, Volume 5, Number 4 (1976), pp. 447–474. © 1976 by the National Bureau of Economic Research, Inc.

The work reported here was supported by NSF grant SOC76-17706 at Columbia University, by NSF grant SOC76-07698 at the University of Wisconsin–Madison, and by funds granted to the Institute for Research on Poverty by the Office of Economic Opportunity pursuant to the Economic Opportunity Act of 1964.

interest in social experimentation, a number of large scale studies have been funded, and sufficient time has elapsed for these investigations to have produced longitudinal files. Indeed, in comparison with even a decade ago, we appear to be moving into an era that will be comparatively rich in the existence of multiwave panel data on large population samples. Important examples of currently available data sets of this sort are the Michigan Panel Study on Income Dynamics (Morgan and Smith, 1969), the National Longitudinal Study of Labor Force Experience (Parnes, 1972), the Panel on Wisconsin Youth (Hauser and Sewell, 1975), and files from several negative income tax studies (for example, Rees and Watts, 1976).

The expansion in availability of these sorts of files raises questions about proper analytic methodology for exploiting the richness and unique properties of panel data, especially in instances where more than two waves of interviews have occurred. Sociologists frequently ask questions about *distributional* change and are interested in forecasting the evolution of a population among system states, as well as in understanding the structure of the dynamic process. The most common examples of such studies concern occupational mobility (for example, Hodge, 1966; Lieberson and Fuguitt, 1967) and geographic migration (for example, Rogers, 1966; Tarver and Gurley, 1965). Some economists (for example, McCall, 1973; Smith and Cain, 1967) have viewed income dynamics from the same perspective.

The mathematical framework that has been used in these investigations is discrete-time Markov chains. We shall discuss a number of limitations of this structure as a description of social processes; at this point, though, we wish only to motivate our investigation by focusing on one discrepancy between forecasts from a Markov model and observations on the empirical process. In applications of Markov chains to industrial mobility, Blumen, Kogan, and McCarthy (1955) (hereafter referred to as BKM) discovered an empirical regularity that has subsequently been observed in many other sociological investigations and that has motivated a rich and diverse research effort. In particular, they noted the tendency for the main diagonal entries of observed stochastic matrices to be underpredicted by the main diagonal entries in powers of one-step Markov transition matrices. This has led to the formulation of a variety of alternative stochastic process models which might plausibly account for the regularity. Furthermore, there has been a critical reevaluation of the substantive and statistical issues involved in estimation and comparison of several models fitted to the rather fragmentary longitudinal data that is usually available on an empirical process.

The purpose of this chapter is to review some of the methodological developments that were an outgrowth of BKM's pioneering investigation. Particular attention will be paid to parsimony of models relative to multi-wave panel data, and to the testing and identification of multiple models that may be compatible with a given set of observations. In the section entitled "Movers and Stayers—A Review" we outline BKM's study and describe some conceptual difficulties that can arise when discrete-time structures are applied to social processes that evolve continuously in time. The section entitled "Other Explanations of High Diagonals" contains an overview of the alternative explanations that have been proposed to account for the empirical regularity observed by BKM; namely, the underprediction of diagonal entries in observed transition matrices by diagonal entries in powers of Markov transition matrices. Models of heterogeneous populations that extend BKM's formulation to continuous time and that incorporate more diverse forms of heterogeneity are described under the heading "Parsimonious Models and Fragmentary Data." In the section that follows we illustrate the companion issues of *embeddability* and *identification* for continuous-time Markov chains. This is the prototype of a set of methodological problems that are central to the analysis of panel data and that have received remarkably little attention.

Generally speaking, *embeddability* tests refer to the task of ascertaining whether or not an empirical process is compatible with the conceptual assumptions (mathematical structure) underlying a particular class of models (for example, general Markov, mixtures of Markov, semi-Markov). Where the answer is affirmative, *identification* procedures refer to techniques for recovering the specific set of structural parameters from the model class that should be associated with the empirical process. One indication of the difficulties involved with identification is the fact that empirically determined stochastic matrices based on data collected at evenly spaced time points may be embeddable in the class of continuous-time Markov models, but a unique structure from that class may not be identifiable.

Finally, the section entitled "Strategies for Discriminating among Competing Models" illustrates a rudimentary procedure for discriminating among four classes of stochastic process models using multiwave panel data. That discussion is intended to illustrate the flavor of the kinds of strategies that are in serious need of development. Indeed this is the place where the greatest methodological challenges lie, and foremost among them is the specification of designs for panel studies that will facilitate discrimination among multiple plausible models.

Movers and Stayers—A Review

MODEL SPECIFICATIONS AND AN EMPIRICAL REGULARITY

In attempting to describe the propensity of persons in particular age and sex cohorts to move between pairs of industrial categories, BKM first fit a discrete-time Markov chain with stationary transition probabilities to quarterly data on the industries of persons listed in the Social Security Administration's Work History File (1972). By a discrete-time Markov chain we mean a stochastic process $\{X(k), k = 0, 1, 2, \ldots\}$ describing state transitions by an individual where the system states might be geographic regions, occupations, industries, or income categories, depending on the particular substantive problem. Probability statements about the process are governed by the analytical recipe

$$\text{Prob}\{X(k + n) = j | X(0), X(1), \ldots, X(n - 1), X(n) = i\}$$
$$= \text{Prob}\{X(k + n) = j | X(n) = i\} = m_{ij}^{(k)} \qquad (1)$$

for $k = 0, 1, 2, \ldots n = 0, 1, 2, \ldots$. Thus the fundamental assumption of a Markov process is that future system state is not a function of past history, once current state is specified. The element $m_{ij}^{(k)}$ is the (i, j) entry in the stochastic matrix $\mathbf{M}^k$ (k-fold matrix multiplication of $\mathbf{M}$). This specifies the k-step transition matrix under a Markov chain, that is, $\mathbf{P}(0, k) = \mathbf{M}^k$. $\mathbf{M}$ is itself a stochastic matrix whose entry m_{ij} has the interpretation,

m_{ij} = probability that an individual in category i will move to category j in one unit of time.

This mathematical structure describes the evolution of a *homogeneous* population because it is assumed that all individuals evolve according to the same transition mechanism (namely, the matrix $\mathbf{M}$).

BKM's estimation method was simply to identify an average of the observed one-quarter (that is, 3-month interval) transition matrices with the matrix of 1-step Markov chain transition probabilities $\|m_{ij}\|$. With this estimate in hand, they tested the model by comparing $\mathbf{M}^k$ with $\hat{\mathbf{P}}(0, k)$, the empirically determined transition matrix[2] based on observations taken at

---

[2] Empirically determined stochastic matrices will be designated by $\hat{P}(u, v)$ with entries

$$\frac{n_{i,j}^{(u,v)}}{n_{i,+}^{(u,\cdot)}} = \frac{\left(\begin{array}{l}\text{number of individuals starting in state } i \\ \text{at time } u \text{ who are in state } j \text{ at time } v\end{array}\right)}{\left(\begin{array}{l}\text{number of individuals starting in state } i \\ \text{at time } u\end{array}\right)}$$

the beginning of the initial quarter and at the end of the kth quarter. BKM carried out this comparison for $k = 4, 8$, and 11 and found that

$$\hat{\mathbf{P}}_{ii}(0, k) > m_{ii}^{(k)}, \qquad k = 4, 8, 11; \quad 1 \le i \le r = \text{number of states;} \quad (2)$$

that is, the main diagonal elements in the k-step matrix predicted by a Markov process underrepresent the main diagonal elements in the observed k-step matrix. They also noted that the magnitude of the inequality increased together with k.

BKM suggested that one plausible explanation for the discrepancy summarized in Inequality (2) was that a socially *heterogeneous* population was being treated as though it was homogeneous. They proposed an alternative model to accommodate heterogeneity, in which the population was viewed as consisting of two kinds of individuals. They assumed that a nondirectly observable fraction s_i of the individuals in industry category i—called stayers—never moved, and that their evolution was described by the degenerate Markov chain $\{X_1(k), k = 0, 1, 2, \ldots\}$ with one-step transition matrix given by the identity I. In addition, the evolution of a nondirectly observable fraction, $1 - s_i$, of the individuals—called movers—who were in industry category i at the beginning of the initial quarter was described by a discrete-time Markov chain $\{X_2(k), k = 0, 1, 2, \ldots\}$ with one-step transition matrix $\mathbf{M}$. The diagonal entries m_{ii} were not required to be zero, thereby allowing for within-industry job change. It was also assumed that the mover population evolved independently of the stayers, and that the same transition matrix $\mathbf{M}$ governed the evolution of movers who started in each category at the beginning of the initial quarter.

The *observable process* $\{Z(k), k = 0, 1, 2, \ldots\}$ describing the evolution of individuals who start out in each industry category in the initial quarter is thus a mixture of the components of the bivariate process $(X_1(k), X_2(k))$. Its transition probabilities are given by

$$\text{Prob}\{Z(k) = j | Z(0) = i\} = \begin{cases} (1 - s_i)m_{ij}^{(k)} & \text{for } i \ne j \\ s_i + (1 - s_i)m_{ii}^{(k)} & \text{for } i = j \end{cases} \quad (3)$$

$$k = 1, 2, \ldots ; 1 \le i, \ j \le r = \text{number of states.}$$

---

where $u < v$. BKM's estimate of $\mathbf{M}$ can thus be written as

$$\frac{1}{12} \sum_{k=0}^{11} \hat{P}(k, k + 1)$$

where the unit of time is 3 months ($=1$ quarter).

In matrix notation, this may be written as

$$\mathbf{P}(k) = \mathbf{SI} + (\mathbf{I} - \mathbf{S})\mathbf{M}^k$$

where

$$\mathbf{S} = \begin{pmatrix} s_1 & & \mathbf{0} \\ & \ddots & \\ \mathbf{0} & & s_r \end{pmatrix}.$$

The formulation (3) has come to be known as the "mover–stayer" model, and a variety of simultaneous estimation methods for the structural parameters $(s_1, \ldots, s_r)$ and $\mathbf{M}$ are given in a paper by L. Goodman (1961), who improved considerably on BKM's initial procedures. BKM found that this model of a heterogeneous population provided a better description of job mobility, as measured by the quarterly observations, than the original Markov chain model of a homogeneous population. Furthermore, the mover–stayer model accounted for much of the empirical regularity (2) and thus has motivated subsequent attempts to develop more refined models of heterogeneous populations.

A DIFFICULTY WITH DISCRETE-TIME MODELS

Despite the initial success of the mover–stayer formulation there are conceptual difficulties with the basic strategy of fitting discrete-time models to mobility data. In particular, when *structural*[3] information about a population is the primary goal of an investigation, then the substantive interpretation attached to estimates of the matrix $\mathbf{M}$—in either the pure Markov or mover–stayer model—is

> m_{ij} = probability that an individual in state i
> will move to state j *when a change occurs.*

If you regard $\mathbf{M}$ as a matrix of structural change parameters and fit discrete-time models to evenly spaced observations, then you are tacitly assuming that the natural time unit between, say, industry or occupational changes coincides with the sampling interval (3 months in the Social Security Administration's Work History File). Since there is no substantive basis for such an identification, the parameters estimated by BKM cannot be interpreted legitimately as structural information about the population of workers; alternate choices of the sampling interval will yield different matrices $\mathbf{M}$. Indeed, BKM were aware of this difficulty and noted that during a given quarter some persons will have moved twice, others will have moved three times, and so on. For these unidentifiable persons you

---

[3] By "structural information" we mean quantities that characterize a population, irrespective of the observation interval used for data collection.

are really estimating $\mathbf{M}^2$, $\mathbf{M}^3$, and so on. Nevertheless, even by dropping any attempt to identify $\mathbf{M}$ as a matrix of structural parameters and just fitting a discrete-time model to quarterly data, BKM found an empirical regularity of considerable importance. In fact, as we will indicate in the section entitled "Parsimonious Models and Fragmentary Data," even when continuous-time Markov models—whose parameters can legitimately be interpreted as structural coefficients[4]—are fit to a variety of longitudinal data sets, the regularity observed by BKM still appears.

The ambiguity in specifying an appropriate time scale for intra-generational mobility processes has also been pointed out by White (1970, pp. 319–320) and Singer and Spilerman (1974, pp. 360–362). However, a facet of this ambiguity that seems to have been overlooked by BKM, as well as by subsequent users of the mover–stayer formulation (for example, McCall, 1973), is the fact that conclusions about compatibility of data with a discrete-time model can depend entirely on an ad hoc choice of unit–time interval. To see this in the simplest possible setting, recall BKM's initial fitting of a discrete-time Markov chain to quarterly observations.

Suppose, for illustrative purposes, that you agree that a natural time unit for job mobility in a particular population cohort is 6 weeks. Then an attempt to fit an observed one-quarter (12-week) transition matrix $\hat{\mathbf{P}}(0, 1)$ to a Markov chain consists of asking whether there exists a stochastic matrix $\mathbf{M}$ such that

$$\hat{\mathbf{P}}(0, 1) = \mathbf{M}^2.$$

An affirmative answer would require that $\hat{\mathbf{P}}(0, 1)$ have at least one stochastic square root, $[\hat{\mathbf{P}}(0, 1)]^{1/2}$. That this is by no means automatic can be seen if you consider a two-state process with observed one-quarter transition matrix

$$\hat{\mathbf{P}}(0, 1) = \begin{pmatrix} \dfrac{1}{4} & \dfrac{3}{4} \\ \dfrac{5}{8} & \dfrac{3}{8} \end{pmatrix}.$$

This matrix has no stochastic square roots, and it is therefore incompatible with a discrete-time Markov structure if the natural time unit is believed to equal 6 weeks. However, if you use a 4-week time unit then you find that $\hat{\mathbf{P}}(0, 1)$ does have a stochastic cube root given by

$$[\hat{\mathbf{P}}(0, 1)]^{1/3} = \begin{pmatrix} .0611 & .9389 \\ .7824 & .2176 \end{pmatrix}.$$

---

[4] As the reader will see, these parameters are independent of the sampling interval.

More generally, $\hat{\mathbf{P}}(0, 1)$ has no stochastic roots of any even order, while it does have a stochastic cube root, a stochastic fifth root, but no odd stochastic root of order greater than five.

A consideration of high order roots (say, greater than four) is not really an issue with quarterly observations of job mobility; however, it certainly could be for annual observations or more widely spaced data. The essential point to be made here, however, is that for processes such as intragenerational occupational mobility, which are both intrinsically nonsynchronous[5] and lack any substantive basis for a choice of unit time interval, a more natural strategy is to fit continuous-time models (in which the waiting times between moves are viewed as random variables) to the data, and carry out systematic discrimination among alternative models in that setting.[6] This kind of extension of the mover–stayer framework was first carried out by Spilerman (1927a) with further generalizations indicated in Singer and Spilerman (1974). These developments will be reviewed together with a variety of other models in the section entitled "Parsimonious Models and Fragmentary Data."

Other Explanations of High Diagonals

BKM's introduction of the mover–stayer model to explain "clustering on the main diagonal," that is, the empirical regularity[7]

$$\hat{p}_{ii}(0, k) > m_{ii}^{(k)}, \qquad i = 1, \ldots, r; \qquad k = 2, 3, \ldots \qquad (4)$$

has led to the development of a variety of qualitatively different kinds of models, all capable of accounting for Inequality (4). The five principal features of social processes that are not taken into account in univariate time-stationary Markov models[8] and that have motivated the construction of alternative models are:

---

[5] By "nonsynchronous" we mean that persons do not all change state simultaneously.

[6] In instances where a substantively meaningful unit time interval exists, a discrete-time model would indeed be appropriate (for example, explaining presidential election outcomes).

[7] $\hat{p}_{ii}(0, k)$ is a diagonal entry in the observed k-step matrix, and $m_{ii}^{(k)}$ is the corresponding entry in the k-step matrix predicted by a discrete-time Markov chain.

[8] We have replaced the usual mathematical terminology "time-homogeneous Markov chain" by the phrase "time-stationary Markov chain." This change of terminology has been incorporated in order to avoid confusion with our use of the word "homogeneous" to describe a population of individuals possessing a common set of transition probabilities. It should also be emphasized that we do not assume that the initial distribution of individuals among system states is the equilibrium distribution for a Markov process. Such an assumption would imply that the Markov process is also a "stationary" process in the usual mathematical sense of the word.

1. Population heterogeneity
2. Time-varying propensities to change system states (e.g., income categories, occupations, industries)
3. Nonexponential waiting times between changes of state
4. Strong dependence on past history
5. Latent variables

Features 1, 2, and 3 have received the most attention in attempts to develop stochastic process models that can account for Inequality (4) and that also mirror other widely observed empirical phenomena, such as the increasing propensity with the passage of time for persons in a particular occupation to remain there. For a nice empirical study of manpower flows in British labor markets where this behavior occurs, see Kuhn *et al.* (1973). Since our primary concern in the next three sections will be with specification, estimation, and identification issues involving models based on 1–3, a few remarks about 4 and 5 are in order.

In a review of BKM's study, Feller (1956) suggested that for processes such as job mobility, dependence on past behavioral patterns probably was so pronounced that it would be essential to develop detailed models incorporating past history in order to have a satisfactory description of the observed empirical patterns. Indeed, Feller suggested the use of higher order Markov processes for this purpose. As a strategy for understanding social phenomena such as mobility among occupation, industry, or income categories, this kind of program has never been seriously followed up and has in fact been criticized on several grounds. Coleman (1964a, pp. 9–11), in particular, has emphasized that the intrinsically heterogeneous nature of most populations is largely ignored by an introduction of higher order Markov models, and that such an exercise is more akin to blind curve fitting of successively higher order polynomials to irregular data.

One might argue that models incorporating both heterogeneity and long-range dependence should be introduced; however, the fragmentary nature of the data that can be collected in most surveys—particularly the small number of time points at which persons involved in panel studies can be reinterviewed—makes judgments as to the relative importance of phenomena that are to be incorporated in parsimonious models essential. In fact, a primary reason for the emphasis on population heterogeneity and the neglect of long range dependence is the greater importance for the development of sociological theory attached to an understanding of the components of heterogeneity. The strategies of introducing independent variables into Markov chain models developed by Coleman (1964a), McFarland (1970), and Spilerman (1927b) as well as the mixture models introduced in Spilerman (1972a) and Singer and Spilerman (1974) are all based on considerations of parsimony of models relative to the available data and on the judged importance of population heterogeneity.

Concerning item 5, many of the observed attitudinal responses in panel studies, such as opinions about political issues, career aspirations, and so on are related to a variety of nondirectly observable (or latent) social and psychological variables. In addition, there are often several competing theories about the relationships which may exist between latent and manifest (that is, observable) variables. An important research objective with panel data is to discriminate among *dynamic* models incorporating a variety of latent and manifest variable relationships. Despite its importance, this aspect of the analysis of longitudinal surveys is largely undeveloped. The major attempts to consider both the substantive and methodological issues have been by Coleman (1964a), Lazarsfeld and Henry (1968), and Wiggins (1973). The last of these contains a superb collection of examples and lucid statements on the enormous range of unresolved mathematical, statistical, and social–theoretic problems. In the remainder of this chapter we will concentrate on models that incorporate population heterogeneity, time-varying propensities to change state, and general classes of waiting times between moves. However, it should be noted that the same methodological issues arise in dealing with latent structure models but with a considerable increase in complexity.

Parsimonious Models and Fragmentary Data

In the context of panel studies, Coleman (1964b) introduced continuous-time Markov chains as an initial baseline class of models. However, in fitting these models to observed data, he noted the same kind of empirical regularity—underprediction of diagonals of observed matrices—which BKM and others had found using discrete-time models. This finding has motivated the development of a variety of formal models of heterogeneous populations that are both moderately realistic and simple enough so that parameters can be estimated and the models falsified using rather fragmentary data. The strategies for introducing heterogeneity have basically been of two distinct types: Individuals (or subpopulations) are classified either according to the *rate* at which they move (Spilerman, 1972a; Singer and Spilerman, 1974) or according to their *propensity* to move between pairs of states when a transition occurs (McFarland, 1970; Spilerman, 1972b; Singer and Spilerman, 1974). These subpopulations are not always directly observable, and mixtures of Markov and semi-Markov processes provide simple, readily interpretable models of the observed population-level processes. Explicit descriptions of models of these types, suited to intragenerational mobility studies, are given in the following subsections.

MODEL SPECIFICATIONS

In order to illustrate some explicit models of heterogeneous populations and clarify the substantive assumptions that accompany their use, we first recall the basic mathematical structure of continuous-time Markov chains with stationary transition probabilities. In particular, consider a stochastic process with a finite number of states whose transition probabilities are governed by the system of ordinary differential equations

$$d\mathbf{P}(t)/dt = \mathbf{Q}\mathbf{P}(t), \qquad \mathbf{P}(0) = \mathbf{I} \tag{5}$$

where $\mathbf{P}(t)$ and $\mathbf{Q}$ are $r \times r$ matrices. It is well known (Chung, 1967, pp. 251–257; Coleman, 1964b, pp. 127–130) that if $\mathbf{Q}$ has the structure

$$q_{ij} \geq 0 \quad \text{for } i \neq j, \quad q_{ii} \leq 0, \quad \sum_{j=1}^{r} q_{ij} = 0, \quad i = 1, \ldots, r \tag{6}$$

then the functions $\mathbf{P}(t)$, $t > 0$ that are solutions of Equation (5) comprise the transition matrices of continuous-time stationary Markov chains. A typical element, $p_{ij}(t)$, of $\mathbf{P}(t)$ has the interpretation,

> $p_{ij}(t)$ = probability that an individual starting in state i at time 0 will be in state j at time t.

The **Q**-arrays, which are known as *intensity matrices*, represent structural information about the population:

1. $q_{ij}/-q_{ii}$ = probability that an individual in state i will move to state j, given the occurrence of a transition

2. $1/-q_{ii}$ = expected length of time for an individual in state i to remain in that state

We will denote the class of intensity matrices [arrays of the form of Equation (6)] by $\mathcal{Q}$.

Solutions of Equation (5) are given by the exponential formula

$$\mathbf{P}(t) = \exp(\mathbf{Q}t), \qquad t > 0 \tag{7}$$

where the matrix exponential $\exp(\mathbf{A})$ ($\mathbf{A}$ being an arbitrary $r \times r$ matrix) is defined by

$$\exp(\mathbf{A}) = \sum_{k=0}^{\infty} \frac{\mathbf{A}^k}{k!}.$$

A Simple Factored Representation of **Q**

The previous general formulation of continuous-time Markov transition matrices has been used in numerous sociological contexts (for example, Bartholomew, 1973; Coleman, 1964b, pp. 177–182). However, the analysis of social processes, particularly in a heterogeneous population, is greatly facilitated by an alternative formulation which provides the basis for a classification of individuals (or subpopulations) according to their rates of movement, their propensities to move to particular states, or both simultaneously. A starting point for this development was Spilerman's (1972a) extension of the mover–stayer formulation to continuous-time, with a more general classification of subpopulations than the simple mover–stayer dichotomy. The basis for this extension was simply the introduction of a factored representation for **Q**-matrices of the special form $\mathbf{Q} = \lambda(\mathbf{M} - \mathbf{I})$, where λ is a positive constant signifying the expected rate of movement, and **M** is the transition matrix that each individual in the population follows at a move.

Classification according to *rate* of movement means assigning a number λ to each individual (or subpopulation), thereby designating what we will call type-λ individuals. The value $1/\lambda$ can be interpreted as an individual's mean waiting time before moving (or before making a decision to possibly move). Similarly, classification according to propensity to transfer to particular states means assigning a stochastic matrix **M** to an individual, thereby designating what we will call type-**M** individuals. If persons are to be classified in both of these ways simultaneously, we would speak of type-$(\lambda, \mathbf{M})$ individuals.

Using this classification scheme, the random variables $\{Y(t), t > 0\}$ that describe a type-λ individual's history may be constructed from two separate processes: (1) a sequence of independent positive random variables $\tau_0, \tau_1, \ldots$ describing waiting times between moves and satisfying

$$\mathrm{Prob}(\tau_i > t) = \exp(-\lambda t), \qquad i = 0, 1, 2, \ldots ; \quad t > 0$$

and (2) a discrete-time Markov chain $\{X(k), k = 0, 1, 2, \ldots\}$ having one-step transition matrix **M** that describes moves when they occur. You can then think of an individual whose transition probabilities are governed by $e^{t\lambda(\mathbf{M}-\mathbf{I})}$ as evolving according to the following prescription:

1. Starting in state i at time 0, the individual stays there for an exponentially distributed length of time τ_0 with

$$\mathrm{Prob}(\tau_0 > t) = \exp(-\lambda t), \qquad t > 0.$$

   Thus $Y(t) = X(0) = i$ for $0 \leq t < \tau_0$.

2. At the end of this time he makes a decision to move to state j with probability m_{ij}. (In general, $m_{ii} \neq 0$.) Thus $Y(\tau_0) = X(1) = j$.
3. Now he waits in state j for an exponentially distributed length of time τ_l that is independent of τ_0, $X(0)$, and $X(1)$; especially,

$$\text{Prob}(\tau_1 > t | X(0), \tau_0, X(1)) = \text{Prob}(\tau_1 > t) = e^{-\lambda t}$$

and

$$Y(t) = X(1) \qquad \text{for} \quad \tau_0 \leq t < \tau_0 + \tau_1.$$

4. Then he makes another decision to move to state h with probability m_{jh}; hence,

$$Y(\tau_0 + \tau_1) = X(2) = h.$$

5. The sequence is repeated. In general,

$$Y(t) = X(k) \qquad \text{for} \quad \sum_{i=0}^{k-1} \tau_i \leq t < \sum_{i=0}^{k} \tau_i$$

with $\tau_0, \tau_1, \ldots$ independent of $\{X(k), k = 0, 1, 2, \ldots\}$ and of each other.

Spilerman's (1972a) extension of the mover–stayer model was a mixture of Markov processes of the previous sort in which individuals associated with the parameter λ were assumed to occur in the total population with a frequency described by the gamma density

$$g(\lambda) = \frac{\beta^\alpha \lambda^{\alpha-1} \exp(-\beta\lambda)}{\Gamma(\alpha)} \qquad \alpha > 0, \quad \beta > 0, \quad \lambda \geq 0.$$

Type-λ individuals are considered to be nondirectly observable, and all types of individuals are treated as having the same propensity to move among the states, prescribed by the matrix $\mathbf{M}$. The *population-level process* $\{Z(t), t > 0\}$, which is observable, then has transition probabilities given by

$$\mathbf{P}(t) = \int_0^\infty \exp[t\lambda(\mathbf{M} - \mathbf{I})]g(\lambda)\, d\lambda$$

$$= \left(\frac{\beta}{\beta + t}\right)^\alpha \left[\mathbf{I} - \frac{t}{\beta + t}\mathbf{M}\right]^{-\alpha}. \tag{8}$$

The choice of a gamma density in this specification is based on the ability of that functional form to describe a variety of unimodal curves, unimodality being a reasonable characterization of the frequency of occurrence of different types of persons, with respect to rate of movement, in heterogeneous populations (Palmer, 1954, p. 50; Taeuber *et al.*, 1968, p. 46).

Two other mixtures of some importance for intragenerational occupational mobility are processes with transition probabilities governed by

$$\mathbf{P}(t) = s\mathbf{I} + (1 - s)\exp[t\lambda_0(\mathbf{M} - \mathbf{I})] \tag{9}$$

and

$$\mathbf{P}(t) = s\mathbf{I} + (1 - s)\int_0^\infty \exp[t\lambda(\mathbf{M} - \mathbf{I})]g(\lambda)\,d\lambda$$

$$= s\mathbf{I} + (1 - s)\left(\frac{\beta}{\beta + t}\right)^\alpha\left(\mathbf{I} - \frac{t}{\beta + t}\mathbf{M}\right)^{-\alpha}. \tag{10}$$

Equation (9) is a continuous-time analog of the mover–stayer model in which the fraction of stayers is the same for all states, and $1/\lambda_0$ is the expected waiting time between moves in the mover population. Equation (10) combines the mover–stayer model with the more general form of heterogeneity in the mover population which was specified in Equation (8). Because this mixture adds a concentration of stayers to the gamma density, it is known as the spiked gamma (with vodka, please).

A More General Factored Representation of **Q**

From a substantive point of view, a principal defect of the individual-level description in "A Simple Factored Representation of **Q**" is the requirement that a person's waiting time distribution be the same in every state. It is desirable to eliminate this constraint and retain the flexibility of the full Markov model, since there are many instances in which rate of movement is a function of system state. For example, if the system states are industry categories we know that industries differ in their rates of employee separation (Blauner, 1964, pp. 198–203).

We therefore classify a person according to the diagonal matrix

$$\Lambda = \begin{pmatrix} \lambda_1 & & \mathbf{0} \\ & \cdot & \\ & & \cdot & \\ \mathbf{0} & & \lambda_r \end{pmatrix}, \qquad \lambda_i \ge 0, \quad i = 1, 2, \ldots, r$$

where $1/\lambda_i$ has the interpretation, "average waiting time in state i." A type-Λ individual's history $\{Y(t), t > 0\}$ is now governed by the transition matrices

$$\mathbf{P}(t) = \exp[t\Lambda(\mathbf{M} - \mathbf{I})], \qquad t \ge 0 \tag{11}$$

and these individuals are viewed as occurring in the total population with a proportion specified by a joint probability density $g(\lambda_1, \ldots, \lambda_r)$. The previous construction of individual histories $\{Y(t), t > 0\}$ out of random waiting times $\tau_0, \tau_1, \ldots$ and a discrete-time Markov chain $\{X(k), k = 0,$

1, 2, . . .} must now be modified by allowing the distribution of τ_k to depend on the current state $X(k)$.

In particular, we define

$$Y(t) = X(k) \quad \text{if} \quad \sum_{i=0}^{k-1} \tau_i \le t < \sum_{i=0}^{k} \tau_i$$

where

$$\text{Prob}(\tau_k > t | X(0), \tau_0, X(1), \tau_1, \ldots X(k-1), \tau_{k-1}, X(k) = i)$$
$$= \text{Prob}(\tau_k > t | X(k) = i) = \exp(-\lambda_i t)$$
$$\text{for} \quad 1 \le i \le r; \quad k = 0, 1, 2, \ldots . \quad (12)$$

It should be pointed out that this formulation requires more complicated estimation techniques than the simple factored representation described in the previous section. However, a full discussion of these issues in the context of panel studies lies outside the scope of the present chapter.

More General Waiting Time Distributions than Exponential

Despite the more diverse form of heterogeneity that is formalized in the previous section, the increasing tendency of persons to remain in a particular state (occupation, geographic region, and so on) the longer they have been there is an empirical regularity that is not captured by any time-stationary Markov model. McGinnis (1968) refers to this phenomenon as cumulative inertia, and empirical evidence of its presence in intragenerational mobility is provided, for example, by Kuhn et al. (1973); Land (1969); and Myers et al. (1967). This phenomenon is also known in the demography literature as "duration-dependence," and a nice review of formal models which incorporate it is provided by Hoem (1972).

In order to formalize duration–dependence and simultaneously classify individuals according to rate of movement and propensity to transfer to particular states, it is convenient to retain the decomposition of individual histories $\{Y(t), t > 0\}$ discussed in the previous sections. The only modification is the introduction of special nonexponential distributions, $F_i(t)$, $1 \le i \le r$, which describe duration-dependent waiting times in state i. In particular, we define

$$Y(t) = X(k) \quad \text{for} \quad \sum_{i=0}^{k-1} \tau_i \le t < \sum_{i=0}^{k} \tau_i \quad (13)$$

where $\tau_0, \tau_1, \ldots$ are positive random variables satisfying

$$\text{Prob}(\tau_k > t | X(0), \tau_0, X(1), \tau_1, \ldots , X(k-1), \tau_{k-1}, X(k) = i)$$
$$= \text{Prob}(\tau_k > t | X(k) = i)$$
$$= 1 - F_i(t) \quad 1 \le i \le r. \quad (14)$$

To incorporate the notion of duration–dependence (or cumulative inertia) we restrict $F_i(t)$ to be of the form

$$F_i(t) = 1 - \exp\left(-\int_0^t h_i(u)\, du\right), \qquad 1 \le i \le r \tag{15}$$

where $h_i(u)$ is a positive decreasing function such that

$$\int_0^\infty h_i(u)\, du = +\infty.$$

The assumption that h_i be decreasing implies that the longer an individual stays in state i, the less likely he is to move in the immediate future. In particular, the probability that an individual known to be in state i at time t will exit from that state in the next dt units of time is given by

$$h_i(t)\, dt = \frac{f_i(t)\, dt}{1 - F_i(t)}$$

where $f_i(t)$ is the probability density corresponding to $F_i(t)$.

The process $\{Y(t),\ t > 0\}$ defined here is a special form of *semi-Markov* process[9] whose transition probabilities

$$\text{Prob}(Y(t) = j \,|\, Y(0) = i) = p_{ij}(t), \qquad 1 \le i \le r$$

are the unique solutions of the system of integral equations

$$p_{ij}(t) = \delta_{ij}[1 - F_i(t)] + \sum_{k=1}^{r} \int_0^t f_i(s) m_{ik} p_{kj}(t - s)\, ds.$$

In this equation,

$$\delta_{ij} = \begin{cases} 1 & \text{if } i = j \\ 0 & \text{if } i \ne j \end{cases} \tag{16}$$

and $\|m_{ik}\| = \mathbf{M}$ is the one-step transition matrix governing the discrete-time Markov chain $X(k),\ k = 0, 1, 2, \ldots$ used to specify $Y(t)$ in Equation (13).[10] Now classification of an individual evolving according to a semi-

---

[9] For a rigorous mathematical discussion of the special semi-Markov construction defined by Equations (13) and (14), see Kurtz (1971).

[10] The specification of semi-Markov processes in Equations (13), (14), and (16) does not describe the most general process of this kind as treated in the mathematics literature. In particular, the original semi-Markov framework allowed for waiting time distributions that could depend on the next future state as well as on the current state of the process. In order to utilize models incorporating this kind of detail, a more extensive data base would be required than is currently available in most multiwave panel studies. Hence, considerations of parsimony have led us to restrict our attention to a subclass of semi-Markov processes which requires the estimation of fewer parameters.

Markov process would mean to characterize him by the family of distributions $\mathcal{F} = \{F_1(t), \ldots, F_r(t)\}$ describing the waiting times in any state, and by the stochastic matrix $\mathbf{M}$ describing his propensity to move to particular states.

In specifying a population-level process $\{Z(t), t > 0\}$ as a mixture of this kind of semi-Markov process, parametric families of distributions are usually used to define $F_i(t)$ and then a suitable mixing distribution is defined on the parameters. For example,

$$F(t) = 1 - \exp(-\gamma_1 t^{\gamma_2}) \quad \text{with} \quad \gamma_1 > 0, \quad 0 < \gamma_2 < 1$$

can be expressed in the form of Equation (15) with

$$h(u) = \gamma_1 \gamma_2 \, u^{\gamma_2 - 1}$$

and a reasonable initial choice of mixing distribution can be defined by

$$\int_0^{\gamma_1} \int_0^{\gamma_2} g(u, v) \, du \, dv = \int_0^{\gamma_1} \frac{\beta^\alpha u^{\alpha-1} \exp(-\beta u)}{\Gamma(\alpha)} \, du \cdot \int_0^{\gamma_2} dv.$$

Thus γ_1 and γ_2 are treated as independent parameters with γ_1 being gamma distributed and γ_2 being uniformly distributed on $[0, 1]$. This mixture specification is meant to be only a suggestion of a reasonable starting point for the fitting of semi-Markov mixtures to multiwave panel data. A series of empirical investigations comparing a variety of mixture models remains to be carried out.

A final point that should be mentioned concerning the semi-Markov models (13) is the basically regenerative nature of these processes. In particular, individuals evolving according to Equations (13)–(15) have an increasing propensity to remain in each state the longer they are there. However, once a change in state occurs, an individual may be much more likely to move again in the immediate future than he was before the change occurred. Although the cumulative inertia behavior occurs in each state separately, it need not, according to these models, hold throughout a career involving changes of state (that is, there is no explicit notion of individual aging). This raises the question of finding alternative models to the previous semi-Markov formulation in which the propensity to move in the immediate future decreases *throughout* an individual's history. This is the subject of the next section.

A Non-time-stationary Markov Model

Consider a population in which an individual's history $\{Y(t), t > 0\}$ is defined by

$$Y(t) = X(k) \quad \text{for} \quad \sum_{i=0}^{k-1} \tau_i \leq t \leq \sum_{i=0}^{k} \tau_i \tag{17}$$

where $\{X(k),\ k = 0, 1, 2, \ldots\}$ is again a discrete-time Markov chain, governed by M and describing moves when they occur. $\tau_0, \tau_1, \ldots$ are waiting times between moves (or decisions to possibly move), and they satisfy

$$
\begin{aligned}
&\mathrm{Prob}(\tau_k > t | X(0), \tau_0, \ldots, X(k-1), \tau_{k-1}, X(k)) \\
&\quad = \mathrm{Prob}(\tau_k > t | \tau_0 + \cdots + \tau_{k-1}) \\
&\quad = 1 - \exp\left(-\int_{(\tau_0 + \cdots + \tau_{k-1})}^{t + (\tau_0 + \cdots + \tau_{k-1})} h(u)\,du\right)
\end{aligned}
\tag{18}
$$

where $h(u)$ is positive, decreasing, and satisfies

$$
\int_0^\infty h(u)\,du = +\infty.
$$

The specification of Equation (18) implies that after each successive move, an individual's propensity to remain in his new state is not only greater the longer he stays, but it is also greater than at any time prior to his last move. In particular, this formulation captures the notion of cumulative inertia throughout a career, such as might result from aging, and seems more appropriate than some of the previous semi-Markov models for investigations of intragenerational occupational mobility. See, in particular, Kuhn *et al.* (1973) for some empirical evidence supporting this position; see also Sørensen (1975) for additional details on this sort of formulation.

The stochastic process specified by Equations (17) and (18) is a special non-time-stationary Markov process[11] where

$$
\begin{aligned}
\mathrm{Prob}(Y(t) = j | Y(0) = i) &= p_{ij}(0, t) \\
&= \left(\exp\left[\left(\int_0^t h(u)\,du\right)(M - I)\right]\right)_{ij}.
\end{aligned}
\tag{19}
$$

In principle, heterogeneous population models could be constructed from mixtures of this kind of non-time-stationary model of individual behavior. However, the fragmentary nature of the data that are usually available in multiwave panel studies makes judgments about the relative importance of nonstationarity versus heterogeneity essential if parsimonious models are to be fit to the data. In terms of the discussion of high diagonals in the section entitled "Other Explanations of High Diagonals," the difficult conceptual point that such judgments raise is that each of the following qualitatively different interpretations is capable of accounting for that empirical regularity.

---

[11] For a nice mathematical treatment of non-time-stationary Markov chains, see Goodman and Johansen (1973).

    i. A *homogeneous* population described by the nonstationary model in Equations (17) and (18)

    ii. A *heterogeneous* population described by mixtures of stationary Markov models such as the mover–stayer extensions in Equations (8), (9), and (10)

    iii. A *homogeneous* population described by a semi-Markov model such as Equations (13)–(15)

    iv. A *heterogeneous* population described by mixtures of interpretations i and iii

Procedures for discriminating among alternative conceptual models, such as these, in a panel study are outlined in the section entitled "Strategies for Discriminating among Competing Models." The discussion there is designed to illustrate a general strategy of fitting several models to the same data, each of which emphasizes a qualitatively different behavioral pattern. Highly structured residuals from such models usually represent the most suggestive information about factors that have not been formally incorporated in a model. (The empirical regularity found by BKM is a simple instance of residuals from a base-line model being suggestive about alternative descriptions of an empirical process.) One of the principal research directions that this approach suggests is the intensive development of fitting and identification procedures for a variety of realistic models using limited longitudinal information.

FRAGMENTARY DATA

From the outset we have emphasized the limited number of time points at which panel data usually are obtained. It is important for a proper understanding of the estimation and identification strategies discussed in the next two sections that some explicit instances of longitudinal data be described, together with an indication of precisely what, in each instance, is meant by the phrase "fragmentary."

Example 1. Let $\{Y^{(i)}(t), 0 \le t \le t^*, t^* = $ duration of the study$\}$ represent the history of the ith individual in a panel study (for example, occupational career pattern, succession of brand preferences, and so on), and let $0 = t_0 < t_1 < \cdots < t_n$ represent the times at which the waves of the panel are scheduled (that is, the reinterview times). Although changes of state can occur at any time t, the observed process is

$$\{Y^{(i)}(t_k), \quad k = 0, 1, 2, \ldots, N\}, \qquad 1 \le i \le N \tag{20}$$

where $N = $ number of persons in the closed population under study. Thus the transitions between sampling instants as well as their times of occurrence are not observed. It is because of this missing information that we refer to data of the form of Expression (20) as fragmentary.[12] It should be noted that this was precisely the sampling situation in BKM's study where $t_{i+1} - t_i = \Delta = 3$ months, $i = 0, 1, 2, \ldots$.

Example 2. In a residence history study (Taeuber *et al.*, 1968), observations were taken retrospectively on current residence, first, second, and third prior residences and birth place of individuals in particular age cohorts. This kind of data represents an instance of fragmentary information about a migration process in that gaps are present in the residence histories.

Example 3. Let $T^{(i)}(t) = \{$number of transitions by the ith individual between time 0 and time $t\}$, and consider observations of the form $\{Y^{(i)}(t_k),$ $T^{(i)}(t_k), 0 \le k \le n, 1 \le i \le N\}$. This kind of information was obtained in the social mobility studies of Palmer (1954), Lipset and Bendix (1959), and in the much longer study of Parnes (1972). It is fragmentary due to the fact that the times of occurrence of the transitions are missing.

From the perspective of estimation and identification with any of the mathematical models mentioned previously, the ideal situation would be to have complete histories of moves among states, as well as durations in each state for a long time interval. However, because of cost considerations in conducting many reinterviews over a long time span, and because of low response reliability when detailed retrospective questions are asked, only fragmentary data have been obtained in such major investigations as the OCG-1 survey (Blau and Duncan, 1967), the OCG-2 survey (Hauser and Featherman, 1973), Michigan's Income Dynamics Panel (Morgan and Smith, 1969), and the National Longitudinal Study of Labor Force Experience (Parnes, 1972). This raises the question of what sorts of partial information to gather if the data are to be used to discriminate among alternative theories using formal mathematical models. For example, if the study concerns occupational mobility and the collection design is a retrospective survey, we might collect any of the following kinds of data:

1. A complete history of all jobs held and durations in the jobs
2. First occupation and current occupation
3. First occupation, current occupation, and number of intervening occupations held

---

[12] Another reason why we might consider data to be fragmentary is if the duration of the study is too brief for significant amounts of movement to have occurred. We do not address this issue in the present discussion.

4. First occupation, current occupation, and previous occupation (possibly together with duration times in each occupational state)

Clearly, the combinations can be elaborated. What is consequential about this decision is that once the first alternative—complete histories—is rejected as a research design, it becomes crucial which pieces of data one decides to collect. Different estimation procedures must be employed according to the kinds of information gathered, and some procedures will yield more efficient estimates of the parameters than will others. The choice of data collection strategy must also reflect the classes of mathematical models that a researcher intends to apply, because certain information that is not required to fit one model type is crucial to the estimation of another.

The simplest setting in which to illustrate estimation and identification with fragmentary data is the fitting of continuous-time Markov chains to data of the form described in Example 1; that is, observations on individuals' locations at a few points in time. The essential steps are described in the next section.

Embeddability and Identification

Suppose observations on a closed population have been collected at the evenly spaced time points $t_0 = 0$, t_1, t_2, . . . , t_n where $t_{k+1} - t_k = \Delta > 0$, for $k = 0, 1, \ldots, n$, and assume that the number of observations on the population is small, say, $n \leq 8$. Furthermore, consider the observations to include only information on current system states; namely, $\{Y^{(i)}(t_k), \quad k = 0, \ 1, \ 2, \ldots, \ n\}$ for $1 \leq i \leq N$, $N =$ number of persons in the closed population under investigation. This is a standard data collection situation in multiwave panel studies (for example, BKM used this type of data), and it provides the simplest setting in which to illustrate embeddability and identification issues.

Embeddability refers to the question of whether observations on an empirical process are compatible with the conceptual assumptions (theoretical structure) underlying a particular class of mathematical models (for example, time-homogeneous Markov, mixture of Markov, semi-Markov). Where the answer is affirmative, *identification* procedures refer to techniques for recovering the particular set of structural parameters from the model class that should be associated with the empirical process. Both issues are central to the analysis of panel data. Identification, in particular, can be difficult to accomplish due to the fact that qualitatively different sets of structural parameters may be consistent with data from evenly spaced observations.

To fix the ideas in the simplest setting, consider fitting a continuous-time Markov chain with stationary transition probabilities to data of the sort just described. A procedure for carrying out this task consists of two principal steps:

1. Form the stochastic matrices $\hat{\mathbf{P}}(k\Delta, l\Delta)$ with entries

$$\frac{n_{ij}^{(k\Delta,l\Delta)}}{n_{i+}^{(k\Delta,\cdot)}} = \frac{\left\{\begin{array}{l}\text{number of persons in state } i \text{ at time } k\Delta \\ \text{who are also in state } j \text{ at time } l\Delta\end{array}\right\}}{\{\text{number of persons in state } i \text{ at time } k\Delta\}}$$

and check that

$$\hat{\mathbf{P}}(k_1\Delta, k_2\Delta) = \hat{\mathbf{P}}(k_3\Delta, k_4\Delta) \tag{21}$$

for $k_1 < k_2 \le n$; $k_3 < k_4 \le n$ with $k_2 - k_1 = k_4 - k_3$
and that

$$\hat{\mathbf{P}}(k_1\Delta, k_2\Delta) = \hat{\mathbf{P}}(k_1\Delta, l\Delta)\hat{\mathbf{P}}(l\Delta, k_2\Delta) \tag{22}$$

where $0 \le k_1 < l < k_2 \le n$.

Equation (21) is a test of time stationarity; and Equation (22) is a primitive test of the Markov assumption (that is, independence of future state from past history, given current state). Formal tests of this kind are described by Anderson and Goodman (1957) and Billingsley (1961).

2. Compute

$$[(l - k)]^{-1} \log \hat{\mathbf{P}}(k\Delta, l\Delta), \qquad 0 \le k < l \le n \tag{23}$$

and observe that if the data are compatible with a time stationary Markov model, then *at least* one branch of the logarithm of any given matrix in the list (23) should be roughly equal to some branch of the logarithm of any other matrix in the list. In addition, this common logarithm should be an intensity matrix (that is, it should belong to the class

$$\mathscr{Q} = \left\{\mathbf{Q}: \ q_{ii} \le 0, q_{ij} \ge 0 \qquad \text{for } i \neq j, \sum_{j=1}^{r} q_{ij} = 0\right\}).$$

The process of verifying that $\hat{\mathbf{P}}$ can be represented in the form $\exp(\mathbf{Q})$ for at least one $\mathbf{Q} \in \mathscr{Q}$ is a test for *embeddability* of the data in a continuous-time Markov model. Although this step is seemingly straightforward, it should be pointed out that some surprisingly subtle phenomena are involved in the embeddability test. In particular, due to the multiple valued nature of the logarithm function, it is not immediately apparent that one can find an effective computation algorithm to check for the existence of even one branch of log $\hat{\mathbf{P}}$, which is an intensity matrix. Indeed, it would appear that infinitely many branches of the logarithm might have to be checked to decide on embeddability.

Fortunately, however, any matrix that can be represented as $\exp(\mathbf{Q})$ with $\mathbf{Q} \in \mathcal{Q}$ must have eigenvalues of a rather restrictive nature. In fact it is the existence of sharp upper and lower bounds on the eigenvalues that leads to a practical computation strategy for deciding embeddability. The explicit eigenvalue restrictions and associated computation scheme are outlined here. However, for a detailed discussion of this point and further indication of its role in the analysis of panel data, the reader should consult Singer and Spilerman (1976).

Closely related to the problem of deciding embeddability with a finite number of tests is the fact that in the course of such a computation, there may be several branches of the logarithm of a stochastic matrix that are intensity matrices. *Identification* refers to the task of deciding which of these intensity arrays should be associated with the empirical process. In particular, it is possible to have

$$\hat{\mathbf{P}}(k\Delta, l\Delta) = \exp[(l - k)\Delta\mathbf{Q}_1]$$

and

$$\hat{\mathbf{P}}(k\Delta, l\Delta) = \exp[(l - k)\Delta\mathbf{Q}_2] \tag{24}$$

$$0 \le k < l \le n$$

where $\mathbf{Q}_1 \ne \mathbf{Q}_2$ but $\mathbf{Q}_1 \in \mathcal{Q}$ and $\mathbf{Q}_2 \in \mathcal{Q}$. (See Singer and Spilerman, 1975, 1976 for explicit examples of this behavior.) The phenomenon in Equation (24) is an instance of aliasing for Markov transition matrices, and it is entirely analogous to the aliasing of structural coefficient matrices in continuous-time econometric models (see, in particular, Phillips, 1973). In this situation, the set of underlying structural parameters (that is, the unique intensity matrix that should be associated with an empirical process) is not identifiable. A researcher confronted with matrices such as $\mathbf{Q}_1$ and $\mathbf{Q}_2$ would either have to adjudicate between them on substantive grounds or collect additional data at a time that is not a multiple of the sampling interval Δ. Then the underlying transition mechanism could be identified since only one of the matrices ($\mathbf{Q}_1$ or $\mathbf{Q}_2$) could be consistent with the nonevenly spaced observations.

The computation scheme outlined here recovers all branches of the logarithm of a stochastic matrix $\hat{\mathbf{P}}$, which are intensity matrices, provided $\hat{\mathbf{P}}$ has distinct eigenvalues. This is clearly the situation in most applications. However, it should be noted that repeated eigenvalue matrices do play an important role in sensitivity analyses, and they can be associated with a continuum of intensity matrices (that is, a stochastic matrix $\bar{\mathbf{P}}$ may be within error distance of the observed array $\hat{\mathbf{P}}$ and be representable as $\bar{\mathbf{P}} = \exp(\mathbf{Q})$ for an uncountably infinite set of matrices in $\mathcal{Q}$: See Singer and Spilerman, 1976 and Cuthbert, 1973 for details on this point). This raises difficult questions of both interpretation and reliability of estimates of structural parameters based on evenly spaced data. Extensive reanalyses of data from a variety of panel studies would be necessary in order to assess whether the possible instability just described is in fact a frequently occurring empirical phenomenon.

A COMPUTATION STRATEGY TO DECIDE EMBEDDABILITY

Step 1. Compute the eigenvalues of $\hat{\mathbf{P}}$ and check whether or not they each satisfy

$$\pi\left(\frac{1}{2} + \frac{1}{r}\right) \le \arg(\log \lambda) \le \pi\left(\frac{3}{2} - \frac{1}{r}\right) \tag{25}$$

where r = order of the matrix, and λ is an eigenvalue of $\hat{\mathbf{P}}$. The inequalities (25) were established by Runnenberg (1962). In particular, he used the inequalities of Karpelevitch (1951)

$$\pi\left(\frac{1}{2} + \frac{1}{r}\right) \le \arg(\lambda - 1) \le \pi\left(\frac{3}{2} - \frac{1}{r}\right) \tag{26}$$

—which restrict the eigenvalues, λ, of an arbitrary $r \times r$ stochastic matrix—together with the representation $\mathbf{P}(t) = \exp(t\mathbf{Q})$ for Markov transition matrices, to obtain (25) as a restriction on the eigenvalues of $\exp(\mathbf{Q})$. The shaded zone in Figure 12.1 depicts the region defined by the inequalities (25) and exhibits a typical set of logarithms of the eigenvalues associated with an embeddable matrix.

Step 2. If all eigenvalues of $\hat{\mathbf{P}}$ are real and positive, then their logarithms are real and negative and they automatically satisfy (25). In this situation there can be at most one branch of $\log \hat{\mathbf{P}}$ in $\mathcal{Q}$. To compute it—and thereby check embeddability—reduce $\hat{\mathbf{P}}$ to diagonal form (that is, represent $\hat{\mathbf{P}}$ as $\hat{\mathbf{P}} = \mathbf{H}\Lambda\mathbf{H}^{-1}$ where

$$\Lambda = \begin{pmatrix} \lambda_1 & & & 0 \\ & \cdot & & \\ & & \cdot & \\ 0 & & & \lambda_r \end{pmatrix}$$

and $\mathbf{H}$ is a nonsingular similarity transformation). Then calculate

$$\log \hat{\mathbf{P}} = \mathbf{H} \log \Lambda H^{-1} \tag{27}$$

where

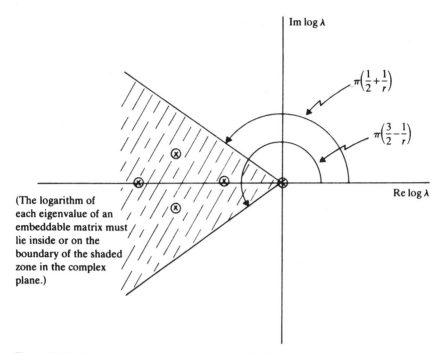

Figure 12.1. Eigenvalue restrictions for embeddable matrics.

$$\log \Lambda = \begin{pmatrix} \log \lambda_1 & & & \underline{0} \\ & \log \lambda_2 & \cdot & \\ & & \cdot & \\ & & & \cdot \\ \underline{0} & & & \log \lambda_r \end{pmatrix}.$$

If the matrix (27) is in $\mathcal{Q}$, then $\hat{\mathbf{P}}$ is embeddable in the unique continuous-time Markov model with intensity matrix given by (27). If (27) is not in $\mathcal{Q}$, then $\hat{\mathbf{P}}$ is simply not embeddable in any continuous-time Markov model.

Step 3. If $\hat{\mathbf{P}}$ has complex eigenvalues they must occur in conjugate pairs. For each such pair $(\lambda = \rho \exp(i\theta), \overline{\lambda} = \rho \exp(-i\theta))$ determine all branches of their logarithms that satisfy (25); especially,

$$\pi \left(\frac{1}{2} + \frac{1}{r} \right) \le \arg(\log_k \lambda) \le \pi \left(\frac{3}{2} - \frac{1}{r} \right)$$

where r = order of the matrix $\hat{\mathbf{P}}$,

$$\arg(\log_k \lambda) = \tan^{-1} \left(\frac{\theta + 2\pi k}{\log \rho} \right),$$

and k specifies a branch of $\log_k \lambda$ according to

$$\log_k \lambda = \log \rho + i(\theta + 2\pi k); k = 0, \pm 1, \pm 2, \ldots ; \quad 0 < \theta < \pi \quad (28)$$

Now select one of the branches for each complex conjugate pair, and compute $\log \hat{\mathbf{P}}$ using (27). Check the resulting matrix for membership in $\mathcal{Q}$. Then repeat this calculation for all branches satisfying (25). The basic importance of Runnenberg's inequalities (25) is revealed at this step, because they guarantee that only *finitely many* branches need be checked. Furthermore, all intensity matrices compatible with the data [the aliases mentioned in (24)] are recovered in these calculations. If multiple matrices $\mathbf{Q} \in \mathcal{Q}$ have been found, the researcher should collect additional information to discriminate among them in the manner described in conjunction with (24).

Strategies for Discrimination among Competing Models

Many of the issues involved in attempting to discriminate among competing models can be illustrated in the relatively simple setting of testing data for compatibility with one of the following four classes of models:

   (i)   Time-stationary Markov chains
   (ii) A restricted class of mixtures of (i)
  (iii) A restricted class of non-time-stationary Markov chains
  (iv) A restricted class of semi-Markov processes

To fix the ideas, assume that observations

$$\{Y^{(i)}(t_k), T^{(i)}(t_k)\}, \quad 1 \le i \le N, \quad 0 \le k \le n \quad (29)$$

have been collected at the evenly spaced time points $0 = t_0 < t_1 < \cdots < t_n$ where $t_{k+1} - t_k = \Delta = $ (spacing between successive observations) > 0; $k = 0, \ldots, n - 1$; $Y^{(i)}(t_k)$ denotes the state of the ith individual in the survey at time t_k; and $T^{(i)}(t_k)$ equals the total number of transitions by the ith individual in the time interval $(0, t_k)$. This is precisely the data collection situation described in Example 3 (see p. 280).

Now introduce models in which individual histories are represented in the form

$$Y(t) = X(T(t)), \quad t \ge 0 \quad (30)$$

where $X(k)$ is a discrete-time Markov chain with stationary transition probabilities having one-step transition matrix $\mathbf{M}$, and $T(t)$ is one of the four kinds of stochastic processes listed here.

A. A time-stationary Poisson process with parameter $\gamma > 0$ [special case of (i)]
B. A mixture of A [special case of (ii)]
C. A non-time-stationary Poisson process with expected number of jumps in the time interval (s, t) given by $\int_s^t h(u)\, du$, where h is a continuous, positive, decreasing function such that $\int_0^\infty h(u)\, du = +\infty$ [special case of (iii)]
D. A renewal process defined by

$$T(t) = \max\left\{n: \sum_{i=0}^{n-1} \tau_i \le t\right\} \qquad \text{if} \quad \tau_0 \le t$$

$$T(t) = 0 \qquad \text{if} \quad \tau_0 > t$$

where $\{\tau_i\}$, $i = 0, 1, \ldots$ i, are independent identically distributed positive random variables such that

$$\text{Prob}\{\tau_i > t\} = 1 - \exp\left(-\int_0^t h(u)\, du\right)$$

and h satisfies the same hypotheses as in C [special case of (iv)].

In each of these models mobility between states is governed by a single stochastic matrix **M**. The models differ only in the assumptions that are made about the waiting times between moves. It should also be observed that the representation of Equation (30) provides an alternative description of some of the models presented in the sections entitled "A Simple Factored Representation of "**Q**," "More General Waiting Time Distributions than Exponential," and "A Non-time-stationary Markov Model."

In particular, when $T(t)$ is a time-stationary Poisson process with parameter $\gamma > 0$ (Model A), then $X(T(t))$ is simply the time-stationary Markov chain described in the section entitled "A Simple Factored Representation of **Q**," where the intensity matrix **Q** has the factored representation $\mathbf{Q} = \gamma(\mathbf{M} - \mathbf{I})$. The advantage of the representation in Equation (30) in the present context (that is, with fragmentary data of the special form of Equation (29)) is that it explicitly describes the relationship between the observable quantities $(Y(t_i), T(t_i))$, $i = 0, 1, 2, \ldots, n$ and the nondirectly observable process $\{X(k), k = 0, 1, 2, \ldots\}$. The latter process describes transitions when they occur, and is governed by the matrix of structural parameters **M**.

When $T(t)$ is a mixture of time-stationary Poisson processes (Model B), then $X(T(t))$ can be any one of the mixtures in Equations (8)–(10) depending on the choice of mixing distribution. Population heterogeneity is introduced only through a classification of persons according to their *rate* of movement, and $T(t)$ describes the number of moves by a type-γ individual. Such individuals are assumed to occur in the total population with a probability specified by the mixing distribution.

When $T(t)$ is a nonstationary Poisson process (Model C), $X(T(t))$ is the nonstationary Markov chain constructed in the section entitled "A Non-time-stationary Markov Model." The following intuitive description is intended to clarify the manner in which this kind of process evolves.

Consider a homogeneous population in which an individual starting in state i at time zero stays there for a random length of time τ_1 with

$$\text{Prob}(\tau_1 > t) = \exp\left(-\int_0^t h(u)\, du\right)$$

The assumption that h be decreasing implies that the longer an individual stays in state i, the less likely he is to move in the immediate future. At the end of the initial waiting time, the individual moves to state j with probability m_{ij}. Then he stays in his new state for a random length of time τ_2 whose distribution depends on τ_1 according to

$$\text{Prob}(\tau_2 > t | \tau_1 = s) = \exp\left(-\int_s^{s+t} h(u)\, du\right)$$

Since h is decreasing, the propensity of the individual to remain in this new state is not only greater the longer he stays, but it is also greater than at any time prior to his first move. At time $\tau_1 + \tau_2$, the individual moves again according to M, and waits there a length of time τ_3 governed by

$$\text{Prob}(\tau_3 > t | \tau_1 + \tau_2 = s) = \exp\left(-\int_s^{s+t} h(u)\, du\right)$$

This process is repeated, and with each change of state the individual has less and less propensity to move than at any previous time.

Finally, we consider processes of the form $X(T(t))$ where $T(t)$ is a renewal process (Model D). With this specification, $X(T(t))$ is a special semi-Markov process as defined in the section entitled "More General Waiting Time Distributions than Exponential." In order to clarify the manner by which these processes evolve, consider a homogeneous population in which an individual's *initial* move is regulated exactly as in the nonstationary Markov model just described. However, his waiting time τ_2 is assumed to be independent of τ_1 and governed by

$$\text{Prob}(\tau_2 > t) = \exp\left(-\int_0^t h(u)\, du\right).$$

After each successive move, the individual's new waiting time is governed by the same probability law as τ_1 and τ_2. The assumption that h is decreasing still implies that the longer the individual remains in a particular state, the less likely he is to move in the immediate future. However, in contrast to the nonstationary Markov model, each time a move is made the propensity to move again starts over at a high value and then decreases. In particular, the *continual* decrease in propensity of the non-stationary Markov model no longer holds for the present semi-Markov processes. Thus while the former process may be identified with "aging of an individual," the latter is akin to "cumulative inertia in an occupation," as described by McGinnis (1968).

In attempting to identify which of the four kinds of models—if any—is compatible with data of the form (29), the following strategy may be utilized.

Plot cumulative number of moves versus t and check whether this is approximately linear (Figure 12.2) or concave downward (Figure 12.3). It is the case that Models A and B are consistent with the linear picture where the principal trend is described by a regression line through the origin. Model D is consistent with the linear picture but with the main trend— (away from $t = 0$)—described by a straight line having a possibly non-zero intercept. Only Model C is consistent with a pattern of the form described by Figure 12.3.

If the empirical picture corresponds to Figure 12.2, then the slope, b, of

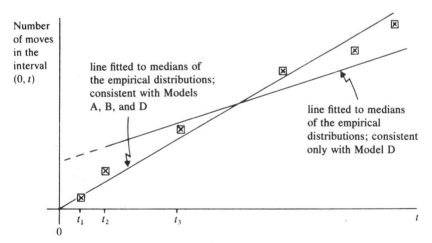

Figure 12.2. Cumulative number of moves versus t for data consistent with Models A, B, and D. The cross above t_i reports the median number of moves by all persons in the panel study during the time interval $(0,t_i)$.

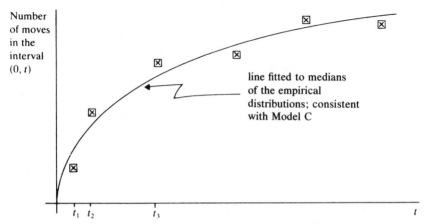

Figure 12.3. Cumulative number of moves versus t for data consistent with Model C. The cross above t_i reports the median number of moves by all persons in the panel study during the time interval $(0,t_i)$.

a straight line fitted to the linear pattern would have the following *alternative* interpretations on the basis of the above data:

1. $b = \gamma =$ time-homogeneous Poisson parameter

2. $\displaystyle\int_0^\infty \gamma \, d\mu(\gamma) = b$ for the mixture of Poisson models[13]

3. $\displaystyle b = \frac{1}{\displaystyle\int_0^\infty \left[\exp\left(-\int_0^t h(u) \, du \right) \right] dt}$

    $\displaystyle = \frac{1}{\text{(expected waiting time between}}$
    moves in a renewal process)

If this linear picture is observed, we would solve—using numerical inversion formulas—the following equations for $\mathbf{M}$:

1. $\hat{\mathbf{P}}(0, t_1) = \exp(t_1\gamma(\mathbf{M} - \mathbf{I})).$

Call the solution $\mathbf{M}_1$; it corresponds to Model A,

---

[13] When the density function $\mu'(\gamma)$ exists, this expression reduces to the familiar formula for a weighted average, $\displaystyle\int_0^\infty \gamma\mu'(\gamma) \, d\gamma$. By the text expression, however, we mean integration with respect to a general probability measure.

$$2. \quad \hat{\mathbf{P}}(0, t_1) = \int_0^\infty \exp(t_1\gamma(\mathbf{M} - \mathbf{I})) \, d\mu(\gamma).$$

Call the solution $\mathbf{M}_1'$; it corresponds to Model B.

$$3. \quad \hat{\mathbf{P}}(0, t_1) = \sum_{n=0}^\infty (F_n(t_1) - F_{n+1}(t_1))\mathbf{M}^n.$$

Call the solution $\mathbf{M}_1^*$; it corresponds to Model D. (*Note:* $F_n(t)$ denotes the n-fold convolution of the waiting time distribution $F(t) = 1 - \exp(-\int_0^t h(u) \, du)$ with itself.)

Now check whether the M-matrix obtained in each case is a bonafide stochastic matrix. This is really an embeddability test for all three model types. If any one of the above calculations yields a matrix that is *not* stochastic then that model is inconsistent with the data $\hat{\mathbf{P}}(0, t_1)$. If one or more of these calculations yields a stochastic matrix, then we test its ability to predict the observed matrices $\hat{\mathbf{P}}(0, t_2)$, $\hat{\mathbf{P}}(0, t_3)$ . . . using the appropriate equation. In particular, prepare tables of the form

$$1'. \quad \hat{\mathbf{P}}(0, t_2) - \exp(t_2\gamma(\mathbf{M}_1 - \mathbf{I})), \qquad \hat{\mathbf{P}}(0, t_3) - \exp(t_3\gamma(\mathbf{M}_1 - \mathbf{I})), \ . \ . \ .$$

$$2'. \quad \hat{\mathbf{P}}(0, t_2) - \int_0^\infty \exp(t_2\gamma(\mathbf{M}_1) - \mathbf{I}) \, d\mu(\gamma),$$

$$\hat{\mathbf{P}}(0, t_3) - \int_0^\infty \exp(t_2\gamma(\mathbf{M}_1' - \mathbf{I})) \, d\mu(\gamma), \ . \ . \ .$$

$$3'. \quad \hat{\mathbf{P}}(0, t_2) - \sum_n [F_n(t_2) - F_{n+1}(t_2)](\mathbf{M}_1^*)^n,$$

$$\hat{\mathbf{P}}(0, t_3) - \sum_n [F_n(t_3) - F_{n+1}(t_3)](\mathbf{M}_1^*)^n, \ . \ . \ .$$

that represent residuals of observed matrices from predictions based on Models 1, 2, and 3, respectively. One instance of the informative nature of such comparisons is the fact that many data sets reveal a discrepancy in comparison ($1'$) in that the diagonal entries in the observed matrices $\hat{\mathbf{P}}(0, t_2)$, $\hat{\mathbf{P}}(0, t_3)$, . . . , and so on, are substantially larger than the time-homogeneous Markov predictions. Both of the model classes 2 and 4 can account for this kind of discrepancy, despite the fact that they have very different substantive interpretations. Further discrimination requires a more detailed consideration—on both substantive and numerical grounds—of the residual matrices.

Finally, if the concave picture, Figure 12.3, occurs, then prepare the comparisons.

$$\hat{\mathbf{P}}(0, t_2) - \exp\left[\left(\int_0^{t_2} h(u) \, du\right)(\mathbf{M}_+ - \mathbf{I})\right],$$

$$\hat{\mathbf{P}}(0, t_3) - \exp\left[\left(\int_0^{t_3} h(u) \, du\right)(\mathbf{M}_+ - \mathbf{I})\right], \ldots$$

where $\mathbf{M}_+$ is a solution of the equation

$$\hat{\mathbf{P}}(0, t_1) = \exp\left[\left(\int_0^{t_1} h(u) \, du\right)(\mathbf{M} - \mathbf{I})\right].$$

Sharp discrepancies here might be revealing about alternative classes of models that should be added to the original list as candidates to describe the empirical process.

We emphasize that the preceding discussion is by no means complete, and is designed only to communicate to the reader, in concise form, the flavor of the sorts of considerations which seem appropriate for the analysis of multiwave panel data.

Conclusions

We have described a number of issues that arise in fitting models of distributional change to fragmentary data, and in attempting to discriminate among alternative structures fitted to the same fragmentary data. The univariate Markov framework has been applied to advantage in the physical sciences in situations where the notion of population heterogeneity is not especially pertinent, and where the number of observations in time available to a researcher is reasonably large. However, both of these factors are crucial considerations in modeling social phenomena, and we have therefore focused on some variants of the univariate Markov framework that were developed for the expressed purpose of incorporating assumptions about the nature of social processes into mathematical models.

There are additional important issues, closely related to the ones we have discussed, which must be addressed if a routine methodology is to be developed regarding the application of these model types to social processes. These issues have not been considered in the present review because they are largely undeveloped research areas.

1.   The introduction of substantive theories into Markov models and their variants via restrictions on the structural parameters, such as by prohibiting certain transitions (for example, occupation or industry shifts) from occurring directly. Some exploratory work on this issue may be found in Coleman (1964a, 1964b).

2. Strategies for sensitivity analyses to assess the nature of the dependence of parameter estimates on small perturbations in the data. This topic is discussed within the context of time-stationary Markov models in Singer and Spilerman (1976), but must be extended to other model types.

3. Specification of formal error structures, and the development of techniques for setting confidence limits on parameter estimates which derive from fragmentary data.

4. The specification of data collection designs for panel studies that will facilitate discrimination among several models fitted to the same fragmentary data. This should include a detailed consideration of the reliability of retrospective interrogation versus the cost and time delays attendant upon reinterview in a panel study. Furthermore, an investigation of the optimal frequency of reinterview in a panel study is required in order to optimize the amount of useful information about change collected per research dollar.

References

Anderson, T. W., and L. A. Goodman
 1957   "Statistical inference about Markov chains." *Annals of Mathematical Statistics* 28: 89–109.
Bartholomew, D. J.
 1973   *Stochastic Models for Social Processes,* 2nd ed. New York: John Wiley and Sons.
Billingsley, P.
 1961   *Statistical Inference for Markov Processes.* Chicago: University of Chicago Press.
Blau, P., and O. D. Duncan
 1967   *The American Occupational Structure.* New York: John Wiley and Sons.
Blauner, R.
 1964   *Alienation and Freedom.* Chicago: University of Chicago Press.
Blumen, I., M. Kogan, and P. J. McCarthy
 1955   *The Industrial Mobility of Labor as a Probability Process.* Cornell Studies of Industrial and Labor Relations, vol. 6. Ithaca, New York: Cornell University.
Chung, K. L.
 1967   *Markov Chains with Stationary Transition Probabilities.* Berlin: Springer.
Coleman, J. S.
 1964a *Models of Change and Response Uncertainty.* Englewood Cliffs, N. J.: Prentice-Hall.
 1964b *Introduction to Mathematical Sociology.* New York: Free Press.
Cuthbert, J. R.
 1973   "The logarithm function for finite-state Markov semi-groups." *Journal of the London Mathematical Society* 6: 524–532.
Feller, W.
 1956   Book Review of Blumen, Kogan, and McCarthy (1955). *Psychometrika* 21: 217.

Goodman, G. S., and S. Johansen
  1973   "Kolmogorov's differential equations for non-stationary, countable state Markov
          processes with uniformly continuous transition probabilities." *Proceedings of the
          Cambridge Philosophical Society* 73: 119–138.
Goodman, L. A.
  1961   "Statistical methods for the mover–stayer model." *Journal of the American
          Statistical Association* 56(296): 841–868.
Hauser, R., and D. Featherman
  1973   "Trends in the occupational mobility of U. S. men, 1962–1970." *American
          Sociological Review* 38 (June): 302–310.
Hauser, R., and W. Sewell
  1975   *Education, Occupation, and Earnings.* New York: Academic Press.
Hodge, R. W.
  1966   "Occupational mobility as a probability process." *Demography* 3: 19–34.
Hoem, J.
  1972   "Inhomogeneous semi-Markov processes, select actuarial tables, and duration-
          dependence in demography." Pp. 251–296 in T. N. E. Grevelle (ed.), *Population
          Dynamics.* New York: Academic Press.
Karpelevitsch, F. I.
  1951   "On the characteristic roots of a matrix with non-negative elements." *Isvestija,
          Serie Mathematique* 15: 361–383.
Kuhn, A., A. Poole, P. Sales, and H. P. Wynn
  1973   "An analysis of graduate job mobility." *British Journal of Industrial Relations* 11:
          124–142.
Kurtz, T. G.
  1971   "Comparison of semi-Markov and Markov processes." *Annals of Mathematical
          Statistics* 42(3): 991–1002.
Land, K.
  1969   "Duration of residence and prospective migration." *Demography* 6: 133–140.
Lazarsfeld, P. F., and N. W. Henry
  1968   *Latent Structure Analysis.* Boston: Houghton Mifflin.
Lieberson, S., and G. V. Fuguett
  1967   "Negro-white occupational differences in the absence of discrimination," *Ameri-
          can Journal of Sociology* 73: 188–200.
Lipset, S. M., and R. Bendix
  1959   *Social Mobility in Industrial Society.* Berkeley: University of California Press.
McCall, J. J.
  1973   *Income Mobility, Racial Discrimination, and Economic Growth.* Lexington,
          Mass.: D. C. Heath.
McFarland, D. D.
  1970   "Intra-generational social mobility as a Markov process: Including a time-
          stationary Markovian model that explains observed declines in mobility rates over
          time." *American Sociological Review* 35: 463–476.
McGinnis, R.
  1968   "A stochastic model of social mobility." *American Sociological Review*
          33(October): 712–722.
Morgan, J. N., and J. D. Smith
  1969   *A Panel Study of Income Dynamics.* Institute for Social Research, Ann Arbor,
          Michigan.

Myers, G. C., R. McGinnis, and R. Masnick
  1967 "The duration of residence approach to a dynamic stochastic model of internal migration: A test of the axiom of cumulative inertia." *Eugenics Quarterly* 14: 121–126.
Palmer, G.
  1954 *Labor Mobility in Six Cities.* New York: Social Science Research Council.
Parnes, H. S.
  1972 "Longitudinal surveys: Prospects and problems." *Monthly Labor Review* (February): 11–15.
Phillips, P. C. B.
  1973 "The problem of identification in finite parameter continuous time models." *Journal of Econometrics* 1: 351–362.
Rees, A., and H. Watts
  1976 *The Urban Negative Income Tax Experiment.* New York: Academic Press.
Rogers, A.
  1966 "A Markovian analysis of migration differentials." Proceedings of the American Statistical Association, Social Science Section Washington, D. C.: American Statistical Association.
Runnenberg, J. T.
  1962 "On Elfving's problem of imbedding a time-discrete Markov chain in a continuous time one for finitely many states." *Kroninklijke Nederlandse Akademie van Wetenschappen* Proceedings, Series A, Mathematical Sciences, vol. LXV, no. 5: 536–541.
Singer, B., and S. Spilerman
  1974 "Social mobility models for heterogeneous populations." Pp. 356–401 in Herbert Costner (ed.), *Sociological Methodology 1973-74.* San Francisco: Jossey-Bass.
  1975 "Identifying structural parameters of social processes using fragmentary data." *Proceedings, 40th Session of International Statistical Institute,* Warsaw, Poland, vol. 2—Invited papers, pp. 681–697.
  1976 "The representation of social processes by Markov models." *American Journal of Sociology* 82(July): 1–54.
Smith, J. O., and G. Cain
  1967 "Markov chain applications to household income distributions." Unpublished paper, University of Wisconsin–Madison.
Social Security Administration
  1972 "Basic statistical data files available to outside researchers." U. S. Department of Health, Education, and Welfare.
Sørensen, A.
  1975 "Growth in occupational achievement: Social mobility or investments in human capital." Pp. 335–360 in K. Land and S. Spilerman (eds.), *Social Indicator Models.* New York: Russell Sage Foundation.
Spilerman, S.
  1972a "Extensions of the mover–stayer model." *American Journal of Sociology* 78: 599–627.
  1972b "The analysis of mobility processes by the introduction of independent variables into a Markov chain." *American Sociological Review* 37(June): 277–294.
Taeuber, K. E., L. Chiazze, Jr., and W. Haenszel
  1968 *Migration in the United States.* Washington, D. C.: U. S. Government Printing Office.

Tarver, J. O., and W. R. Gurley
　　1965　"A stochastic analysis of geographic mobility and population projections of the census divisions in the United States." *Demography* 2: 134–139.
White, H. C.
　　1970　"Stayers and movers." *American Journal of Sociology* 70(2): 307–324.
Wiggins, L. M.
　　1973　*Panel Analysis—Latent Probability Models for Attitude and Behavior Processes.* San Francisco: Jossey-Bass.

IV
EMERGING ISSUES

13

The Next Fifteen Years
in Demographic Analysis

SAMUEL H. PRESTON

Demography is conventionally defined as the study of determinants and consequences of the size and structure of human populations. Because population size can change only through the birth of new members, the death of old ones, or the movement of people across the boundaries that define the population, demographic analysis necessarily comprises the study of fertility, mortality, and migration. The major indeterminacy in the definition of demographic analysis is the elements of population structure that are to be objects of study. Every demographer's list of eligible targets includes the biological characteristics of age, sex, parity, and race and the social characteristics of marital status and place of residence. Except for marital status, the distribution of each of these variables is uniquely determined by the cumulative history of fertility, mortality, and migration in a population, and marital status usually has a powerful influence on fertility, and to a lesser extent on mortality and migration. At a maximum, the list extends to any item included in a census or nationally representative survey.

Definitions of a scholarly discipline will differ and it is pointless to attempt to specify precisely the boundaries of a field. But those who define

299

Social Demography

demography in terms of variables rather than of data seem to have the stronger case. The data are generated principally for nondemographic consumption and under procedures and authorities that are largely beyond demographers' control. This review will emphasize projected research on the core demographic variables. It starts with some general remarks about research performed by persons prominently identified as demographers, and then deals more specifically with the analysis of core demographic variables, much of which is performed by nondemographers.

Trends in Demographers' Analyses

There are four principal traditions in demographic research in the United States, each of them associated loosely with one or two major universities, although all coexist at each of the institutions that will be mentioned.

The Princeton Tradition.   The Princeton tradition emphasizes international population developments and is the most strictly demographic, focusing especially on analyses of fertility and mortality at the aggregate level. It is more concerned than other traditions with estimation and decomposition of birth and death rates and with monitoring of demographic trends. This orientation is partly a product of a substantive interest in the economic consequences of population growth and concern for the shape of the future. By its nature, this mode of research tends to involve the largest quantity of formal mathematical treatment.

The Chicago–Berkeley Tradition.   The Chicago–Berkeley tradition attempts to view population processes within a broad social context, stressing interrelations between populations and societies, again with focus at the aggregate level. Population is viewed as one of several social systems, and research is directed toward understanding and explaining the behavior of this system as a whole. It is the most theoretical of the traditions in the sense of trying to deduce propositions about population from principles presumed to govern the behavior of groups.

The Pennsylvania–Brown Tradition.   The emphasis here is on using census volumes to paint a picture of the changing character of populations, particularly with respect to spatial distribution and labor force size and structure. Because the raw analytic material is aggregated, analysis is usually carried out at the aggregate level. As a result of its emphasis on spatial distribution, this research tradition is more heavily involved in migration research than the others. Its emphasis on census materials has lent itself gracefully to the coordinated function of training many foreign demographic statisticians.

The Michigan–Wisconsin Tradition. The Michigan–Wisconsin tradition is that most concerned with studying the demographic behavior of individuals and the individual-level processes that determine, in the aggregate, population structure. The principal mode of analysis is survey research, and in the analysis of survey data it necessarily becomes most concerned with problems of statistical inference. It has traditionally devoted more attention to the study of socioeconomic composition than have the other traditions, and tends to have the most inclusive definition of the field.

During the last decade, the fourth approach has become relatively more prominent and the second and third relatively less. The reasons may be in large part technological, a change in the relative costs of pursuing the different approaches as a result of technical change. Especially noteworthy are the development of high-speed and high-capacity computers and of canned software programs of statistical analysis, together with the widespread dissemination of data tapes containing results of surveys. The U. S. Census Bureau has cooperated in this trend by creating and distributing sample tapes from the U. S. Census, and other nations and organizations are now following suit. Since there have been no equivalent developments in social theory or in the material published in basic census volumes themselves, the result has been the relative emergence of data-intensive work of the fourth type.

While this development is perfectly understandable and undoubtedly desirable, the adjustment to these technical changes may be nearly completed, at least in the United States. Population processes cannot be completely understood in terms of individual-level characteristics that come in the form of discrete vectors of observations. Levels of fertility, mortality, and migration all depend upon relations among individuals and especially on relations between the individual and the various aggregates of which he or she is a part. Demographers have not been successful in ascribing variation in vital rates to variation in the characteristics of members of populations generating those rates. The mortality decline in the twentieth century cannot be understood by reference to, say, increasing educational levels of the population but only by reference to broader systemic factors. The postwar marriage and baby boom or the 19% decline in American fertility between 1970 and 1972 were not primarily products of the changing social or residential composition of the American population. The decline in female marriage during the late 1960s cannot be analyzed without reference to the changing sex ratio of marriage eligibles, a property of an aggregate rather than of individuals. The structure of opportunities at origin and prospective destinations is clearly a critical variable in migration analysis.

It seems clear that the occurrence or nonoccurrence of birth, death, and migration is a product of an individual's response to a complex set of environmental signals. An individual's *responsiveness* is a product of unique social experiences and biological endowments, and is reflected very imperfectly in such census-type characteristics as educational attainment. The environmental signals themselves, extraneous to the individual, are often untapped in survey research; the best we sometimes do is to record whether the person lives in an urban or rural setting. Environmental properties such as the sex ratio, the distribution of jobs and wages available, the penetration of mass media and the message it presents, laws governing divorce and sexual conduct, migration opportunities, the cost and types of contraceptives available, and so on, must be suspected of powerfully influencing family-building behavior, but many such variables are excluded at the outset from survey research. Similar exclusions often apply to health technology in the study of mortality, changing modes of production in the study of occupational distribution, and potential wages and environmental amenities in the study of migration.

A powerful integration of the second and third traditions is provided by what has become known in sociology as contextual analysis. Operationally, this usually takes the form of merging information on individuals with that on characteristics (and not simply categories) of the areas in which they live, the social classes to which they have belonged or do belong, the households in which they reside, the period in which the observation was recorded, and so on. This integration seems fundamentally important for the advance of the field because, on the one hand, all variables must influence vital processes through events occurring to individuals, but on the other hand, many of those influential variables are properties not of individuals but of their environmental context. Such a treatment is almost axiomatic to economists who are used to thinking in terms of individual utility maximization under environmentally imposed constraints. But it has made relatively few inroads into demography. (For a review of the limited work in fertility that uses contextual analysis, see Freedman, 1974.) Contextual analysis is a prime candidate for expansion in the next 15 years and should provide the instrument for a revitalized application of social theory to demographic analysis. Such an expansion would not entail a decomputerization of demography, although it would direct more attention to research design and less to technical virtuosity in the analysis of "found" data sets. But fundamentally it would require even larger data sets in order to accommodate and represent an exceedingly complex reality.

Future Developments in Demographic Analysis

In order to deal in somewhat more detail with possible developments, it is convenient to divide demographic analysis into three parts:

1. *Models,* used to identify variables that play a critical role in demographic processes, to demonstrate the implications of changes in the value of variables, and to make clearer the interactions that exist among them
2. *Measurement and estimation,* used to establish the values of those variables
3. *Inference,* the socioeconomic-biological study of why those variables take on the values they do and the quantitative assignment of responsibility for their variation

Work done in any of these categories by no means develops independently of that done in others. Until mortality was measured carefully enough to show it to be highly dependent upon age, it was pointless to develop a life table and the stationary population model. Only after the stable population model had demonstrated the sensitivity of growth rates to changes in the length of generation was demographic attention directed toward the substantive study of age at marriage. But it is convenient for expositional purposes to treat the different modes of analysis separately.

POPULATION MODELS

The basic purpose of a population model is to demonstrate the implications of a certain combination of necessary or assumed relationships and parameter values for population processes. The most notable model developed in demography has been that of the stable population, a closed one-sex model that assumes constancy over time in age-specific mortality and fertility rates. This model was developed and elaborated primarily by Alfred Lotka and Ansley Coale and receives its most detailed and accessible exposition in Coale (1972). It is well known that the stable population assumptions ultimately produce a population whose age composition, birth, death, and growth rates are fixed through time and independent of the characteristics of the initial population to which those rates are applied. Thus it becomes meaningful to speak of an actual population's *intrinsic* characteristics, uniquely implied by its current regime of age-specific vital rates. This model produces relatively simple analytic expressions of the interdependence of demographic variables and thereby clarifies what might otherwise remain remote: for example, that mortality decline has relatively little impact on population age distribution, and can often make a population younger.

It appears that the analytic potential of the stable population model has been largely exhausted. Coale (1972) considered in detail the convergence of populations to their stable form, the most important related topic whose coverage had been incomplete. The usefulness of the model for estimation and measurement has been impaired by the major mortality changes that have occurred throughout most regions of the world since 1940, rendering its assumptions seriously invalid for most populations. The search for equally concise analytic expressions of population relations in simplified situations of instability (for example, linear decline in age-specific fertility rates) seems worthwhile but has been largely unsuccessful. One notable exception is the elegant closed-form expression that emerges to represent the "momentum" factor in population growth that would pertain in a previously stable population on which a zero-growth fertility regime is suddenly imposed (Keyfitz, 1971). The value of such expressions is largely heuristic; an alternative technique, population projection, offers a flexibility and power that cannot be surpassed for practical application and illustration in individual populations.

Age, the basic variable in stable population models and in projection procedures, is only one source of variation in vital rates. While it probably remains the single most important individual-level factor to consider in the analysis of mortality, fertility models that are exclusively age-dependent are obviously incomplete. Developments in population modeling during the next decade will probably continue to feature the explicit introduction of other endogenous variables into fertility analysis. There are three types of efforts currently underway that will probably flourish in the near term. One is simply the integration of new variables into the basic stable population model. For example, Das Gupta (1976) derives the intrinsic growth rate for the U. S. population implied by its current marriage rates and marital age–parity-dependent fertility rates. The point is that fertility rates vary not only with age but also with marital status and parity and that current marriage–parity distributions may be distorted relative to those implied by current behavior, just as current age distributions can be distorted. The intrinsic growth rate implied by a marriage–parity–age-specific fertility regime is typically different from that implied by the age schedule alone and probably provides a somewhat more accurate measure of current conditions, one that better reflects cohort-specific influences on fertility. Other factors such as marital dissolution and sterility could be introduced in the same way, and undoubtedly will be.

A second area, where advance in modeling is more important but much more problematic is in the demography of sex. One-sex models like the stable population assume that fertility is a function of the size and composition of that sex's population alone. It is well known that the male intrinsic rate of increase computed under this assumption is often very different from the rate of females in the same population. For example, the U. S. male rate for 1969 was 8.64/1000 and the female rate only 5.63 (Preston, 1974). Obviously, such a situation could not long persist; the assumption of constancy for at least one of the sexes is not just empirically incorrect but logically invalid. The direction of the solution is obvious: Make reproduction a function of couples rather than of a woman or man and build into the model a submodel that converts the distribution of men and women into a distribution of couples. The search for a marriage function that would accomplish this conversion has been largely unavailing (Pollard, 1977). Appropriate mathematical formulations are difficult to specify and, once specified, the parameter values will be very hard to estimate because so many factors affect marriage other than the population's age–sex distribution. But the solution is important. According to one crude estimate, a majority of the recent major decline in female nuptiality is attributable to an increasingly deformed sex distribution of marriage eligibles (Preston and Richards, 1975); undoubtedly a substantial proportion of the recent female fertility decline is attributable to declining marriage.

The third important development in fertility models will be the continued elaboration of the interbirth interval model pioneered by Henry, Sheps, and Potter (Sheps and Menken, 1973). In its simplest expression, this model divides the reproductive years of a fecund women into components representing periods of pregnancy, sterile periods associated with pregnancy, and intervals spent in the stage of susceptibility to conception, with the latter represented as a random variable depending on biological fecundability and use–effectiveness of contraception. The length of the total reproductive period and fetal mortality can be readily incorporated into the model. Expressions for the expected number of live births in the course of a woman's life, or the expected birth rate for a group of women, can then be derived as a function of all of these variables. The model incorporates all of the intervening variables identified by Davis and Blake (1955–1956) 20 years ago and has the added virtue of demonstrating explicitly how sensitive fertility should be to variation in parameter values and how variables interact. This model has been very informative for understanding the sources of variation in fertility in noncontracepting populations and is quite valuable in the design and evaluation of fertility control programs. For example, the basic model shows that there are strikingly increasing returns to improvements in contraceptive use–effectiveness in terms of births averted, suggesting that programs should be highly focused rather than diffuse. It has also been shown that abortion has a more important proportionate effect on fertility the higher the population's level of use–effectiveness; that is, contraception and abortion act synergystically (Keyfitz, 1972).

The needed developments of the model are again in the form of building in realism: allowing fecundability, contraceptive effectiveness, sterility and fetal mortality to vary with age and parity and from one women to the next. An integration of assumptions about family size goal-directed behavior is clearly needed in populations where such behavior is prevalent. Most of these complications render analytic expressions exceedingly awkward to apply or interpret. As a result, simulation is required, which reduces the generality of results. Fertility is one area where simulation has clearly paid off, and its successful application has not been confined to biological processes. One useful behavioral application occurs in the analysis of relations between fertility and child mortality. Heer and Smith (1968) showed by simulation that if parents bore children until they were 95% certain that a son would be alive when the father reached age 65, net reproduction rates would decline as mortality improved. Simulation has also proven useful to anthropologists interested in the effect of marital and reproductive customs on social survival in small groups (Hammel and Hutchinson, 1974).

MEASUREMENT AND ESTIMATION

The most fundamental problem in demographic measurement continues to be the identification within reasonably narrow confidence intervals of the value of vital rates in nations and regions where vital registration is poor. Such areas still represent more than half of the world's population: most of Asia and Latin America and almost all of Africa. Reasonably reliable rates are essential in order to identify the demographic situation with which an area is confronted and to gauge the impact of various policies that have been implemented. In general, the nations with the poorest data are the ones that are most in need of good data for policy and planning purposes.

There are two basic approaches to filling gaps in registration systems, and each has vigorous proponents. One can be called indirect estimation by reference to presumed quantitative regularities in human vital processes. If one assumes that age patterns of mortality in a particular nation belong to a particular one- or two-parameter system of mortality functions, then vital rates can be estimated readily (though not necessarily reliably) from two consecutive census age distributions. Other useful assumptions are that age-specific vital rates have been constant for a long period, that death registration completeness is invariant with age, or that the age curve of fertility can be accurately fit by a second-degree polynomial (United Nations, 1967; Brass *et al.*, 1968; Brass, 1975). The accompanying methods are some of the most ingenious developments the field of demography has to offer, they are inexpensive to apply, and they often produce reasonable looking estimates. The disadvantage is that there is usually no way of externally validating the estimates or of testing the assumptions on which they are based. The overarching need in this area is for a systematic evaluation, involving both deterministic and stochastic elements, of the sensitivity of estimates to errors in data or assumption. Many are probably quite robust to error but this has not been demonstrated except through isolated illustrations.

The second major approach, which is vastly more expensive, is a direct attempt to estimate the extent of error in existing or specially devised sample registration schemes by matching records with those from another source, usually a household survey. On the assumption of independence of error in the two systems, the total number of events that should have been recorded can be estimated. The technique is identical to capture–recapture experiments that have been employed in animal ecology. This approach has now been applied in a dozen or so populations and is the subject of a review volume by Marks *et al.* (1974). The problem with this technique is that errors in the two systems are rarely independent, both being subject not only to differential omission by social characteristics but also to the migration of households after an event and willful omission in order to circumvent legal requirements. In addition,there is the problem of attaining accuracy in the matching process itself—knowing what events were in fact unrecorded in either system. Brass (1971) points out specific instances where the technique gives badly distorted estimates and recommends trying out a third procedure: a single system with reliability checks built in, through careful resurvey of a sample of those initially contacted. This technique is still subject to errors induced by migration, willful omission, and consistent recall lapse, and unlike the second technique, it provides no way of estimating the extent of double omissions because the assumption of independence is intrinsically untenable. It is a special case of multi-round surveys, which present an increasingly important third alternative.

In short, there are no clearly preferred techniques for taking demographic inventory in most of the world. No one can deny the importance of the task, and the currently unsettled methodology portends a good deal of activity in the near term. The problems are magnified because much of the interest is in establishing trends. A drop of 5 points in the birth rate would imply resounding success for a family planning program but is less than one standard error of estimate for some of the techniques used to monitor levels.

More developed countries, of course, have their own measurement problems, although birth, death, and reproduction rates are not prominent among them. One area in serious need of attention is the estimation of the distribution of the biological variables necessarily underlying fertility levels, especially exposure, fecundability, frequency and effectiveness of contraception, and extent of spontaneous and induced abortion. Biological, social, and legal factors differentially impinge on these intervening variables, and a thorough understanding of how fertility levels are determined requires their separate recognition. To quote Ryder and Westoff's (1971, p. 358) ringing last sentence in *Reproduction in the United States, 1965:*

> The subtleties of complex explanatory systems, employing sophisticated social, economic, and psychological concepts, will provide meagre returns unless and until we learn to measure more accurately the dependent variables at the core of the analysis of fertility.

Such measurement is practically impossible from single-round retrospective surveys. It is essential that nationally representative panels of women and men, married and unmarried, be followed prospectively and closely. The same statement can be made with equal validity for mortality. What we need is a sample national population register with monthly updating and more detail on life events, personal characteristics, and ecological circumstances than is currently available in other nations' registers. This is one area where the U. S. lags behind certain less developed countries. Large monthly visit household surveys with considerable information on the biological variables related to fertility are now being conducted by the Cholera Research Lab in Bangladesh and by INCAP in Guatemala. Such systems may not be necessary to measurement of vital rates themselves but they are critically important for measuring the biological parameters that underlie the demographic processes.

An important estimation problem that arises in analysis of longitudinal data has been identifying the influence of characteristics on the risk that an event, such as marriage, divorce, or childbirth, will occur. One can, of course, compute life tables separately for persons falling into certain categories of a variable, but this procedure requires making discrete what may be a continuous relationship and becomes very tedious and subject to small Ns when more than one characteristic is considered at a time. In the analysis of longitudinal data, there is no equivalent in power and convenience to multiple classification analysis. Fortunately, this problem seems well on its way to solution by biostatisticians. Cox (1972) has developed and Kalbfleisch and Prentice (1973) modified a procedure that permits the estimation of a linear regression equation where the chance of an event is the dependent variable and data come in the form of truncated life histories of individuals. The procedure does not require prior specification of the time path of the risk function. The procedure in effect joins regression and life table analysis, a wedding that should prove quite fruitful. The availability of this analytic technique makes even more compelling the advantages of large scale nationally representative longitudinal studies. Whether or not they evolve, this technique seems destined to become prominently featured in the next decade.

There are important new developments underway not only in the measurement of biological processes but also of individual motivations that bear on those processes. Perhaps most significant are new measures of fertility attitudes and increased attention to the reliability and validity of old ones. A technique for measuring fertility attitudes, which requires individuals to make pairwise comparisons between different family size outcomes, produces a function that describes the shape of preferences for all possible outcomes (Coombs *et al.*, 1975). This approach may yield more successful predictions of childbearing behavior than do standard measures such as desired family size, although this remains to be demonstrated. Knowing the approximate shape of the preference function should prove especially useful in countries where child mortality is still high and consequently where parents have a high likelihood of attaining a completed family size other than their most-preferred target.

INFERENCE

The study of why demographic variables take on the values that they do in a particular population involves at a minimum all of the behavioral sciences as well as economics and the biological and health sciences. The contribution that each of the disciplines can make probably varies with the type of population under study. Bourgeois-Pichat (1967) suggests that fertility in preindustrialized societies is strongly determined if not completely controlled by biological factors and rather rigid social norms. It is reasonable to suggest that the relevant norms are not those for families of different sizes but those which govern exposure to intercourse: age at marriage and number of partners, postnatal intercourse taboos, remarriage after widowhood, and so on (Polgar, 1972). Such strict social control is presumably functional where the size of the group is small and where conditions change little from year to year. In the course of socioeconomic modernization, he argues, childbearing comes more and more to be the result of decisions made by a couple within marriage. On the other hand,

Easterlin (1973) suggests that childbearing was always under the conscious control of couples but that the advantages of having a large number of births were formerly so great that it merely appeared to be uncontrolled. And there are some who deny that rigid social control has diminished (Blake, 1972).

There are four rather distinct disciplines that study the reproductive behavior of individuals:

1. *Demography,* which seeks to explain differences in fertility by differences in broad, census-type characteristics of couples of reproductive age, such as age, marital status, parity, and educational attainment
2. *Social psychology,* which seeks to explain differences in fertility by differences in attitudes and mental traits of individuals, and sometimes to explain how those traits come to be developed
3. *Microeconomics,* which assumes that couples behave rationally out of some appreciation of the costs and benefits associated with a particular act, with economic costs and benefits featured in the analysis
4. *Public health,* which tends to ascribe fertility variation to differentials in access to and use of fertility control devices

The degree of integration of these different approaches is unfortunately rather limited. Consider explanations of the widely observed inverse relation between cumulative fertility and woman's educational attainment. A demographer will first apportion this relationship into marital fertility and age at marriage, and then perhaps show how many of the effects remain after controlling husband's income, race, and labor force participation. A social psychologist will argue that education has opened new vistas to women, increased their sense of efficacy thereby making them more "planful," and increased their relative power in the family. The microeconomist *knows* that higher education has reduced fertility by increasing the opportunity cost of such time-intensive activities as childraising. The health viewpoint may stress the effect of education on a woman's efficiency in contraception and her exposure to alternative devices.

Probably all of these factors are usually operating to some extent. Clearly, their relative importance cannot be established without researchers' stepping over the disciplinary barriers and testing the predictive power of the alternatives. The study of fertility today is highly fractioned, a problem throughout the social sciences but one which is enormously magnified here. An appropriate division of labor among the fields may occur along the following general lines. If childbearing is to an important extent the outcome of individual decisions to have or not to have a child—and most couples in the U. S. are under the impression that it is—then the economists' cost and benefit framework logically must be invoked to study the decision. There is no other conceivable basis for deciding whether to have a child or to use a particular form of contraception than a weighing of the advantages and disadvantages of the act. But it is obvious that many of the relevant costs and benefits are not economic. Social psychologists and anthropologists have an important role to play in studying the process by which the parameters in the decision-making function are determined: how much the various features of children (or of measures required to avoid them) are valued and how they came to be that way. The Value of Children project currently being directed by Fawcett (1974) is investigating some of these questions in six countries, with promising initial results. It remains for sociologists and economists to link the individual perceptions and decision-making functions with socially imposed reality through some variant of contextual analysis. Once the decision is reached, whether or not a child is born is a probabilistic process that depends on fecundability, contraceptive effectiveness, and fetal mortality—factors that epidemiologists and biostatisticians are best equipped to study. All of this takes place in populations whose composition is constantly changing in ways that affect responsiveness and the signals received, changes which demographers are in the best position to describe.

Much the same framework can be employed to study voluntary migration, although it has less applicability to the study of mortality simply because individual motivation is so uniformly and powerfully to avoid death. Some kind of integration of the approaches is likely to occur, simply because the discipline cannot afford to have its members keep talking past one another and misappropriating even the limited explanatory power that can be generated by segmented approaches.

References

Berelson, B.
    1974   *Population Policy in Developed Countries.* New York: McGraw-Hill.
Blake, J.
    1972   "Coercive pronatalism and American population policy." Pp. 85–114 in U. S. Commission on Population Growth and the American Future, *Aspects of Population Growth Policy.* Vol. VI. Washington, D. C.: U. S. Government Printing Office.
Bourgeois-Pichat, J.
    1967   "Social and biological determinants of human fertility in nonindustrial societies." *Proceedings of the American Philosophical Society* 3(3): 160–163.

Brass, W. *et al.*
  1968   *The Demography of Tropical Africa.* Princeton, N. J.: Princeton University
         Press.
Brass, W.
  1971   "A Critique of methods for estimating population growth in countries with limited
         data." *Bulletin of the International Statistical Institute* 44 Book 1: 397–412.
  1975   *Methods for Estimating Fertility and Mortality from Limited and Defective Data.*
         Laboratories for Population Statistics Occasional Publication. University of North
         Carolina, Chapel Hill.
Coale, A. J.
  1972   *The Growth and Structure of Human Populations.* Princeton, N. J.: Princeton
         University Press.
Coombs, C. H. L., C. Coombs, and G. H. McClelland,
  1975   "Preference scales for number and sex of children." *Population Studies* 29(2):
         275–298.
Cox, D. R.
  1972   "Regression models and life tables." *Journal of the Royal Statistical Society. B.*
         34: 187–220.
Das Gupta, P.
  1976   "Age-parity-nuptiality-specific stable population model that recognizes births to
         single women." *Journal of the American Statistical Association* 71(354): 308–314.
Davis, K. and J. Blake
  1955– "Social structure and fertility: An Analytic framework." *Economic Develop-*
  1956   *ment and Cultural Change* 4: 211–235.
Easterlin, R. A.
  1973   "The economics and sociology of fertility: A synthesis." Unpublished manu-
         script.
Fawcett, J. T. *et al.*
  1974   "The value of children in Asia and the United States: Comparative perspec-
         tives." Papers of the East–West Population Institute, No. 32. Honolulu.
Freedman, R.
  1974   "Community-level data in fertility surveys." In K. Williams (ed.), Occasional
         Paper No. 8 of the World Fertility Survey, London.
Hammel, E. A., and D. Hutchinson
  1974   "Two tests of computer microsimulation: The effect of an incest taboo on popula-
         tion variability." Pp. 1–14 in *Computer Simulation in Human Population Studies.*
         New York: Academic Press.
Heer, D. M., and D. O. Smith
  1968   "Mortality level, desired family size, and population increase." *Demography*
         5(1): 104–121.
Kalbfleisch, J. D., and R. L. Prentice
  1973   "Marginal likelihoods based on Cox's regression and life model." *Biometrika*
         60: 267–278.
Keyfitz, N.,
  1971   "On the momentum of population growth." *Demography* 8(1)(February): 71–80.
  1972   "How birth control affects births." *Social Biology* 18(2): 109–121.
Marks, E. S., W. Seltzer, and K. J. Krotki
  1974   *Population Growth Estimation.* New York: The Population Council.

McFarland, D. D.
   1972   "Comparison of alternative marriage models." Pp. 89–106 in T. N. E. Greville
          (ed.), *Population Dynamics*. New York: Academic Press.
Parlett, B.
   1972   "Can there be a marriage function?" Pp. 107–136 in T. N. E. Greville (ed.),
          Population Dynamics. New York: Academic Press.
Polgar, S.
   1972   "Population history and population policies from an anthropological perspective."
          Current Anthropology 13(2): 203–11.
Pollard, J.
   1977   "The continuing attempt to incorporate both sexes into marriage analysis," In-
          ternational Union for the Scientific Study of Population, International Popula-
          tion Conference. Mexico City. August. *Proceedings*. Vol. 1:291–309.
Preston, S. H.
   1974   "Demographic and social consequences of various causes of death in the United
          States." *Social Biology* 21(2): 144–162.
Preston, S. H., and A. T. Richards
   1975   "The influence of women's work opportunities on marriage rates." *Demography*
          12(2): 209–222.
Ryder, N. B., and C. F. Westoff
   1971   *Reproduction in the United States, 1965*. Princeton, N. J.: Princeton Univer-
          sity Press.
Sheps, M. C., and J. Menken
   1973   *Mathematical Models of Conception and Birth*. Chicago: Chicago University
          Press.
United Nations, Department of Economic and Social Affairs
   1967   *Methods of Estimating Basic Demographic Measures from Incomplete Data*.
          Population Study No. 42. New York.
Venkatacharya, K.
   1975   "Influence of variations in child mortality on fertility: A simulation model study."
          Proceedings of the Seminar on Infant Mortality in Relation to Level of Fertility.
          Bangkok, May 6–12, 1975. Committee for International Coordination of National
          Research in Demography. Paris: 87–102.

14

Organization of Demographic Research: Problems of the Next Decade

HALLIMAN H. WINSBOROUGH

The task for this chapter is to make a forecast about the organization of demographic research in the United States over the next decade. The word *forecast,* with its implication of a statement about the future which involves many judgments, is used intentionally. It is wise to begin such an exercise with an assessment of trends in factors that impinge on demographic research. I shall address trends in four such areas. They are:

1. Trends in the availability of data
2. Trends in the availability of "technology"
3. Trends in the place of demography in the social sciences
4. Trends in the demand for demographic knowledge

Trends in these areas have important implications for the organization of demographic research: They suggest that an increasingly heterogeneous group of skills, knowledge, and abilities must be applied to the individual research effort. They also imply an increasing dependence on shared physical and intellectual facilities by most demographers addressing most topics. These trends and implications suggest a set of necessities and possibilities for the organization of the research effort in demography.

Social Demography

Trends in the Availability of Data

It is a commonplace observation that the last decade has seen a revolution in the amount and kind of data available to demographers. Ten years ago the major data source for demographic research was the published tabulations from the census and vital statistics systems. Ten years ago some demographers were beginning to use the one-in-a-thousand sample from the 1960 Census; some demographers had access to the GAF and FAGMA files and the fertility survey tradition was active in work on the 1965 National Fertility Study. By and large, however, access to these tapes and these survey data was limited. By 1975 we had access to a remarkable wealth of data including the several one-in-a-hundred samples from the 1970 Census, the comparable one-in-a-hundred sample from the 1960 Census, a growing number of publicly released CPS files and supplements, codified files from the GAF surveys, and all of the wonderfully complex and difficult summary tapes from the 1970 Census.

During the upcoming decade, the increase in the volume of available data is likely to be even greater than in the last decade. Two aspects of this increase are likely to be especially important.

The first aspect has to do with the potentials of the data base for cross-temporal analysis. This potential exists in the continuation of data release policies presently in existence. By 1985 it seems certain that one will be able to construct the same table from the 1960, 1970, and 1980 Public Use Samples. By 1985 it seems likely that scholars will routinely exploit the rotation group aspect of the CPS to construct panel data on households.

Not only does the continuation of present release policies imply more cross-temporal data, but also the recent successes of projects designed to produce new cross-temporal data is likely to spawn the further collection of such data. It seems likely that the success of such panel studies as the Panel Study of Income Dynamics, the National Fertility Survey followback, and the National Survey of Labor Market Experience will prompt further national surveys having an explicit panel design.

Increasing experience with the error structure of retrospective questions and the likely success of explicit replication studies—both are aspects of the OCG II project—will motivate the collection of new retrospective replicative material.

Finally, and this is a good deal less certain, the demographer's need to push his series of census-based microdata further back in time and the demographic historian's need to use the manuscript censes may result in a program to process samples of the archival data in order to make "public use" data available for earlier censuses.

Concurrent with the trend toward increasing amounts of cross-temporal data, I expect that the next decade will see the release of increasing amounts of cross-national machine readable data. A review of the present availability and future plans for release of such data can be found in an article by J. S. Rowe (1974). Although it is clear from the survey reported in Rowe's article that a number of countries have not yet settled their policy about releasing machine readable data, some 43 countries declare their data are, or will be, available in this form. Rowe's survey did not distinguish between microdata on individuals or households and aggregate data in their tabular form. The author, however, believes that many responses pertain only to aggregate data and notes that several countries have explicit laws prohibiting release of microdata. Nonetheless, I imagine that the internal demand for microdata will be very high and that such data will be increasingly available.

The possibility of simultaneously manipulating microdata for several countries will certainly generate a good deal of cross-national research. This capacity may permit solutions to some of the difficulties which have bedeviled us for some time. For example, Rindfuss (1975) has made concurrent use of the U. S. and the Puerto Rican censuses to unravel difficult questions about international migration.

Despite these and other possibilities it is clear that cross-national comparisons using data not specifically designed for that purpose are difficult. Witness, for example, the complex analysis in Freedman and Coombs (1974). The World Fertility Survey is a project specifically designed for cross-national comparability. This survey will not only yield invaluable cross-nationally comparable data, but will also serve as an example of what can be done and hence may spawn additional explicitly cross-national studies. Another source of both data and example will come from the collection of comparable surveys of intergenerational mobility, many of which are now in the field. Comparability among these surveys is being attempted by communication among the principal investigators with limited coordination performed through the Research Committee on Social Stratification of the International Sociological Association. A description of these efforts can be found in Featherman *et al.* (1974). It may be that a very important aspect of these efforts will be to demonstrate the limitations of voluntary and informally coordinated efforts as contrasted with the formality of the World Fertility Survey.

By 1985, then, working demographers will have an awesome amount of data at their disposal. Not only will these data be extensions of the sorts of data we have now, but also they will provide the opportunity for two styles of research which are close to most of our hearts. They will increasingly permit full blown cross-temporal studies. They will increasingly permit comparative cross-national research.

Both of these kinds of research are very difficult. Each kind will require the development of complex models, use sophisticated statistical estimation and testing, and require that the demographer have access to wide knowledge of the times or places that are his units of analysis.

Trends in the Availability of Technology

Under the general rubric of trends in "technology," I want to group several sorts of things. First are those trends in computing and data processing that will influence our ability to deal with the increasing volume of data. Second are trends in the development of retrieval systems to make use of the mechanical possibilities extant in the hardware. Finally, there are trends in the development and use of complicated analytic methods.

Let us begin our discussion by considering trends in computing. There seem to exist two trends in this fast-moving area which are contradictory in their implications for demography.

On the one hand, the greatest recent innovation in computing is the dramatically decreasing cost of minicomputers. A recent article in *Datamation* forecasts the day when it will be possible to provide small, very powerful machines tailor-made to fit the specific needs of a user at quite modest cost. This possibility suggests that computing and data management facilities for demographic research may become quite decentralized.

On the other hand, there are trends in the manufacture of very large mass data storage units. These devices have been in existence for some years, but their price has recently dropped to the point where customers other than the Defense Department can think about acquiring them. Nonetheless, they will remain at an acquisition cost and are of such a size as to require centralized and shared use. All of the data likely to be available to demographers in the next several decades can, I am told, fit into a small fraction of one of these units and be "on line" at all times for a modest price. Some of these units are designated as "archival" ones indicating, as I understand it, that the stored information is quite stable over long periods of time.

On the one hand, then, the technology seems to be moving in the direction of decentralized computing, while on the other hand some of the hardware of special interest to demographers must be part of a central utility to be cost effective.

This anomaly may be less of a problem for us if one considers yet a third trend within the computing arena, that of the computer network. Networks permit one computer "on" the system to freely make use of the facilities of other computers which are also tied in. The archtypical ARPA network connects Defense Department computers around the country and is also available at some universities. A number of smaller interuniversity networks are presently up and functioning with a large number of others being planned. Such networks allow one to take advantage of the cost savings of minicomputers while retaining access to central utilities of various kinds. They also make possible some division of labor among demographic computing sites. I shall discuss subsequently how demographers may choose to utilize these networking possibilities.

Let us now turn our attention to trends in retrieving information from the massive data base to be available to demographers. In the world at large a great deal of attention is currently being given to the question of how to organize very large data bases, how to add to and modify them, and how to get information from them quickly.

There is a good deal of knowledge in the computer science field on these issues. There is a great demand for such systems from business, government agencies, and even university administrations. All of us deal regularly with existing systems when we pay our monthly bills, buy an airline ticket, or try to get students registered.

To date only a modest amount of this developing expertise in the world at large has been very useful to the demographer. The success of the retrieval systems that exist depends on the data existing on some random access device, there being some way of computing or looking up the address for the record desired, and then going directly to that address to get the record. For most of the files demographers want to use there has simply not been enough space on extant random access devices to store the whole file. Thus the demographer has had to process every record on a file to retrieve the ones he wants. That is why the development of very large mass storage devices is likely to be so important to us. The demographer's problem is even more complicated, however, when it comes to finding the address of the records he wants to look up. The demographer is not interested in finding a single record—Winsborough's water bill or McFarland's airline reservation. The demographer usually wants all of the records of a certain type—for example, records for husband–wife families with each spouse married only once or records for black female household heads between the ages of 14 and 45. Furthermore, the type of record to be retrieved changes with each run and varies over a large number of types.

Now there exist ways of dealing with these problems. They require relatively complicated methods for finding the addresses of the desired records, and of course they require that the data be arrayed on the storage devices appropriately and perhaps have some additions made to their contents. Constructing retrieval systems of this kind is a rather expensive business. Once accomplished, however, the task pays off in a markedly reduced cost of extracting a working file. For commonly used data files—for example, the Public Use Sample—the effort would probably be cost effective for federal support under present circumstances. For the very large data base demographers will want to access in the future, the organization of the data base for direct access and the construction of software to manage the system are probably crucial.

As the amount of data used by demographers expands, it will also become necessary to have a greatly expanded control over the information *about* the data base. Retrieval systems for this information *about* data will become necessary because the volume of such information will rapidly overwhelm the presently informal method for finding out from widely scattered sources which data file contains a useful set of variables. Methods for creating retrieval systems for information about the data are presently extant. The raw material for their construction could be easily, and perhaps necessarily, a by-product of the establishment of random access retrieval systems on a centralized data utility. It may be, however, the price of setting up all the data on a single utility is too high to be practical. In that case, construction of a number of partial systems for retrieval of information about some of the data may be necessary. That route will ideally entail a good deal of cooperation among the several sites undertaking the task for parts of the data base.

To summarize these aspects of computing and data management, we can observe that trends exist in both hardware and software that may permit demographers to access their growing data base with reasonable cost and time efficiency. These developments, however, will mean that the demographic research enterprise in the future will need to include people representing many more kinds of computing, information, and data retrieval specialities than is presently the case.

To complete our discussion of trends in technology, let us turn now to the issue of trends in model construction, data analysis, and parameter estimation. Not only are demographers going to have access to a large volume of data, but the variety of things they are likely to want to do with those data is sure to increase in scope and complexity. Four books published since 1973 indicate something of the range of potential methods of analysis available to demographers.

1. Bartlett and Hiorns, *The Mathematical Theory of the Dynamics of Biological Populations.* New York: Academic Press, 1973
2. Goldberger and Duncan, *Structural Equation Models in the Social Sciences.* New York: Seminar Press, 1973
3. Dyke and MacCluer, *Computer Simulation in Human Population Studies.* New York: Academic Press, 1974

4. Bishop *et al.*, *Discrete Multivariate Analysis*. Cambridge, Mass: MIT Press, 1975

Each of these books represents a rapidly developing style of analytic work. The strength of each of these separate styles of analysis is evident in the fact that it would be fairly easy to choose a contemporary alternate for each; for example, Haberman (1974) for Bishop *et al.* (1975), and Pollard (1973) or Sheps and Meken (1973) for Barlett and Hiorns (1973).

Beyond these, there may well be additional styles in the offing which will also become important to demographers. For example, the importance of the Tukey (1971) and Mosteller–Tukey (1968) work on exploring data analysis is yet to be assayed in relation to demography.

Few demographers are likely to be capable of working independently in more than a couple of the previously mentioned styles. Yet many of us are likely to find that the problems we want to address can be most profitably approached at one time from one of these styles and at another time from another. Thus most of us are going to need access to colleagues capable of providing guidance and tutoring. Because each of these styles requires computational work that rapidly becomes quite difficult, even the experts among us are likely to require the assistance of skillful numerical analysts. The outcome of all of this is that the body of colleagues accessible to the working demographer must increasingly include capable statisticians and numerical analysts, as well as colleagues practiced in the research use of each style of model building.

The likely result, then, of all these trends in "technology" is fairly consistent. Research in demography is going to require the application of increasing amounts of highly specialized skills, abilities, and knowledge in the course of a single research project.

Trends in the Place of Demography in the Social Sciences

The two previous sections have discussed trends in the availability of some factors in the production of demographic research. This and the following section are related to the demand for demographic knowledge. This section discusses some aspects of what seems to me to be the unfolding place of demography within the social sciences. The demand for demographic research discussed in this section can be seen as deriving from the scholarly effort to shed light on the operation of society. The next section will turn its attention to demands for the fruits of demographic research in terms of its utility for policy making and guidance.

In this section I want to argue that there exists a unique demographic view of society which, I believe, is becoming increasingly evident and attractive to social scientists. In the 1940s and 1950s, many demographers seemed to feel somewhat uneasy about the place of theory in demography. During that period of time, social scientists' notions of how a science should proceed were primarily drawn by analogy from physics with a good deal of proscription from the logical positivists' position in the philosophy of science. Aspects of theory construction in economics, psychology, and even sociology had some pretentions to fitting within this mold. But demography did not seem to fit very well. In the ensuing decades, two things have happened. First, there seems to have developed a decreasing infatuation with theoretical structures in other parts of the social sciences. Second, as the philosophy of science has paid more attention to the progress of other—notably biological—sciences, considerable difficulties with logical positivism and the strict adherence to the physics analogy have become apparent. A position has appeared, sometimes designated as the realist or super realist or realist–pluralist position, which seems a good deal more appropriate to the way good demographers go about their work. [For discussions of the realist position in the philosophy of science, see Hesse (1974) and Harré (1970).]

Two aspects of this realist position seem especially appropriate to demography. The first is the notion that some of the conceptual entities described in the theory must be thought to actually exist and to be demonstrable. Second is the idea that there may be more than one coherent way of describing the reality. Thus a single, monolithic theory and set of coherent categories is not required. Both aspects seem to fit demography fairly well. The central idea of demography is the idea of a population (Ryder, 1964). Populations, like molecules or viruses, actually exist. There are clear ways for pointing them out. Whatever else a society may be—a class structure, a value system, ways of choosing how to use scarce resources to produce and distribute commodities—it is also a population. A population is a persistent aggregate of individuals. Although individuals enter and leave the population by birth, death, and migration, the population as a real entity survives these gains and losses of individuals except for the death or departure of the last member.

A population, then, has an existence that is separate from that of any of its members taken singly. The population also has attributes that are separate and different from those attributes of individual members. Processes pertain to populations that are different from the processes that pertain to individuals. Populations may grow, decline, and grow again; indeed, they may do so with a specific periodicity. Once an individual has "declined" by death it is not generally useful to think of him reappearing.

There also exist in demography some quite strong laws about how a population changes its size and characteristics. These laws state how a population "works." Individuals are born into the population at age zero. Every year they get a year older. For both biological and social reasons the likelihood of events occurring to individuals is strongly conditional on their age. The patterns of these changing likelihoods is so strong that it is useful to think of a given society as having a life cycle through which cohorts of individuals move on their way to extinction through mortality. Changes in the characteristics of the population as a whole, then, can be seen as a translation of these cohort-specific processes into rates for the society as a whole.

Now, perhaps, we can state the place of the demographic view of society in the social sciences. The demographic view of society focuses on that which is true of the society because it is a population. Clearly, most demographers believe there are many other aspects of society that are worthy of investigation and that constitute alternative views. One can focus on society as a set of institutions, as a set of changing sustenance arrangements, as a set of rules, norms, and laws governing behavior, as a set of beliefs about the ultimate value of things and actions. No doubt all of these views and still others are necessary for a total picture of society. Aspects of many of these other views are often assumed in demographic research. Aspects of these other views often are seen as interacting with populational aspects of the society.

The important and attractive thing about the demographic view of society, then, is that it takes a realist position with respect to the construction of its science. This realist aspect of the demographic view of society seems to me to have two important features that are now and will increasingly make it attractive to scholars trying to figure out parts of the social world. For those scholars whose basic concern is trying to understand specific social events and who are casting around for a frame of reference within which to pursue this specific understanding, the demographic perspective is likely to be attractive both because of its concreteness and clear context and because almost every phenomenon at the societal level has a population component. Thus assumption of the demographic view of society is likely to be a strategic decision for someone pursuing understanding of specific social events. Within that view it is fairly clear what one is up to. Some of one's basic concepts refer to things that are clearly real. The outcome is quite likely to shed light on a part of the puzzle one has in hand. I hazard the guess that the growing interest in demography by historians has aspects of such a decision process.

On the other hand, I believe that an excursion into the demographic view of society is also likely to be useful and interesting to scholars whose basic concern is working out some alternate view of society. The truth of the assertion that "whatever else a society is it is also a population" implies that other views of society must come to grips with the interaction between those things and processes, which they have defined, and populational ones. It seems to me particularly the case that views of society that begin with individuals or collections of individuals as their basic unit are likely to look to the demographic view of society as a way of dealing with the problem of aggregating the effects of individual behaviors into change at the societal level. Perhaps examples of such situations can be seen in Keyfitz (1973) on the effects of changes in fertility rates on the internal structure of bureaucratic organizations and in Becker and Ghez (1975) on earnings over the life cycle.

If any of the preceding argument is true, then the increasing interest of scholars from quite diverse social science fields is not simply a result of the availability of funds for work related to population problems but also results in part from the logic of the demographic view of society. The implication, then, is that we are likely to see an expansion of the demands the social sciences in general will place on the facilities and data for demographic research. Individuals coming to these facilities and data are likely to be quite heterogeneous in terms of their knowledge and their interests. At the same time that these newcomers represent increasing demands on the facilities and data for demographic research, they also may represent an important supply of labor for the production of demographic research. They may become a source for some of the specialized substantive knowledge that increasingly will be required in our field.

Trends in the Demand for Demographic Knowledge

In the last section I focused on demand for the light demography can shed on society. In this section I shall focus on the demand for the fruits of demographic research. By and large, the demand which currently exists is related to the issue of population growth. The most certainly true assertion one can make about the policy implications of continued growth is that "There is hardly any social problem confronting this nation whose solution would be easier if our population were larger [Duncan, 1971]." It is probably the case that this truth is sufficient to make persistent some policy concern about the balance of fertility and mortality rates. Although recent declines in U. S. fertility and fertility expectations probably reduce the felt urgency of the population problem, the very precipitousness of the decline calls to mind the potential volatility of these variables and suggests the importance of "control" over them at least in the sense of understanding their likely patterns in the future. Indeed, the possibility of rapid increases in fertility, whether chimera or not, combined with the vivid image from the Population Commission report of the python swallowing the pig has probably led thoughtful policy makers to a concern about paths toward, as well as the eventual achievement of, population stability.

In the next several years, then, although it may be that we will see a diminution in the intensity of concern about growth rates, we are unlikely to witness a disappearance of that concern and the interest that remains may, indeed, be more sophisticated than in the past.

Although the demand for demographic knowledge deriving from concern about population growth is likely to diminish somewhat, I would expect that the demand for knowledge deriving from concern about equity may well rise. For many years demographic research has been of interest to, and supported by, policy concern about equity by race, region, ethnicity, and more recently by sex. Consider, for example, work by demographers on residential segregation, status attainment, education, poverty, and female labor force participation. As the federal government expands its domain over the delivery systems for services and as its concern for equal treatment is forced to expand, it seems almost certain that demographic research on issues related to equity problems will expand. For example, the increasing involvement of the federal government in paying for the delivery of medical care surely will generate new concerns about equity and equal treatment. In this arena, careful demographic studies of changes in differential mortality and morbidity are likely to be strongly desired. One also might imagine that in the next several years we are likely to see an increasing concern with equity by age, especially as it pertains to disadvantages accruing to the elderly. In another vein, the concern for finding equitable methods for the redistribution of taxes to state and local governments is one from which we are likely to see an increasing demand for demographic information, and forecasts.

In balance, then, it seems likely to me that demographic research is sufficiently useful for policy purposes that the demand for such research will remain at a fairly high level. It also seems likely, however, that there may be some redistribution of demand over topics in demography with a less acute concern for problems of growth and an increasing concern for problems of equity.

Implications for the Organization of Research

In the foregoing discussion I have tried to outline trends in several areas that seem likely to influence the organization of demographic research in the next decade. Let me summarize these trends briefly.

The first assertion is that in the next 10 years demographers are going to have lots more data then they do now. Additions of particular note are increasing amounts of cross-temporal and cross-national data. The second assertion is that the price of processing these data will decline but the task of managing it—keeping it organized and retrievable—will become a good deal more complicated. The third assertion is that the demographic view of society is so attractive as to draw an increasing number of social scientists into the field. Finally, the assertion is made that the demand for demographic knowledge deriving from policy issues will hold up but will be redistributed between concern for growth and concern for equity.

The following implications for the process of demographic research seem to me likely to constitute a series of robust forecasts because each depends on a similar implication from several trends just discussed.

1. The array of topics addressed under the general rubic of demographic research is likely to expand markedly:
   A. Because the data and methods likely to be available will permit investigation of more subjects
   B. Because social scientists attracted to the demographic view of society are likely to be interested in a wider variety of things than have been traditional in the field
   C. Because the demand for demographic research by policy makers is likely to range over more subjects
2. Pursuit of the typical research project is likely to require application of a wider array of technical, statistical, and substantive expertise than has been the case in the past. This situation will require a more elaborate division of labor within a given project. This multidisciplinary character of the typical project derives:
   A. From the increasing complexity of data retrieval and methods of analysis
   B. From the increasingly likely concern with cross-temporal and cross-national research and the consequent requirement for a greater range of substantive expertise
   C. From the necessity of social scientists who are neophytes to demography to collaborate with an old hand
   D. From the inherently interdisciplinary character of most equity-oriented problems
3. Most demographic research will be increasingly dependent on shared physical and colleagial resources. The quantity and complexity of the data to be available to demographers, the equipment to maintain it, and the personnel to make it useful are all too expensive for one user or a small collection of users to support. Econo-

mies of scale in this area are important indeed. Similar economies of scale exist in the availability of colleagial interaction about substantive problems.

Now to a forecast about the organization of demographic research. I believe that the previously described characteristics of future demographic research suggest that relatively large population centers are likely to become even more important to the pursuit of research than has been the case in the past. This is not to say that I think all demographic research will be carried on in a few centers; indeed, the possibilities for computer networks may make it easier to work in a noncenter location than it has been recently. Rather, I do believe that large centers are increasingly likely to be organizational foci for a somewhat more decentralized effort. Not only is the remote user likely to be tied to a center for data access and retrieval and for more complex estimation programs, but he is also likely to depend upon the professional and technical staff of the center for help. Perhaps increasingly, the remote person will be coprincipal investigator with professionals in the center. Perhaps noncenter scholars will, because of their special knowledge, also become a part of the skill base of the center.

Although I believe that the larger demography centers will increasingly operate as organizational and resource "nodes" for a hinterland of remote users, I do not believe that all of the larger centers will be similar, all-purpose ones. Indeed, a cressive, substantive division of labor among centers seems a likely outcome of the present, relatively unplanned growth and distribution of centers in the United States. Such a division of labor is likely to imply that a member of one center may sometimes need to behave like a remote user of another center. Thus centers are likely to be interconnected in a stronger fashion than has been the case in the past.

The nature of this interconnection between centers will, of course, depend greatly on how we go about organizing the demographic data base. If each center organizes the data and the retrieval system for that part of the data base most pertinent to its substantive interests, the pattern of connections between centers is likely to be fairly evenly distributed and fairly informal. The volume of interactions will depend upon the degree to which the various centers choose to organize their data and retrieval systems in a similar way. If each center goes its own way, the volume will be relatively low because of the burden of learning a new retrieval language each time one wants to use the facilities of another center. On the other hand, if centers can agree on some common procedure and language the volume of interaction could be quite large.

There exists, of course, an alternative to each center organizing its own data: the alternative of a centralized data utility. Such a utility would force a common retrieval method on each center. Even if the utility did not contain the whole of the data base, the existence of a common language would probably constrain the designers of center-specific data systems to conform. Thus the existence of a centralized utility might make interaction among substantively focused centers easier to accomplish. By and large, however, the existence of a data utility would leave interactions among substantive centers to the arena of sharing analytic programs and substantive expertise.

In the foregoing I have made no distinction between university and nonuniversity centers. It is not clear to me that the past tendency for most demography centers to be in a university will persist. Universities typically have rather flat organizational charts and norms of independent and coequal authority. But a number of the computer and data base management problems facing the field are of the sort that require well-defined levels of hierarchy and a fairly complex vertical division of labor. Such tasks may well find more fertile ground outside of the university environment.

If any of the foregoing arguments are correct, I suppose the question arises of what needs to be done to maximize the productivity of demographic research in the near future. Let me conclude with a suggestion. Many of the most important problems thar arise seem to me to be supracenter ones. They pertain to how centers will interact with one another and with remote users to accomplish the access to data, method, and colleagueship that will be necessary.

Two steps seem to me appropriate. The first is a meeting of the directors of demographic population centers, without regard to who supports their centers, to discuss ways in which they can usefully provide mutually supportive facilities. The second step is to begin exploration of the possibility of computer network links between interested centers.

I suspect that neither of these suggestions is likely to seem too attractive to center directors themselves. Most center directors have enough problems simply keeping things going internally and getting their own work done. They are likely to be uninterested in accepting a very large responsibility for provision of services to "outsiders," unless they can be convinced that the fairly immediate returns to their own center will outweigh the costs of operation.

Overall, then, I believe the next decade will be a productive one for demographic research. Difficult challenges will exist to master the new data, methods, and topics that will be forthcoming. Even more difficult challenges may present themselves in the tasks of organizing within demography an infrastructure capable of permitting the full realization of the possibilities of the decade.

References

Bartlett, M. S., and R. W. Hiorns, Eds.
   1973 *The Mathematical Theory of the Dynamics of Biological Populations.* New York: Academic Press.
Becker, G. S., and G. R. Ghez
   1975 *The Allocation of Time and Goods over the Life Cycle.* New York: National Bureau of Economic Research.
Bishop, Y. M. M., S. E. Fienberg, and P. W. Holland
   1975 *Discrete Multivariate Analysis.* Cambridge, Mass.: MIT Press.
Duncan, O. D.
   1971 "Observations on populations." *The New Physician* 20 (April): 243–245.
Dyke, B., and J. W. MacCluer, Ed.
   1974 *Computer Simulation in Human Population Studies.* New York: Academic Press.
Featherman, D. L., R. M. Hauser, and W. H. Sewell
   1974 "Toward comparable data on inequality and stratification: Perspectives on the second generation of national mobility surveys." *The American Sociologist* 9 (February): 18–25.
Freedman, R., and L. C. Coombs
   1974 "Cross-cultural comparisons: Data on two factors in fertility behavior." An Occasional Paper of the Population Council. New York: The Population Council.
Goldberger, A. S., and O. D. Duncan
   1973 *Structural Equation Models in the Social Sciences.* New York: Seminar Press.
Haberman, S. J.
   1974 *The Analysis of Frequency Data.* Chicago: University of Chicago Press.
Harré, R.
   1970 *The Principles of Scientific Thinking.* Chicago: University of Chicago Press.
Hesse, M.
   1974 *The Structure of Scientific Inference.* Berkeley and Los Angeles: University of California Press.
Horn, B. K. P., and P. H. Winston
   1975 "Personal computers." *Datamation* 21(May): 111–115.
Keyfitz, N.
   1973 "Individual mobility in a stationary population," *Population Studies* 27(July): 335–352.
Mosteller, F., and J. W. Tukey
   1968 "Data analysis, including statistics." In G. Lindzey and E. Aronson (eds.), *Revised Handbook of Social Psychology.* Reading, Mass.: Addison-Wesley.
Pollard, J.
   1973 *Mathematical Models for the Growth of Human Populations.* Cambridge, England: University Press.
Rindfuss, R. R.
   1975 "Fertility and migration: The case of Puerto Rico." University of Winsconsin–Madison, Center for Demography and Ecology Working Paper 75-18.

Rowe, J. S.
   1974   "Census data in machine readable form." *Population Index* 40(October): 623–635.
Ryder, N. B.
   1964   "Notes on the concept of a population." *American Journal of Sociology* 69(March): 447–463.
Sheps, M. C., and J. Menken
   1973   *Mathematical Models of Conception and Birth*. Chicago: The University of Chicago Press.
Tukey, J. W.
   1971   *Exploratory Data Analysis* Vol. 3. Reading, Mass.: Addison-Wesley.

INDEX